Multidisciplinary Approach to Obesity

Andrea Lenzi • Silvia Migliaccio
Lorenzo Maria Donini
Editors

Multidisciplinary Approach to Obesity

From Assessment to Treatment

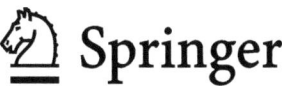

Editors
Andrea Lenzi
Department of Experimental Medicine
Section of Medical Pathophysiology,
Endocrinology and Nutrition
Sapienza University
Rome
Italy

Lorenzo Maria Donini
Department of Experimental Medicine
Section of Medical Pathophysiology,
Endocrinology and Nutrition
Sapienza University
Rome
Italy

Silvia Migliaccio
Department of Movement, Human
and Health Sciences
Unit of Endocrinology
Foro Italico University
Rome
Italy

ISBN 978-3-319-09044-3   ISBN 978-3-319-09045-0   (eBook)
DOI 10.1007/978-3-319-09045-0
Springer Cham Heidelberg New York Dordrecht London

Library of Congress Control Number: 2014956547

© Springer International Publishing Switzerland 2015
This work is subject to copyright. All rights are reserved by the Publisher, whether the whole or part of the material is concerned, specifically the rights of translation, reprinting, reuse of illustrations, recitation, broadcasting, reproduction on microfilms or in any other physical way, and transmission or information storage and retrieval, electronic adaptation, computer software, or by similar or dissimilar methodology now known or hereafter developed. Exempted from this legal reservation are brief excerpts in connection with reviews or scholarly analysis or material supplied specifically for the purpose of being entered and executed on a computer system, for exclusive use by the purchaser of the work. Duplication of this publication or parts thereof is permitted only under the provisions of the Copyright Law of the Publisher's location, in its current version, and permission for use must always be obtained from Springer. Permissions for use may be obtained through RightsLink at the Copyright Clearance Center. Violations are liable to prosecution under the respective Copyright Law.
The use of general descriptive names, registered names, trademarks, service marks, etc. in this publication does not imply, even in the absence of a specific statement, that such names are exempt from the relevant protective laws and regulations and therefore free for general use.
While the advice and information in this book are believed to be true and accurate at the date of publication, neither the authors nor the editors nor the publisher can accept any legal responsibility for any errors or omissions that may be made. The publisher makes no warranty, express or implied, with respect to the material contained herein.

Printed on acid-free paper

Springer is part of Springer Science+Business Media (www.springer.com)

Preface

Obesity has reached epidemic proportions all over the world. In the last 25 years, epidemiological research and national surveys confirm this tendency.

From children to older adults, much attention has been given to this health problem by researchers, politicians, the media, and the public. In fact, obesity is the most common chronic disorder in the industrialized societies, with an important impact on individual lives as well as on health economics (medical expenses, lost income as a result of disability, and complications of adult obesity), and therefore, obesity has already become a major factor in health care planning systems.

There is also controversy regarding the role of the different identified determinants, the importance of the components necessary for successful prevention and management of obesity weight loss, and the strategies to address common barriers, which need to be changed.

Most reports agree that a lack of physical activity plays a role in obesity, while dieting (in particular unhealthful and repeated) may actually contribute to obesity and eating disorders. Psychological issues (e.g., anxiety, depression and other mood disturbances, body image disturbance, social stigma) are considered important in determining obesity and/or in making it more difficult to treat. The genetic basis of obesity has been studied analyzing the role of different gene products and through the increasing knowledge of the role of different neuropeptides, hormones, and their receptors, suggesting that approximately 50 % of the tendency toward obesity is inherited.

Currently, many actions with a correct planning of diet and exercise have been proposed to prevent obesity. While these procedures might have some benefit at an individual level, they have made only little impact on halting the rise of obesity at a national level. This may be due, at least in part, to the significant differences in existing services among nations.

Moreover, many advices and programs are offered to the public. There is consensus among all that programs centered on nutritional intervention, physical activity, and cognitive behavioral therapy are considered vital to improve the quality of life and to reduce the comorbidity, disability, and mortality of obese individuals. However, the best way to combine these interventions between them and with other methods of treatment (e.g., pharmacological approach, bariatric surgery) is still under discussion. Similarly, methods of managing health services in tackling obesity, comorbidity, and disability are still under debate.

In this book, the authors' contributions address the spectrum of the multidisciplinary approach to obesity, ranging from physiological characteristics to epidemiology and to clinical characteristics. Metabolism and endocrinological aspects of obesity are faced in depth, considering the role of thyroid, adrenal, and ovarian functions, the interaction between obesity and osteoporosis or sarcopenia, and the role of obesity in glucose or lipid metabolism. Clinical aspects are considered, starting from the multidimensional evaluation (clinical, nutritional, functional, and psychological) through the different interventions (therapeutic education and psychotherapy, nutritional counseling and dietetic intervention, physical activity and training prescription, prescription medications, bariatric and reconstructive *plastic* surgery, and nutritional-metabolic-psychological rehabilitation) up to the interdisciplinary management of obesity.

Finally, the book provides an up-to-date review about advances made in the multidisciplinary approach to obesity from the clinical statement to treatment. Involving experts in nutrition, endocrinology and andrology, exercise and sports medicine, psychiatry and bariatric surgery, the multidisciplinary approach that should characterize the clinical care of the obese patient is promoted.

The experts involved in this project have made every effort to produce manuscripts rich in basic research and evidence-based medicine contents underlining the importance of a translational approach "from the bench to the bedside" facing perspectives from multiple disciplines and the multilayered treatment issues involved in the care of obese patients.

The book is therefore useful to physicians, scientists, postgraduate students, and students of various disciplines dealing with obesity.

Rome, Italy
Andrea Lenzi
Silvia Migliaccio
Lorenzo Maria Donini

Contents

Part I Introductory Chapters

1. **Anatomy and Physiology of Adipose Tissue** 3
   Graziana Colaianni, Silvia Colucci, and Maria Grano

2. **Regulation of Energy Intake** 13
   Roberto Vettor, Roberto Fabris, and Marco Rossato

3. **Obesity: Definition and Epidemiology** 31
   Stefania Maggi, Luca Busetto, Marianna Noale,
   Federica Limongi, and Gaetano Crepaldi

Part II Metabolism and Endocrinology

4. **Obesity and Thyroid Function** 43
   Giovanni Ceccarini, Alessio Basolo, and Ferruccio Santini

5. **Hypothalamic Growth Hormone/IGF-1 Axis** 53
   Annamaria Colao, Silvia Savastano, and Carolina Di Somma

6. **Adrenal Function and Obesity** 63
   Laura Proietti Pannunzi, Cecilia Motta, and Vincenzo Toscano

7. **Ovarian Function and Obesity: PCOS, Menopause** 73
   Carla Lubrano, Lucio Gnessi, and Silvia Migliaccio

8. **Obesity and Osteoporosis** 83
   Emanuela A. Greco, Lorenzo M. Donini, Andrea Lenzi,
   and Silvia Migliaccio

9. **Sarcopenic Obesity** 89
   Lorenzo M. Donini, Stefan A. Czerwinski, Audry C. Choh,
   Eleonora Poggiogalle, Silvia Migliaccio, and Andrea Lenzi

10. **Obesity and Testicular Function** 99
    Alessandro Ilacqua, Davide Francomano, and Antonio Aversa

11	**Obesity and Glucose Metabolism**...........................	107
	Nicola Napoli and Paolo Pozzilli	
12	**Dyslipidemia and Cardiovascular Risk in Obesity**...............	121
	Marcello Arca	
13	**Pulmonary Complications of Obesity**	131
	Dinkar Bhasin, Animesh Sharma, and Surendra K. Sharma	
14	**Sexual Distress in Obesity**..................................	145
	Erika Limoncin, Giacomo Ciocca, Daniele Mollaioli, and Emmanuele A. Jannini	

Part III Evaluation of Obese Subjects

15	**Clinical Evaluation**...	157
	Luca Busetto and Fabio De Stefano	
16	**Nutritional Status Evaluation: Body Composition and Energy Balance**...	171
	Massimo Pellegrini and Nino C. Battistini	
17	**Psychiatric and Psychological Evaluation**......................	193
	Massimo Cuzzolaro	
18	**Functional Evaluation (Joint and Muscle Problems, Cardiopulmonary Exercise Testing, Disability Evaluation)**........	205
	Gian Pietro Emerenziani, Federico Schena, and Laura Guidetti	
19	**Impairment of Quality of Life in Obesity**	211
	Carlo M. Rotella and Barbara Cresci	

Part IV Therapeutic Approach

20	**Therapeutic Education and Psychotherapy**	219
	Giovanni Gravina, Monica Palla, Carla Piccione, and Grazia Nebbiai	
21	**Dietary Intervention and Nutritional Counseling**................	233
	Alessandro Pinto, Lucia Toselli, and Edda Cava	
22	**Physical Activity and Training Prescription**	253
	Cosme F. Buzzachera, Marco Meucci, and Carlo Baldari	
23	**Prescription Medications for the Treatment of Obesity**...........	261
	Valentina Lo Preiato, Elena Daniela Serban, Renato Pasquali, and Uberto Pagotto	

24	**Bariatric Surgery**...	271
	Nicola Basso, Emanuele Soricelli, Giovanni Casella, Alfredo Genco, and Adriano Redler	
25	**Reconstructive Plastic Surgery**.............................	301
	Paolo Persichetti, Stefania Tenna, and Pierfranco Simone	
26	**Nutritional, Metabolic, and Psychological Rehabilitation**.........	315
	Paolo Capodaglio and Maria Letizia Petroni	
27	**Increasing Adherence to Diet and Exercise Through Cognitive Behavioural Strategies**............................	327
	Riccardo Dalle Grave, Simona Calugi, and Marwan El Ghoch	
28	**Interdisciplinary Approach to Obesity**......................	337
	Stefania Mariani, Mikiko Watanabe, Carla Lubrano, Sabrina Basciani, Silvia Migliaccio, and Lucio Gnessi	
Index...		343

Part I
Introductory Chapters

Anatomy and Physiology of Adipose Tissue

Graziana Colaianni, Silvia Colucci, and Maria Grano

1.1 Overview of Adipose Tissue

The adipose organ has been traditionally classified into white (WAT) and brown adipose tissue (BAT). WAT is the storage organ of energy in the form of lipids, whereas BAT regulates body temperature by producing heat via the expenditure of stored energy. The morphology of white and brown adipocytes is reasonably different, because these lipids are organized in a unique droplet in white adipocytes (unilocular) and in many droplets in brown adipocytes (multilocular) [1]. Another feature that differs in the morphology of these two cell types is the presence of numerous large mitochondria in brown adipocytes. These latter are also characterized by the expression of uncoupling protein 1 (UCP1), the protein able to uncouple oxidative phosphorylation from ATP synthesis, resulting in the production of heat [2].

Interestingly, UCP1 immunoreactive brown adipocytes are present in all depots of the adipose organ [3]. These adipocytes are also named "beige" [4] or "brite" (brown in white) [5], and their origin is debated [6]. These brown/beige/brite cells in WAT are derived from precursor cells that could be different from classical brown adipocytes and are closer to the white adipocyte cell lineage [7]. However, in response to certain stimuli, these adipocytes can be activated into cells having BAT-like phenotype, as demonstrated by the expression of UCP1 and other BAT-like genes [8]. This process, named browning response, is a transdifferentiation program from white-to-brown phenotype, and it will be discussed below.

Although the presence of adipocytes in the bone marrow is well recognized, the role of these cells has been recently better defined. Traditionally, marrow adipocytes were described as passive cells, occupying space not required for hematopoiesis or

G. Colaianni • S. Colucci • M. Grano (✉)
Department of Basic Medical Science, Neuroscience and Sense Organs, University of Bari, Piazza Giulio Cesare 11, Bari 70124, Italy
e-mail: graziana.colaianni@libero.it; silviaconcetta.colucci@uniba.it; maria.grano@uniba.it

bone formation [9], but it has been finally documented that these cells have an active role in the bone marrow microenvironment. Hence, marrow adipose tissue (MAT) is considered a type of adipose tissue, holding different features from white and brown adipose tissue. At birth, the bone marrow is mostly hematopoietic (the red marrow), but, throughout life, it is progressively transformed to fatty yellow marrow [10]. Therefore, the marrow adiposity expansion is age related in both genders [11]. The earliest fatty conversion of the human marrow begins at birth, accelerates between 4 and 8 weeks of age, and reaches full fatty conversion after 1 year [12]. MAT continues to accumulate in the appendicular skeleton from distal to proximal until age of 20–25, and, throughout life, gradual MAT formation continues in the axial skeleton [13]. Although in young subjects the content of marrow fat appears higher in men than women [14], this trend is reversed in elderly subjects, so that older women have higher bone marrow adiposity [15]. This age-related increases in marrow fat content are defined hypertrophy, if depends on increased size, or hyperplasia, if depends on increased number of adipocytes in the marrow. As physiological role, MAT serves as a local storage for energy. In pathological conditions, such as in state of calorie restriction and anorexia, although there is a considerable reduction in the volume of WAT, the amount of MAT appears strongly increased [15]. For long time, MAT has been considered a negative regulator of bone formation. Hence, MAT accumulation are correlated with osteoporosis and osteopenia [16]. Despite these correlations, it is unclear whether excessive MAT could directly influence bone metabolism or the bone loss occurring provokes changes in the marrow microenvironment that indirectly influence MAT formation.

A fourth type of adipocyte has recently been characterized in mouse subcutaneous fat depots during pregnancy and lactation, when the adipose portion of the mammary gland gradually disappears and an extensive development of milk-secreting lobuloalveolar epithelial glands appears. These newly formed epithelial cells, called pink adipocytes, derive from a direct transdifferentiation of white adipocytes into milk-secreting epithelial cells (adipo-epithelial transdifferentiation) [17]. The formation of pink cells is reversible, and, following end of lactation, they revert into white adipocytes, restoring the adipose component of the mammary gland [17, 18].

1.2 The Anatomy of the Multi-depot Adipose Organ

White and brown adipocytes have different morphology and functions, but numerous studies have shown that, in several locations, both cells cohabit together, forming the multi-depot adipose organ [19]. These depots are located in the subcutaneous space (subcutaneous depots) or close to organs located in the trunk (visceral depots).

The anterior subcutaneous depot is mainly located in the upper dorsal area at the level of the scapulae. It is composed by interscapular, subscapular, axillary, and cervical depots [20]. The posterior subcutaneous depot is located primarily in the lower ventral part of the body, and it is also formed of different parts: dorsolumbar, inguinal, and gluteal depots. The truncal or visceral depots are contained in the mediastinum and abdomen. All truncal depots are intimately associated with the aorta. Furthermore, in females, it has been also described another anatomical form of fat called the abdominopelvic depot, which comprises perirenal, periovarian, parametrial, and perivesical fat [3, 20]. Of note, the subcutaneous tissue in female mice has been found infiltrated by ramified epithelial ducts ending in five symmetrical pairs of nipples. Therefore, it can be considered as part of mammary glands subcutaneous depots [21, 22].

Pericardic, omental, mesenteric, and subcutaneous depots are characterized by the presence of lymphatic tissue [23]. All adipose depots are associated with specific nerve-vascular peduncles [24], enabling the connection with the nervous system in order to respond to physiological and environmental stimuli. Most of nerve fibers in contact with adipocytes express tyrosine hydroxylase (TH), the enzyme marker of noradrenergic fibers [24]. When mammals are exposed to temperatures below thermoneutrality, the sympathetic nervous system is activated because thermogenesis is required. This implies the action of norepinephrine on beta-3 adrenoreceptors, which promotes the molecular pathway for thermogenesis in brown adipocytes [2]. Interestingly, patients affected by pheochromocytoma, a norepinephrine-secreting tumor of the adrenal gland, show increased amount of BAT detectable by positron emission tomography (PET) [25]. Moreover, elegant data have shown that the density of TH-expressing nerve fibers is much higher in the brown adipose tissue than in white, and the density of these fibers increases during cold exposure, as well as increase the number of brown adipocytes [26]. Therefore, adipose tissues exposed to cold temperature appear browner and more innervated than those exposed to a warm environment.

In contrast, aging seems to have an opposite effect on white and brown fat balance. Thus, experiments performed in rats demonstrated an increase in the number of white adipocytes in the anterior subcutaneous depot correlated with the increase of age and with a concomitant progressive reduction in the number of brown adipocytes [27]. In agreement with this, human studies showed that BAT seems to be replaced by WAT in elderly [28]. Interestingly, cold exposure restores the numbers of brown adipocytes to the levels of young animals [29], and similar effects have been found in humans [30].

Large white adipocytes are mainly present in subcutaneous depots, whereas small white adipocytes are mostly located in visceral depots [31]. Brown adipocytes in visceral depots are mainly found near the aorta. Because beige/brite adipocytes were recently defined [32], brown adipocytes are termed classical or constitutive brown adipocytes to distinguish them from brown-like cells in WAT. Constitutive brown fat is predominantly located around interscapular, paravertebral, and perirenal sites. The most classical brown fat depots reside subcutaneously between the shoulders and can be easily excised. In contrast, perirenal BAT is difficult to remove without removing the kidney. Small areas of interscapular BAT could also reside in the supraclavicular region [33]. Conventionally, BAT was thought to be restricted to the neonatal and early childhood periods [33]. However, PET scanning analysis has showed the presence of active BAT in adult humans, particularly in the upper trunk, such as cervical, supraclavicular, paravertebral, pericardial, and to a certain extent, in mediastinal and mesenteric regions [34].

1.3 Adipose Cell Differentiation

The formation of WAT begins shortly after birth. Mesenchymal stem cells become adipoblasts and afterward differentiate into preadipocytes. The primary phase of adipogenesis is characterized by the proliferation of preadipocytes, which move forward into mitosis until they reach growth arrest. At this point, if preadipocytes exit the cell cycle, they change their morphology and accumulate cytoplasmic triglycerides, gaining characteristics of mature adipocytes and loosing the ability to divide [35]. Both white and brown adipocytes originate from the mesoderm, but they derive from different precursor cells. Mesenchymal stem cells can be committed to either a Myf5-negative adipogenic and osteoblastogenic lineage (white adipocytes) or to a Myf5-positive myogenic lineage (brown adipocytes) [36]. Although the adipocytes originate from two different lineages, the differentiation of adipocytes shares common transcriptional pathway involving CCAAT/enhancer-binding proteins (C/EBPs) [37].

In white adipocytes, once differentiation is active, the cAMP response element-binding protein becomes phosphorylated and then induces the expression of C/EBP-β [38]. The mitogen-activated protein kinase and GSK3β phosphorylate C/EBP-β, which leads to dimerization of C/EBP-β, thus inducing a DNA-binding domain. The binding of C/EBP-β to DNA allows preadipocytes either to reenter the cell cycle or to increase levels of transcripton factors C/EBP-α and peroxisome proliferator-activated receptor-γ (PPAR-γ) [37]. PPAR-γ is crucial to promote lipid and glucose metabolism and insulin sensitivity of adipocytes.

BAT develops before birth because it plays role in protecting newborn against cold. The differentiation of brown preadipocytes into mature brown adipocytes is positively and negatively controlled by bone morphogenetic protein (BMP)-7 [39] and myostatin [40], respectively. C/EBP-β and PR domain containing 16 (PRDM16) have been shown to act as key transcriptional factors in the differentiation of brown adipocytes [41]. Thus, when PRDM16 was suppressed in brown precursor cells, the cells differentiated into skeletal muscle cells. Likewise, myoblasts in which PRDM16 was ectopically expressed are able to transdifferentiate into brown fat cells [41]. The fate of BAT from the myogenic lineage depends on transcriptional complex formed between PRDM16 and C/EBP-β [42] that induces the expression of peroxisome proliferator-activated receptor gamma coactivator-1 alpha (PGC-1α) [43], which in turn regulates mitochondrial biogenesis and oxidative metabolism [44, 45]. Furthermore, C/EBP-β is a key transcriptional activator that leads to UCP1 expression, inducing the thermogenesis process [42].

1.4 Transdifferentiation Process

The white adipose depots have the ability to switch between energy storage and energy expenditure. Thus, in specific physiologic conditions, white adipocytes transform into brown adipocytes to contribute to thermogenic needs [46].

As mentioned above the beige/brite cells in WAT are derived from precursor cells that are different from classical brown adipocytes. These depots can shift from a WAT phenotype to a BAT-like phenotype showing morphology, gene expression pattern, and mitochondrial respiratory activity quite identical to those of classical BAT [47]. This induction of the brown adipocyte-like phenotype in WAT is called browning response [7]. Understanding the molecular mechanisms of this process is taking great relevance for human health since it could be used for developing therapeutic strategies to prevent the excessive formation of white adipocytes, in favor of increasing amount of brown adipocytes. The strongest inducer of beige/brite cells activation is cold exposure via several molecular mechanisms. This conversion is principally mediated by the sympathetic nervous system through the beta3AR because it has been shown that browning response can be induced by the administration of beta3AR agonists [48] and, additionally, beta3AR knockout mice do not respond to the browning transdiffrentiation [8].

Transcription factors such as PPAR-γ, its coactivator 1 alpha (PGC-1α), C/EBP beta, and PRDM16 seem to play key roles in regulation of the browning program [43]. The thiazolidinediones, a group of PPAR-γ activator agents, are synthetic ligands used to control glycemia [49], and they have proved effective in transforming WAT into BAT-like tissue in mice, rats, and dogs [50–52]. PGC-1α, originally described as a cofactor of PPARγ, is inducible by cold exposure in BAT [53]. Furthermore, human white adipocytes transfected with PGC-1α express UCP1, the marker gene of brown adipocytes [54]. C/EBPβ and PRDM16 are powerful inducers of the brown phenotype of fat cells. They form a molecular complex that is essential for the brown differentiation of mesenchymal stem cells. Hence, transplantation of skin fibroblasts, in which C/EBPβ and PRDM16 were ectopically expressed, gave rise to functional BAT [42]. Moreover, PRDM16 transgenic expression in all adipose tissues induced browning of WAT, particularly in subcutaneous fat, enhancing energy expenditure and suppressing weight gain in high-fat diet [55].

Fibroblast growth factor 21 (FGF21) is a growth factor produced by the liver and BAT under the control of sympathetic nervous system [56]. It has been recently shown that FGF21 acts in an autocrine/paracrine manner to increase expression of UCP1 and other thermogenic genes in fat tissue through the β-Klotho receptor [57]. FGF21 modulates this process by enhancing PGC-1α protein levels in adipose tissue [58]. Conversely, transforming growth factor beta (TGF-beta) negatively affects the browning process. Thus, the absence of smad3, a downstream molecule of TGF-beta signaling, induces white-to-brown conversion with positive metabolic response on glucose levels in diet-induced obese mice [59]. BMP7 stimulates a full program of brown adipogenesis through PRDM16 and PGC-1α activation and promotes commitment of mesenchymal progenitors to a brown adipocyte lineage. Furthermore, adenoviral-mediated expression of BMP7 in mice induces significant increases in BAT that consequently enhances energy expenditure and reduces weight gain [39].

Cold exposure is not the unique stimulus triggering the browning process. Interestingly, a recently discovered hormone called irisin, which is produced by skeletal muscles during physical exercise, has been proven to be a potent inducer of white-to-brown conversion both in vitro and in vivo [60].

The ability to transform itself according to the need of more energy consumption is defined as plasticity of white adipose tissue. However, this extraordinary plasticity is not solely related to the browning response. During pregnancy and lactation, all subcutaneous depots of the adipose organ can turn into mammary glands [22]. During pregnancy, white adipocytes lose their lipid content, acquire epithelial features, and form glandular structures able to produce and secrete milk. Following lactation, part of the epithelial component of the gland converts into adipocytes, allowing recovery of the adipose component in the subcutaneous depot [22].

The adipose cell plasticity and ability to adapt to environmental stimuli, modifying their phenotype, satisfy important physiological needs of the organism. These new insights in the adipocyte biology establish that these cells have a multipotent differentiation potential in vitro [61] and in vivo [22].

1.5   Adipokines and Cytokines

Considerable evidence shows that molecules secreted by adipose tissue play a key role in metabolic homeostasis, and their deficiency, caused by massive adiposity or adipocyte dysfunction, leads to obesity or several obesity-related pathologies. Therefore, adipose tissue is considered an endocrine organ whose action on target tissues depends on the location of fat depots and may differ according to its functional state. The full understanding of adipose tissue secretome might provide significant insights into the functions of the most important metabolic regulator of the body. Leptin is one of the most potent adipokines in metabolic regulation. It controls body weight by signaling sense of appetite or satiety to hypothalamus, which produces neurotransmitters that adapt food intake and energy expenditure. Leptin also regulates hepatic lipogenesis by suppressing fatty acid synthesis pathway [62] and improves muscle fatty acid oxidation [63]. Adiponectin is the most abundant secreted adipokine. It enhances insulin sensivity and partially reverse insulin resistance in obese mice [64]. Currently, researches for treatment of obesity-induced inflammation and insulin resistance are exploring strategies to increase adiponectin levels or adiponectin receptor activities [65].

Tumor necrosis factor alpha (TNFα) was the first cytokine identified in the adipose tissue of obese mice. This cytokine is involved in obesity-induced insulin resistance because it interferes with insulin signaling and blocks insulin actions [66]. The adipose TNFα pool is produced by macrophages and other immune cells. Interleukin 6 (IL6) is the other pro-inflammatory cytokine whose expression level increases in the adipose tissue of obese mice and patients, but its role in glucose metabolism has not been fully determined. Mice lacking IL6 develop obesity and insulin resistance, which can be rescued by central injection of IL6 [67] suggesting that this interleukine is required for the maintenance of whole-body glucose metabolism and metabolic homeostasis.

References

1. Cinti S (2001) The adipose organ: morphological perspectives of adipose tissues. Proc Nutr Soc 60:319–328
2. Cannon B, Nedergaard J (2004) Brown adipose tissue: function and physiological significance. Physiol Rev 84:277–359
3. Vitali A, Murano I, Zingaretti MC, Frontini A, Ricquier D, Cinti S (2012) The adipose organ of obesity-prone C57BL/6J mice is composed of mixed white and brown adipocytes. J Lipid Res 53:619–629
4. Ishibashi J, Seale P (2010) Medicine. Beige can be slimming. Science 328:1113–1114
5. Waldén TB, Hansen IR, Timmons JA, Cannon B, Nedergaard J (2012) Recruited vs. nonrecruited molecular signatures of brown, "brite", and white adipose tissues. Am J Physiol Endocrinol Metab 302:E19–E31
6. Smorlesi A, Frontini A, Giordano A, Cinti S (2012) The adipose organ: white-brown adipocyte plasticity and metabolic inflammation. Obes Rev 13(Suppl 2):83–96
7. Petrovic N, Walden TB, Shabalina IG, Timmons JA, Cannon B, Nedergaard J (2010) Chronic peroxisome proliferator-activated receptor gamma (PPARgamma) activation of epididymally derived white adipocyte cultures reveals a population of thermogenically competent, UCP1-containing adipocytes molecularly distinct from classic brown adipocytes. J Biol Chem 285:7153–7164
8. Barbatelli G, Murano I, Madsen L et al (2010) The emergence of cold-induced brown adipocytes in mouse white fat depots is determined predominantly by white to brown adipocyte transdifferentiation. Am J Physiol Endocrinol Metab 298:E1244–E1253
9. Rosen CJ, Bouxsein ML (2006) Mechanisms of disease: is osteoporosis the obesity of bone? Nat Clin Pract Rheumatol 2:35–43
10. Moore SG, Dawson KL (1990) Red and yellow marrow in the femur: age-related changes in appearance at MR imaging. Radiology 175:219–223
11. Justesen J, Stenderup K, Ebbesen EN, Mosekilde L, Steiniche T, Kassem M (2001) Adipocyte tissue volume in bone marrow is increased with aging and in patients with osteoporosis. Biogerontology 2:165–171
12. Vande Berg BC, Malghem J, Lecouvet FE, Devogelaer JP, Maldague B, Houssiau FA (1999) Fat conversion of femoral marrow in glucocorticoid-treated patients: a cross-sectional and longitudinal study with magnetic resonance imaging. Arthritis Rheum 42:1405–1411
13. Gimble JM, Zvonic S, Floyd ZE, Kassem M, Nuttall ME (2006) Playing with bone and fat. J Cell Biochem 98:251–266
14. Kugel H, Jung C, Schulte O, Heindel W (2001) Age- and sex-specific differences in the 1H-spectrum of vertebral bone marrow. J Magn Reson Imaging 13:263–268
15. Griffith JF, Yeung DK, Ma HT, Leung JC, Kwok TC, Leung PC (2012) Bone marrow fat content in the elderly: a reversal of sex difference seen in younger subjects. J Magn Reson Imaging 36:225–230
16. Griffith JF, Yeung DK, Antonio GE et al (2005) Vertebral bone mineral density, marrow perfusion, and fat content in healthy men and men with osteoporosis: dynamic contrast-enhanced MR imaging and MR spectroscopy. Radiology 236:945–951
17. Morroni M, Giordano A, Zingaretti MC, Boiani R, De Matteis R, Kahn BB, Nisoli E, Tonello C, Pisoschi C, Luchetti MM et al (2004) Reversible transdifferentiation of secretory epithelial cells into adipocytes in the mammary gland. Proc Natl Acad Sci U S A 101:16801–16806
18. De Matteis R, Zingaretti MC, Murano I, Vitali A, Frontini A, Giannulis I, Barbatelli G, Marcucci F, Bordicchia M, Sarzani R et al (2009) In vivo physiological transdifferentiation of adult adipose cells. Stem Cells 27:2761–2768
19. Cinti S (2005) The adipose organ. Prostaglandins Leukot Essent Fat Acids 73:9–15

20. Frontini A, Cinti S (2010) Distribution and development of brown adipocytes in the murine and human adipose organ. Cell Metab 11:253–256
21. Masso-Welch PA, Darcy KM, Stangle-Castor NC, Ip MM (2000) A developmental atlas of rat mammary gland histology. J Mammary Gland Biol Neoplasia 5:165–185
22. Giordano A, Smorlesi A, Frontini A, Barbatelli G, Cinti S (2014) White, brown and pink adipocytes: the extraordinary plasticity of the adipose organ. Eur J Endocrinol 170(5):R159–71
23. Cinti S (2011) Between brown and white: novel aspects of adipocyte differentiation. Ann Med 43:104–115
24. Giordano A, Frontini A, Cinti S (2008) Adipose organ nerves revealed by immunohistochemistry. Methods Mol Biol 456:83–95
25. Kuji I, Imabayashi E, Minagawa A, Matsuda H, Miyauchi T (2008) Brown adipose tissue demonstrating intense FDG uptake in a patient with mediastinal pheochromocytoma. Ann Nucl Med 22:231–235
26. Murano I, Barbatelli G, Giordano A, Cinti S (2009) Noradrenergic parenchymal nerve fiber branching after cold acclimatisation correlates with brown adipocyte density in mouse adipose organ. J Anat 214:171–178
27. Sbarbati A, Morroni M, Zancanaro C, Cinti S (1991) Rat interscapular brown adipose tissue at different ages: a morphometric study. Int J Obes 15:581–587
28. Zingaretti MC, Crosta F, Vitali A et al (2009) The presence of UCP1 demonstrates that metabolically active adipose tissue in the neck of adult humans truly represents brown adipose tissue. FASEB J 23:3113–3120
29. Morroni M, Barbatelli G, Zingaretti MC, Cinti S (1995) Immunohistochemical, ultrastructural and morphometric evidence for brown adipose tissue recruitment due to cold acclimation in old rats. Int J Obes Relat Metab Disord 19:126–131
30. Nedergaard J, Bengtsson T, Cannon B (2010) Three years with adult human brown adipose tissue. Ann N Y Acad Sci 1212:E20–E36
31. Murano I, Barbatelli G, Parisani V, Latini C, Muzzonigro G, Castellucci M, Cinti S (2008) Dead adipocytes, detected as crown-like structures, are prevalent in visceral fat depots of genetically obese mice. J Lipid Res 49:1562–1568
32. Wu J, Boström P, Sparks LM, Ye L, Choi JH, Giang AH, Khandekar M, Virtanen KA, Nuutila P, Schaart G et al (2012) Beige adipocytes are a distinct type of thermogenic fat cell in mouse and human. Cell 150:366–376
33. Lean ME (1989) Brown adipose tissue in humans. Proc Nutr Soc 48:243–256
34. van Marken Lichtenbelt WD, Vanhommerig JW, Smulders NM, Drossaerts JM, Kemerink GJ, Bouvy ND, Schrauwen P, Teule GJ (2009) Cold-activated brown adipose tissue in healthy men. N Engl J Med 360:1500–1508
35. Otto TC, Lane MD (2005) Adipose development: from stem cell to adipocyte. Crit Rev Biochem Mol Biol 40:229–242
36. Timmons JA, Wennmalm K, Larsson O, Walden TB, Lassmann T, Petrovic N, Hamilton DL, Gimeno RE, Wahlestedt C, Baar K et al (2007) Myogenic gene expression signature establishes that brown and white adipocytes originate from distinct cell lineages. Proc Natl Acad Sci U S A 104:4401–4406
37. Rosen ED, MacDougald OA (2006) Adipocyte differentiation from the inside out. Nat Rev Mol Cell Biol 7:885–896
38. Zhang JW, Tang QQ, Vinson C, Lane MD (2004) Dominant-negative C/EBP disrupts mitotic clonal expansion and differentiation of 3T3-L1 preadipocytes. Proc Natl Acad Sci U S A 101:43–47
39. Tseng YH, Kokkotou E, Schulz TJ, Huang TL, Winnay JN, Taniguchi CM, Tran TT, Suzuki R, Espinoza DO, Yamamoto Y et al (2008) New role of bone morphogenetic protein 7 in brown adipogenesis and energy expenditure. Nature 454:1000–1004
40. Kim WK, Choi HR, Park SG, Ko Y, Bae KH, Lee SC (2012) Myostatin inhibits brown adipocyte differentiation via regulation of Smad3-mediated β-catenin stabilization. Int J Biochem Cell Biol 44:327–334

41. Seale P, Bjork B, Yang W, Kajimura S, Chin S, Kuang S, Scimè A, Devarakonda S, Conroe HM, Erdjument-Bromage H et al (2008) PRDM16 controls a brown fat/skeletal muscle switch. Nature 454:961–967
42. Kajimura S, Seale P, Kubota K, Lunsford E, Frangioni JV, Gygi SP, Spiegelman BM (2009) Initiation of myoblast to brown fat switch by a PRDM16-C/EBP-beta transcriptional complex. Nature 460:1154–1158
43. Kajimura S, Seale P, Spiegelman BM (2010) Transcriptional control of brown fat development. Cell Metab 11:257–262
44. Townsend K, Tseng YH (2012) Brown adipose tissue: recent insights into development, metabolic function and therapeutic potential. Adipocyte 1:13–24
45. Barbera MJ, Schluter A, Pedraza N, Iglesias R, Villarroya F, Giralt M (2001) Peroxisome proliferator-activated receptor alpha activates transcription of the brown fat uncoupling protein-1 gene. A link between regulation of the thermogenic and lipid oxidation pathways in the brown fat cell. J Biol Chem 276:1486–1493
46. Cinti S (2009) Transdifferentiation properties of adipocytes in the adipose organ. Am J Physiol Endocrinol Metab 297:E977
47. Wu J, Cohen P, Spiegelman BM (2013) Adaptive thermogenesis in adipocytes: is beige the new brown. Genes Dev 27:234–250
48. Himms-Hagen J, Melnyk A, Zingaretti MC, Ceresi E, Barbatelli G, Cinti S (2000) Multilocular fat cells in WAT of CL-316243-treated rats derive directly from white adipocytes. Am J Physiol Cell Physiol 279:C670–C681
49. Schoonjans K, Auwerx J (2000) Thiazolidinediones: an update. Lancet 355:1008–1010
50. Toseland CD, Campbell S, Francis I, Bugelski PJ, Mehdi N (2001) Comparison of adipose tissue changes following administration of rosiglitazone in the dog and rat. Diabetes Obes Metab 3:163–170
51. Wilson-Fritch L, Nicoloro S, Chouinard M et al (2004) Mitochondrial remodeling in adipose tissue associated with obesity and treatment with rosiglitazone. J Clin Invest 114:1281–1289
52. Koh YJ, Park BH, Park JH et al (2009) Activation of PPAR gamma induces profound multilocularization of adipocytes in adult mouse white adipose tissues. Exp Mol Med 41:880–895
53. Puigserver P, Spiegelman BM (2003) Peroxisome proliferator-activated receptor-gamma coactivator 1 alpha (PGC-1 alpha): transcriptional coactivator and metabolic regulator. Endocr Rev 24:78–90
54. Tiraby C, Tavernier G, Lefort C et al (2003) Acquirement of brown fat cell features by human white adipocytes. J Biol Chem 278:33370–33376
55. Seale P, Conroe HM, Estall J et al (2011) Prdm16 determines the thermogenic program of subcutaneous white adipose tissue in mice. J Clin Invest 121:96–105
56. Hondares E, Iglesias R, Giralt A et al (2011) Thermogenic activation induces FGF21 expression and release in brown adipose tissue. J Biol Chem 286:12983–12990
57. Hondares E, Rosell M, Gonzalez FJ, Giralt M, Iglesias R, Villarroya F (2010) Hepatic FGF21 expression is induced at birth via PPARalpha in response to milk intake and contributes to thermogenic activation of neonatal brown fat. Cell Metab 11:206–212
58. Fisher FM, Kleiner S, Douris N et al (2012) FGF21 regulates PGC-1alpha and browning of white adipose tissues in adaptive thermogenesis. Genes Dev 26:271–281
59. Yadav H, Quijano C, Kamaraju AK et al (2011) Protection from obesity and diabetes by blockade of TGF-beta/Smad3 signaling. Cell Metab 14:67–79
60. Bostrom P, Wu J, Jedrychowski MP et al (2012) A PGC1-alpha-dependent myokine that drives brown-fat-like development of white fat and thermogenesis. Nature 481:463–468
61. Matsumoto T, Kano K, Kondo D et al (2008) Mature adipocyte-derived dedifferentiated fat cells exhibit multilineage potential. J Cell Physiol 215:210–222
62. Cohen P, Miyazaki M, Socci ND, Hagge-Greenberg A, Liedtke W, Soukas AA, Sharma R, Hudgins LC, Ntambi JM, Friedman JM (2002) Role for stearoyl-CoA desaturase-1 in leptin-mediated weight loss. Science 297:240–243

63. Minokoshi Y, Kim YB, Peroni OD, Fryer LG, Muller C, Carling D, Kahn BB (2002) Leptin stimulates fatty-acid oxidation by activating AMP-activated protein kinase. Nature 415:339–343
64. Berg AH, Combs TP, Du X, Brownlee M, Scherer PE (2001) The adipocyte-secreted protein Acrp30 enhances hepatic insulin action. Nat Med 7:947–953
65. Yamauchi T, Kadowaki T (2008) Physiological and pathophysiological roles of adiponectin and adiponectin receptors in the integrated regulation of metabolic and cardiovascular diseases. Int J Obes 32(Suppl 7):S13–S18
66. Hotamisligil GS, Murray DL, Choy LN, Spiegelman BM (1994) Tumor necrosis factor α inhibits signaling from the insulin receptor. PNAS 91:4854–4858
67. Wallenius V, Wallenius K, Ahren B, Rudling M, Carlsten H, Dickson SL, Ohlsson C, Jansson JO (2002) Interleukin-6-deficient mice develop mature-onset obesity. Nat Med 8:75–79

Regulation of Energy Intake

2

Roberto Vettor, Roberto Fabris, and Marco Rossato

Obesity is considered one of the leading health issues and is becoming a global epidemic that is rising worldwide [1]. Overweight and obesity depend on the unbalance between energy intake and expenditure, and there is no doubt that food intake is controlled by internal signals [2]. Since food and then energy intake is a behaviour, it must be mediated by the brain. Although many different regions of the brain have been shown to be involved in the control of daily intake, several studies have demonstrated that two main regions, the ventromedial hypothalamus (VMN) and the lateral hypothalamus (LH), are critically involved in the control of food intake and body weight [2]. The dual-centre hypothesis in the central control of energy balance originates from the first observations performed more than six decades ago with specific brain regions damage and stimulation experiments. On the basis of these studies the "satiety centre" was located in the ventromedial hypothalamic nucleus (VMN), since lesions of this region caused overfeeding and excessive weight gain, while its electrical stimulation suppressed eating. On the contrary, damage or stimulation of the lateral hypothalamus (LH) elicited the opposite set of responses, thus leading to the conclusion that this region represented the "feeding centre" [3, 4]. The subsequent expansion of our knowledge of specific neuronal subpopulations involved in energy homeostasis has replaced the notion of specific "centres" controlling energy balance with that of discrete neuronal pathways fully integrated in a more complex neuronal network [5].

The advancement of our knowledge on the anatomical structure and the function of the hypothalamic regions reveals the great complexity of this system. In this brief overview, we will focus on the knowledge of the main central and neurohormonal mediators involved in the control of energy balance and their possible role in the pathophysiology of obesity.

R. Vettor (✉) • R. Fabris • M. Rossato
Department of Medicine – DIMED, Internal Medicine 3, School of Medicine,
University of Padova, Clinica Medica 3, Via Giustiniani, 2, 35128 Padova, Italy
e-mail: roberto.vettor@unipd.it; roberto.fabris@sanita.padova.it; marco.rossato@unipd.it

2.1 Control of Energy Metabolism by Circadian Clocks

In the vast majority of living organisms, synchronous oscillations of biological parameters can be detected, most of them paralleling the night and day, sleep and waking, rest and activity and feeding and fasting cycles. This is an intrinsic characteristic of each cell of the body to coordinate and integrate all the metabolic, hormonal, immune, neurological and many other functions of the body with the environmental daily, monthly or yearly rhythmic oscillation and cycles. This finely tuned mechanism in humans and all other living organisms involves an intrinsic machinery that tracks time in approximately 24-h cycles being controlled by a series of genes that are down- and upregulated in a closely coordinated feedback loop. The importance of the circadian clock in the control of energy metabolism has been clearly demonstrated, but the detailed mechanisms are far to be elucidated. The complexity of mammalian circadian system is explained by the presence of multiple cellular clocks located in the different tissues. In the hierarchical organization, the master regulator is the suprachiasmatic nuclei (SCN), which synchronizes the downstream organs and tissue clocks using neuronal, endocrine and metabolic signalling pathways that influence the molecular machinery of cellular clocks. Disruption in this synchronization may contribute to the development of diseases such as obesity. This disruption could arise from insensitivity of the suprachiasmatic nucleus and the pineal clock to sense the light and release melatonin according to the circadian cycle. Peripheral hormones as ghrelin, leptin, insulin, corticosteroids and adrenalin affect or are affected by the master clock and a reciprocal alteration could result in a disruption of the coordinated cycling of the metabolic control during the day. Moreover metabolic fuels as glucose, fatty acids, amino acids, lactate and ketone bodies could act as signals having deep influence in the right functioning of the central clock which in turn could influence peripheral organ metabolism throughout specific neuronal connections. In order to understand the clock systems, a useful distinction in three major steps could be taken into account both at the cellular and at the systemic level: (1) the input to the system, (2) the intrinsic mechanisms linked to the clock function and (3) the output system. The clock mechanism consists of two main parts: (1) a transcriptional–translational feedback loop (TTL) consisting of a positive and a negative branch and (2) oscillating post-translational modification of gene products in the TTL, which regulate degradation and/or nuclear localization of these proteins. The positive and negative branches are intertwined via clock protein-driven nuclear receptors and their interactions with period circadian protein homolog 2 (PER2), a component of the negative limb. Per2 is an integral component of a glucocorticoid regulatory pathway involving peripheral clock selectively required for some actions of glucocorticoids. A metabolic oscillator is driven by the TTL and feeds back on it via SIRT1 which stands for sirtuin (silent mating type information regulation 2 homolog) 1, an enzyme that deacetylates proteins that contribute to cellular regulation. The promoter elements in clock-controlled genes (CCGs) are regulated either directly or indirectly. (1) Direct regulation via Circadian Locomotor Output Cycles Kaput (BMAL/CLOCK) functions as an essential activator of downstream elements in the pathway critical to the generation of circadian rhythms by binding at E-boxes or via the nuclear receptors REV-ERB and retinoic acid receptor-related orphan receptors (RORs), which are involved in many physiological processes, including regulation of metabolism, development and immunity as well as the circadian rhythm, by binding at RORE elements and (2) Indirect regulation via binding of clock-regulated circadian transcription of proline- and acidic amino acid-rich basic leucine zipper (PAR-B-ZIP) transcription factors like Dbp (D-element-binding protein) on D-elements or via protein–protein interactions between period circadian protein homolog 2 (PER2) and nuclear receptors at nuclear receptor elements (NREs) such as ROREs [6]. The light–dark cycle is for sure one of the major determinant of the circadian clock. Light signals are directly conveyed to three units in the brain: (1) centres which control timing, such as the SCN and pineal gland; (2) centres devoted to the metabolic integration, such as the subparaventricular zone (sPVZ); and (3) centres which control rewarding, such as the habenula (HB). Light sensing and the subsequent neuronal messages are indirectly transmitted from the SCN which in turn projects to areas devoted to the metabolic integration including the paraventricular nucleus (PVN), sPVZ, dorsomedial hypothalamus (DMH) and arcuate nucleus (ARC). The pineal gland also transmits light information to the HB. Anorexigenic signals as leptin and orexigenic signals as ghrelin primarily affect the ARC, which is important for the metabolic integration of feeding signals, and the ventral tegmental area (VTA), which is important for the integration of reward. The centres important for metabolic and reward integration exchange information with each other and can affect the SCN and pineal gland timing centres. Light and feeding signals combine and contribute to motor coordination and activity [7]. It is therefore well defined that circadian programming mechanisms regulating food intake are crucial in maintaining energy homeostasis [8] and that the development of most of the metabolic disorders could be due to clock genes disruption [9].

2.2 The Arcuate Nucleus

The arcuate nucleus (ARC) is one of the most important brain regions involved in the control of energy homeostasis. It is located in the mediobasal hypothalamus, adjacent to the floor of the third ventricle. Neurons in the ARC express receptors for a variety of hormones known to affect food intake, such as leptin, cortisol, oestrogen, progesterone and growth hormone [10], and the permeability of blood–brain barrier of this part of the brain [11] allowing the passage of these signalling molecules into the brain. Moreover the ARC, like other hypothalamic nuclei (dorsomedial hypothalamic nucleus [DMH], paraventricular nucleus [PVN], VMH and LH), contains neurons that are thought to represent the central glucose sensor element [12], but their action may also be affected by other circulating metabolites, such as FFA [13]. Then the ARC may be viewed as a "metabolic sensor", since it receives and integrates endocrine and metabolic information arriving from periphery concerning the body nutritional and energetic status.

The ARC houses a number of neurons which can be differentiated on the basis of their signalling molecule expression. A first population of cells co-express two neuropeptides which have been strongly implicated in the control of food intake and energy homeostasis that are NPY and AgRP [14]. Two other important signalling molecules, POMC and CART, are co-localized in a distinct, but adjacent, subset of ARC neurons [15].

2.3 Neuropeptide Y

NPY is a 36 amino acid orexigenic peptide with many other endocrine and behavioural effects [16]. It belongs to the pancreatic polypeptide (PP) family, and it is considered the most abundant neuropeptide in the brain [17], the ARC nucleus being the major hypothalamic site of NPY expression. A dense projection is directed to the PVN, but other less dense projections are directed into other nuclei [18]. PVN also receive afferent NPY-containing fibres from catecholaminergic nuclei in the brainstem [19]. NPY is also released locally in the ARC and regulates the NPY/AgRP neurons in a ultrashort loop feedback acting on NPY-Y2/NPY-Y4 receptors [20].

Four different NPY receptors have been recognized in human named NPY-Y1, NPY-Y2, NPY-Y4 and NPY-Y5 that are widely distributed in the hypothalamus [21]. Selective receptor antagonists and the administration of antisense oligonucleotides directed against the different Y receptor subtypes were recognized to inhibit both NPY-induced food intake and the abnormalities of feeding behaviour present in genetically obese animal models [22] although conflicting results have been obtained with other experimental approaches using different putative selective antagonists [23].

2.4 Neuropeptide YY

Neuropeptide YY (PYY) belongs to the NPY and PP family [24]. It is 70 % identical to NPY in mammals, and it was first identified as a gastrointestinal hormone, but it has subsequently been found to occur in neurons. Peptide YY3-36 (PYY3-36) is released from the gastrointestinal tract postprandially in proportion to the calorie content of a meal [25].

In contrast to the well-established functions of NPY, the role of PYY in the nervous system remains obscure. Experiments carried out in humans by intravenous injection of physiological doses of PYY3-36 lead to a significant reduction of appetite and food intake. All these data taken together lead to hypothesize that the elevation of PYY3-36 observed after a normal meal may act through the ARC Y2 receptor to inhibit feeding, thus suggesting at that time the existence of a new important gut–hypothalamic axis as demonstrated successively (see below).

2.5 Agouti-Related Protein

Agouti-related protein (AgRP) is a peptide with orexigenic properties [26], which mRNA and protein can be found in virtually all NPY-expressing cells of the ARC, but not in any other brain region [18]. As with NPY, AgRP synthesis is increased in response to leptin deficiency and during fasting and is inhibited by leptin treatment [17]. The icv AgRP administration, as well as the overexpression of AgRP in transgenic mice, stimulates feeding and induces obesity, and its expression is significantly elevated in genetic models of obesity in mice [27]. AgRP is thought to influence feeding by blocking the action of α-MSH at the melanocortin receptors MC4 and possibly MC3 [28]. However, AgRP's orexigenic action is still potent at long term after melanocortin receptor blockade, indicating the existence of alternative mechanisms for its orexigenic action.

2.6 Pro-opiomelanocortin

Pro-opiomelanocortin (POMC) is the precursor of a number of peptides, including α-MSH and ACTH. It is expressed in the ARC, and many of its effects on energy balance appear to be mediated by α-MSH, which exerts its action by binding to members of a family of melanocortin receptors [29]. In rodents, stimulation of MC3 and MC4 receptors suppresses feeding behaviour, whereas binding of these receptors with synthetic ligands stimulates eating [30]. Moreover the POMC-null mutant mice progressively develop obesity [31], which can also be obtained by targeted deletion of melanocortin receptor gene MC3 and MC4 [32]. In humans abnormalities in both the MC4-R gene and the POMC gene are associated with severe obesity [33] indicating that tonic signalling by MC4 receptor limits food intake and body fat mass. The deletion of the MC3-R gene leads to a different phenotype, having the mutant mice a weight close to the wild-type animals but an altered body composition characterised by an increased fat mass and reduced lean mass. Thus, contrary to what is observed in the MC4-deficient mice, the obesity due to MC3 receptor gene deletion results more from altered metabolism and energy partitioning than to feeding changes. Current available data suggest that MC3 and MC4 receptors have different nonredundant functions in energy homeostasis. As a matter of fact, mice lacking both types of receptors are more obese than the MC4-R-deficient mice, showing therefore additive effects of the two deletions.

2.7 Cocaine- and Amphetamine-Regulated Transcript

Cocaine- and amphetamine-regulated transcript (CART) is a anorectic factor, which is produced in the ARC but also in the PVN, dorsomedial (DMN) and other hypothalamic nuclei [34] and inhibits feeding when administered icv. Hypothalamic

CART peptide and mRNA levels are decreased in fasted rats, genetically obese ob/ob mice, which are leptin deficient, and fa/fa Zucker rats, characterized by a defective leptin receptor [35]. CART is co-expressed with POMC in a subpopulation of neurons in the ARC and distributed to the LH, PVN and preganglionic sympathetic neurons in the thoracic spinal cord. These neurons respond directly to circulating leptin, and it is possible that CART and POMC mediate the inhibitory effect of leptin on food intake.

A majority of both NPY/AgRP and POMC/CART neurons co-express leptin receptors. NPY/AgRP neurons are inhibited by leptin and activated by low leptin levels. Similarly these neurons seem to be activated also by insulin deficiency [36], and insulin receptors have been found to be highly concentrated in the ARC [37]. On the contrary, conditions characterized by insulin or leptin deficiency inhibit POMC and CART expression in the ARC, while the administration of these hormones can prevent or reduce these neuropeptide responses [38]. Taken together, these data indicate that the ARC represents a major site for transducing peripheral adiposity signals, such as leptin and insulin, into a neuronal response.

2.8 Neurotransmitters and Peptides Mediating Appetite Stimulation

Urocortins are a family of CRH-related peptides identified in humans, rodents and other mammalian species. The administration of urocortin into the PVN decreases feeding [39]. Urocortin III distribution in the brain differs from that of CRH and includes the VMH, lateral septum and other areas known to express high levels of CRH-R2, suggesting that urocortin III is the endogenous ligand for this receptor in these areas [40].

TRH, apart from its role in pituitary–thyroid axis, inhibits feeding and drinking when injected icv; its metabolite cyclo(His-Pro) produces a long-lasting reduction in food intake and body weight in rats [41]. The NPY-TRH connection is thought to be mediated through the Y1 receptor, and it has been shown that icv NPY administration can decrease plasma levels of thyroid-stimulating hormone, which links TRH with the thyroid hormones [42].

Orexins A and B are encoded by the same gene and produced in the same regions by a population of neurons separate from MCH. Icv injection of orexin stimulates feeding, and its gene expression increases in response to fasting and leptin deficiency [43]. On the contrary, icv administration of orexin A had no effect on body weight in rats [44]; moreover genetic ablation of orexin-sensitive neurons in mice caused late-onset obesity despite a decrease in food intake [45]. These results may be explained by the observation that orexin A, beyond its stimulation on food intake, increases oxygen consumption and energy expenditure, thus preventing weight gain [46]. Glucose, another signal that is essential in initiating and terminating feeding [47], also appears to regulate orexin neuronal activity since orexin neurones are stimulated by falling blood glucose levels but are inhibited by feeding-related signals, such as signals from the gut as well as a rise in blood glucose [48].

GABA stimulates carbohydrate-rich food intake after injection in the PVN through interaction with GABA-A receptors [49] and benzodiazepines, which are agonists of GABA, beyond their action on anxiety, increase food consumption by potentiating taste palatability of food [50].

2.9 Neurotransmitters and Peptides Mediating Appetite Suppression

Neurotensin, which is produced in the ARC, PVN and DMN, inhibits food intake after icv injection. Leptin stimulates neurotensin synthesis in the hypothalamus; moreover genetically obese ob/ob mice and fa/fa rats exhibit a decreased neurotensin expression, suggesting that neurotensin could mediate, at least in part, the anorectic effect of the ob gene product.

Bombesin-like peptides include gastrin-releasing peptide (GRP), neuromedin B (NMB) and glucagon-like peptide (GLP)-1. Either peripheral or central administration of bombesin-like peptides inhibits food intake by acting on satiety [51]. This effect appears to be mediated through three different receptors: the GRP receptor, the NMB receptor and the bombesin receptor subtype 3 (BRS-3). These receptors share about 50 % amino acids sequence identity but show different affinities for the bombesin-like peptides [52].

2.10 The Cannabinoid System

Epidemiological evidence reporting an orexigenic activity of cannabinoids and the insights into the molecular mechanisms underlying cannabinoid action have suggested a role for this neuromodulatory system in the pathophysiology of obesity. The observation that exogenous cannabinoid derivatives may influence food intake was extensively studied in the 1970s [53]. However, the demonstration in the 1990s of the existence of a new class of endogenous ligands and of specific receptors binding to cannabinoids led to a substantial advancement of the knowledge of this new pathway of regulation of food intake and other central and peripheral functions. Exogenous cannabinoids act by binding two specific receptors, cannabinoid receptor 1 (CB1), abundantly expressed in brain areas involved in feeding behaviour [54], and cannabinoid receptor 2 (CB2) which is mostly expressed in cells of the immune system.

The endogenous cannabinoids. The most common endogenous ligand binding to cannabinoid receptors are anandamide and 2-arachidonoyl glycerol [55], which are produced within the brain by the phospholipid precursor N-arachidonoyl phosphatidylethanolamine by the action of a phospholipase D. Anandamide binds with a higher affinity to CB1 and is present at highest concentration in the hypothalamus, cortex, thalamus and cerebellum of different species including humans. Other endogenous ligands for CB1 and CB2 are docosatetraenoyl ethanolamide, di-homo-γ-linolenoyl ethanolamide and 2-arachidonyl glyceryl ether. Interestingly all these compounds are polyunsaturated fatty acid derivatives. Anandamide and CB1 are present in the hypothalamus in centres known to regulate food intake and body weight regulation.

Extensive data are available on the effects of cannabinoids on food intake in animals. Anandamide administration was demonstrated to induce overeating in rodents, and this effect was mediated by CB1 receptors [56]. A specific CB1 receptor antagonist (SR141716) has been previously synthesized reducing food intake in rats, mice and marmosets. This effect was selective for sweet food, sucrose and ethanol. Interestingly SR141716 inhibition of food intake was present also in NPY-stimulated food intake, thus indicating a neuronal pathway independent from the hypothalamic NPYergic neuronal circuit [57].

Hypothalamic endocannabinoids are elevated in leptin signalling-deficient rodents (*ob/ob* and *db/db* mice, *fa/fa* rats), while leptin administration in normal and *ob/ob* mice reduces anandamide and 2-arachidonoyl glycerol [58]. Moreover knockout mice for CB1 receptor eat less food than wild-type littermates. Taken together, available data on exogenous and endogenous cannabinoids administration, knockout model and endocannabinoid regulation in experimental obesity is strongly suggestive for a role of this biological system in the regulation of feeding behaviour, and an effective antagonist of the CB1 receptor has been recently marketed for obesity treatment although it has been successively retired due to its side effects.

2.11 Signals from Gastrointestinal Tract

Nutrient ingestion stimulates secretion of numerous gastroenteropancreatic hormones into the bloodstream that regulate digestive function. However, it has been proposed that these hormones may play a role also as feedback regulators of meal ingestion and in particular of meal size.

Cholecystokinin (CCK) is present in the brain and the endocrine cells of the duodenum and jejunum. It is released into the bloodstream in response to the presence of food in the intestinal lumen. In addition to its actions on gastrointestinal system, several experimental evidences in different species show that CCK administration reduces food intake [59]. However, the inhibition of food consumption induced by CCK seems to be limited to the reduction of meal size without any significant effect on daily food intake and body weight. Two CCK receptors have been identified. Type A CCK receptor is more abundant in peripheral tissues including pancreas, pyloric sphincter and afferent vagal fibres but is present also in CNS structures. Type B CCK receptors are widely distributed throughout the brain. Type A receptor inhibition, but not type B, prevents the satiety action of administered CCK and increases basal food intake in rats by inhibiting the action of endogenous CCK [60].

Peripheral CCK administration appears to promote satiety by both inhibition of gastric emptying, that indirectly activates vagal afferent signals, and direct activation of a vagal afferent pathway driving to the hypothalamic effector pathways through specific CCK receptors present on vagus nerve fibres. Both these mechanisms require the integrity of the vagus nerve [61].

Ghrelin is a gastrointestinal peptide with a peculiar structure characterized by an octanoic acid chain esterified on a serine residue. It is synthesized in the stomach, intestine, placenta, pituitary and hypothalamus. Ghrelin binds to a specific transmembrane G-protein linked receptor of 366 amino acids belonging to the rhodopsin family [62]. Circulating ghrelin mainly derives from the stomach, and its plasma concentration is influenced by acute and chronic changes in nutritional state [63]. A postprandial reduction of ghrelin is observed in humans, and infusion of ghrelin leads to short-term increase in hunger [64], thus suggesting that ghrelin inhibition shortly after a meal may be responsible for meal cessation. Moreover in obese humans, ghrelin is markedly reduced compared to lean subjects, but it is not further inhibited by feeding [65]. Low ghrelin levels in human obesity exclude that fat excess is determined by an increased activity of this orexigenic pathway. It is of interest that diet-induced weight loss, but not weight loss obtained by gastric surgery, increases ghrelin thus suggesting a link between the persistence of low ghrelin levels and the more effective and prolonged weight loss after gastric bypass surgery [66]. In summary, available data suggest that ghrelin is an orexigenic signal starting in the stomach and acting on CNS by activating hypothalamic effector mechanisms that induce eating and a positive energy balance although other studies are needed in order to better clarify the role of ghrelin in the pathophysiology of human obesity.

Glucagon-like peptide-1 (GLP-1) is a gut hormone secreted after food intake. This hormone greatly increases glucose-stimulated insulin secretion while inhibiting glucagon production [67]. It is also synthesized in the NTS and released in the PVN and DMH. It has anorexigenic effects after central administration; it also has some important role in the regulation of glucose homeostasis. The majority of these actions are probably mediated by the GLP-1 receptor (GLP-1-R). However, data coming from GLP-1-R-knocked-out mice are consistent with a minor role of GLP-1 in the control of satiety [68].

Glucagon-like peptide-2 (GLP-2) is a newly discovered anorectic hormone that is expressed in the NTS and released in the DMH [69]. It is co-secreted with GLP-1 from enteroendocrine cells in the small and large bowels. GLP-2 secretion is regulated by food nutrients, mainly fat and carbohydrates, and targets receptors in the gastrointestinal tract, from the stomach to the colon. The major known actions of GLP-2 are mucosal growth (especially in the proximal bowel, increasing villous height and crypt cell proliferation and inhibiting apoptosis in both the crypt and villous compartments) and increase of the uptake of intestinal nutrients [70]. GLP-2 also increases mesenteric blood flow, thus providing another mechanism to facilitate digestion and absorption of nutrients [71].

GLP-2 may also influence food intake since icv administration of GLP-2 reduces food intake in rats [72] although to date, studies in humans have not demonstrated a decrease in food intake after peripheral GLP-2 administration [73]. The clear demonstration of GLP-2R expression in the nonrodent brain is still lacking, and then the role of this hormone in the central regulation of food intake is still under consideration.

2.12 Signals from Adipose Tissue

Leptin. Several years ago, Coleman and Hummel first hypothesized the existence of a humoral factor, produced by adipose tissue, involved in the monitoring of lipid stores and regulation of body weight. The discovery of leptin then confirmed the theory of the so-called "adipostatic model". Leptin is synthesized mainly in the adipose tissue at levels proportional to body fat content and enters the CNS via a saturable process [74]. Leptin role in energy homeostasis is critical, since the genetic deficiency of either leptin or its receptor causes profound hyperphagia, morbid obesity and several neuroendocrine and metabolic abnormalities both in rodents and in humans. Leptin receptors are expressed by brain neurons involved in energy intake. Neuronal targets for leptin have been identified in the ARC, VMN, DMH and other brain regions [75]. Leptin receptors are also expressed in many peripheral tissues, implying that the role of leptin is much broader than that of a circulating satiety factor [76]. The dramatic effects of leptin administration to ob/ob mice raised expectations that human obesity might also be a leptin deficient state, and so that the exogenous administration of the hormone might be effective in the treatment of the disease as demonstrated successively [77]. However, most obese subjects have increased leptin levels, indicating that obesity is a leptin-resistant state in the majority of cases. A leptin receptor defect caused by a mutation, similar to that described in some rodent models of obesity, was found in obese members of two unrelated families [78], but the frequency of similar mutations in the general population is thought to be very low. Other potential mechanisms of leptin resistance include impaired transport into the brain and defective intracellular leptin signalling. Saturable transport of leptin through the blood–brain barrier may be a rate-limiting step [79]; however, brain leptin transport appears to be saturated even at the low leptin levels found in lean individuals [80].

Insulin was the first hormonal signal to be implicated in the control of body weight by the CNS, acting there to reduce energy intake [81]. Insulin receptors are expressed by brain neurons involved in energy intake, and the administration of the pancreatic hormone directly into the brain reduces food intake, whereas its deficiency does the opposite [36]. These effects appear to be mediated, at least in part, by NPY, since insulin suppresses NPY mRNA expression, while its deficiency has been associated with increased hypothalamic NPY levels [82]. Finally the disruption of the brain insulin receptor gene produced a modest but significant increase in food intake and body weight in mice [83].

Glucocorticoids exert a permissive effect on feeding and adiposity, as confirmed by the presence of hyperphagia and obesity in Cushing's syndrome and anorexia in Addison's disease. Moreover most experimental obesities in rodents are associated with hypercorticism and prevented by adrenalectomy [84]. The effects of glucocorticoids on food intake could be mediated by orexigenic peptides, such as NPY, and there is significant overlap in neuronal targets of glucocorticoids, leptin and insulin, raising the possibility that these hormones act in a coordinated fashion to regulate feeding and energy balance [85]. Indeed glucocorticoids enhance leptin production both in vitro and in vivo [86]. Moreover glucocorticoids can act at the CNS level by reducing the anorectic action of leptin [87] inducing a relative leptin resistance, which in turn may be responsible for the fat deposition observed in hypercorticism. On the other hand, leptin seems to regulate glucocorticoid levels by directly inhibiting cortisol release, but the existence of a feedback between leptin and glucocorticoids in humans has not been demonstrated [88].

Sex steroids are able to influence food intake, body weight and composition, as well as leptin production; conversely sex steroid are related to body fat. Androgens stimulate appetite and increase lean mass, while oestrogens tend to decrease feeding and body weight. Oestrogen deficiency in rats causes impaired central leptin sensitivity and increased hypothalamic NPY production [89]. Sex steroid effects are probably mediated through the regulation of the synthesis of neuropeptides such as NPY, POMC and MCH in similar hypothalamic targets as leptin [90].

Pro-inflammatory cytokines, such as tumour necrosis factor- α (TNF-α), interleukin (IL)-1 and IL-6, which are produced in response to infections and cancer, have been implicated in anorexia and wasting syndrome associated with these conditions. These cytokines can be transported from periphery to the CNS across the blood–brain barrier, where they can act on neuronal pathways and modulate eating behaviour and energy balance [91]. Moreover TNF-α can directly induce ob gene expression in rodents as well as in man [92]; furthermore IL-1 seems to increase leptin levels both directly and through the increase of the hypothalamus–pituitary–adrenal axis activity [93]. IL-6 is expressed both in adipose tissue and in hypothalamic nuclei that regulate body composition. Mice lacking the gene encoding for IL-6 develop mature-onset obesity, altered carbohydrate and lipid metabolism, increased leptin levels and decreased responsiveness to leptin treatment. Icv, but not ip, IL-6 administration was able to increase energy expenditure, partly reversing obesity [94].

Ciliary neurotrophic factor (CTNF), a neurocytokine, decreases body weight and fat depot by inhibiting food intake and increasing energy expenditure [95]. As for leptin, CTNF acts through the Jak–STAT signal transduction pathway; however, hypothalamic targets of CTNF differ from those of leptin [96].

2.13 Monoamine Neurotransmitters

Aminergic neurotransmitter systems provide important targets for drug treatment of obesity. However, these pathways exert ambiguous effects on food intake and their role is complex.

Noradrenaline is synthesized in dorsal vagal complex and locus ceruleus. These areas project to the spinal cord, hypothalamus, thalamus and cortex. In some of these neurons and particularly in those projecting to the PVN, noradrenaline is co-localized with NPY. Like NPY, icv administration of noradrenaline increases food intake and weight gain [97]. Moreover noradrenaline levels in the PVN of ob/ob mice are elevated, suggesting that leptin may inhibit its release in this brain area, as confirmed by in vitro studies using rat hypothalamus [98, 99].

Dopamine signalling is thought to play a relevant role in the regulation of food intake, since pharmacological depletion or genetic disruption of its synthesis deeply alters food intake [100, 101], even if the interpretation of these finding is complicated by motor impairments associated with dopamine deficiency. Mesolimbic dopamine pathways seem to contribute to the "rewarding" aspects of palatable foods [102], while dopamine signalling in the hypothalamus seems to inhibit food intake [3].

Serotonin (5-HT) is synthesized in the dorsal raphé nucleus (DRN) and is distributed to the PVN, VMN and other forebrain regions [112]. It inhibits eating in spontaneously feeding and food-deprived animals. 5-HT agonists reduce body weight in humans by suppressing appetite and increasing energy expenditure, probably acting at the 5-HT2C receptor subtype level [103].

2.14 Nutrient Sensing in the Hypothalamus

In addition to hormones and neurotransmitters, the brain also directly responds to nutrients, such as glucose, fatty acid and amino acids. Within specific hypothalamic nuclei, subsets of neurons with specific neurobiological phenotypes are responsive to nutrients that act as signalling molecules to engage a complex set of neurochemical and neurophysiological responses, thereby regulating energy intake.

Brain glucose sensing. Two different glucose-responsive neurons have been described within the hypothalamus depending on the effect of altered glucose concentration: glucose-excited (GE) neurons, abundant in the lateral hypothalamus (LH), and glucose-inhibited (GI) neurons which are more abundant in the ventromedial hypothalamus (VMH) [104]. Different nutrient-sensing mechanisms and intracellular signal transduction pathways have been implicated in the ability of nutrient-sensing neurons to monitor the amount of available fuel in the body. ATP production and the associated changes in the ADP/ATP ratio have long been considered as the main metabolic signals of nutrient availability although other mechanisms have been suggested in the last years [98, 105].

Brain lipid sensing. Despite the fact that the brain does not use fatty acids (FA) as a major fuel source, there is growing evidence that FA metabolism within distinct hypothalamic regions can function as a sensor for nutrient availability. It has been previously shown that FA, particularly long-chain FA, activate LH neurons [106] and modify neuronal firing rate in ARC [107]. However, the idea that increases in brain FA levels act as a satiety signal to inhibit feeding contrasts with the fact that plasma FA levels do not rise substantially after food ingestion but rise significantly during fasting [108]. Another problem concerning the view of FA directly acting on neurons as a satiety signal is the fact that the vast majority of FA oxidation in the brain occurs in astrocytes rather than neurons [109]. So there must be a mechanism by which alterations in astrocyte FA metabolism can provide a signal to neurons. Hypothalamic glia responds to increases in extracellular glucose levels through an increase in glycolytic ATP production, which induces lactate release from astrocytes [110], and hypothalamic lactate sensing has been shown to regulate food intake [111].

Brain amino acid sensing. Recent data demonstrate that ARC neurons can also sense changes in amino acid availability and implicate this sensing in the regulation of energy balance. Leucine administration into the mediobasal hypothalamus reduces food intake, both through a rapid reduction in meal size and a longer-term reduction in meal number, leading to a reduction in body weight gain [112]. This effect is blunted by rapamycin, a pharmacological inhibitor of the serine–threonine kinase mammalian target of rapamycin (mTOR) [113], a protein kinase activated by states of positive energy balance that is expressed in POMC and AgRP neurons in the ARC, where they respond to insulin, leptin and nutrient levels and exert potent effects on feeding and energy balance [114].

Conclusions

The survival of higher organisms depends on the ability to efficiently acquire, use and conserve energy. Humans and other mammals have developed complex mechanisms to ensure a constant supply of energy for cellular functions in an attempt to fight against the periods of energy deprivation. Like other biological parameters, body weight is usually maintained within a narrow range of variations for long time periods. To ensure the stability of this parameter, calories intake must equal energy needs, and even small environmental reduction in energy availability, food intake and body weight may be perceived as an emergency situation that activates a wide spectrum of events teleologically directed to the survival of the individuals and of the species. The anatomical and functional structure regulating feeding behaviour evolved in an energy-deficient environment. Therefore, at present time the great and easily available quantity of food present in the western countries may be considered an abnormal situation in evolutionary terms, and the immense complexity of these mechanisms adapts poorly to these conditions, explaining at least in part the overwhelming increase in the prevalence of obesity in our population. The complete understanding of all pathophysiological mechanisms regulating energy metabolism in human will lead to the discovery of new medical approaches to treat obesity and related diseases.

References

1. Caballero B (2007) The global epidemic of obesity: an overview. Epidemiol Rev 29:1–5
2. Koopmans HS (2004) Experimental studies on the control of food intake. In: Bray GA, Bouchard C (eds) Handbook of obesity. Marcel Dekker Inc, New York, pp 373–425
3. Anand BK, Brobeck JR (1951) Hypothalamic control of food intake in rats and cats. Yale J Biol Med 24:123–130
4. Elmquist JK, Elias CF, Saper CB (1999) From lesions to leptin: hypothalamic control of food intake and body weight. Neuron 22:221–232
5. Schwartz MW, Woods SC, Porte D Jr et al (2000) Central nervous system control of food intake. Nature 404:661–671
6. Albrecht U (2012) Timing to perfection: the biology of central and peripheral circadian clocks. Neuron 74:246–260
7. Peek CB, Ramsey KM, Marcheva B et al (2012) Nutrient sensing and the circadian clock. Trends Endocrinol Metab 23:312–318

8. Bechtold DA, Loudon ASI (2013) Hypothalamic clocks and rhythms in feeding behaviour. Trends Neurosci 36:74–82
9. Hatori M, Vollmers C, Zarrinpar A (2012) Time-restricted feeding without reducing caloric intake prevents metabolic diseases in mice fed a high-fatdiet. Cell Metab 15:848–860
10. Baskin DG, Breininger JF, Schwartz MW (1999) Leptin receptor mRNA identifies a subpopulation of neuropeptide Y neurons activated by fasting in rat hypothalamus. Diabetes 48:828–833
11. Broadwell RD, Brightman MW (1976) Entry of peroxidase into neurons of the central and peripheral nervous systems from extracerebral and cerebral blood. J Comp Neurol 166:257–283
12. Muroya S, Yada T, Shioda S (1999) Glucose-sensitive neurones in the rat arcuate nucleus contain neuropeptide Y. Neurosci Lett 264:113–116
13. Williams G, Bing C, Cai XJ (2001) The hypothalamus and the control of energy homeostasis: different circuits, different purposes. Physiol Behav 74:683–701
14. Hahn TM, Breininger JF, Baskin DG et al (1998) Coexpression of AgRP and NPY in fasting-activated hypothalamic neurons. Nature Neurosci 1:271–272
15. Khachaturian H, Lewis ME, Haber SN et al (1984) Proopiomelanocortin peptide immunocytochemistry in rhesus monkey brain. Brain Res Bull 13:785–800
16. Tatemoto K (1982) Neuropeptide Y: complete amino acid sequence of the brain peptide. Proc Natl Acad Sci U S A 79:5485–5489
17. Allen YS, Adrian TE, Allen JM et al (1983) Neuropeptide Y distribution in the rat brain. Science 221:877–879
18. Bai FL, Yamano M, Shiotani Y et al (1985) An arcuate-paraventricular and -dorsomedial hypothalamic neuropeptide Y-containing system which lacks noradrenaline in the rat. Brain Res 331:172–175
19. Sawchenko PE, Swanson LW, Grzanna R et al (1985) Colocalization of neuropeptide Y immunoreactivity in brainstem catecholaminergic neurons that project to the paraventricular nucleus of the hypothalamus. J Comp Neurol 241:138–153
20. Broberger C, Landry M, Wong H et al (1997) Subtypes Y1 and Y2 of the neuropeptide Y receptor are respectively expressed in pro-opiomelanocortin- and neuropeptide-Y-containing neurons of the rat hypothalamic arcuate nucleus. Neuroendocrinology 66:393–408
21. Herzog H, Hort YJ, Ball HJ et al (1992) Cloned human neuropeptide Y receptor couples to two different second messenger systems. Proc Natl Acad Sci U S A 89:5794–5798
22. Schaffhauser AO, Stricker-Krongrad A, Brunner L et al (1997) Inhibition of food intake by neuropeptide Y Y5 receptor antisense oligodeoxynucleotides. Diabetes 46:1792–1798
23. Kanatani A, Fukami T, Fukuroda T et al (1997) Y5 receptors are not involved in physiologically relevant feeding in rodents. Regul Pept 71:212–213
24. Tatemoto K, Carlquist M, Mutt V (1982) Neuropeptide Y: a novel brain peptide with structural similarities to peptide YY and pancreatic polypeptide. Nature 296:659–660
25. Pedersen-Bjergaard U, Host U, Kelbaek H et al (1996) Influence of meal composition on postprandial peripheral plasma concentrations of vasoactive peptides in man. Scand J Clin Lab Invest 56:497–503
26. Hagan MM, Rushing PA, Pritchard LM et al (2000) Long-term orexigenic effect of AgRP-(82-132) involve mechanisms other than melanocortin receptor blockade. Am J Physiol 279:R47–R52
27. Ollman MM, Wilson BD, Yang YK et al (1997) Antagonism of central melanocortin receptors in vitro and in vivo by agouti-related protein. Science 278:135–138
28. Fong TM, Mao C, MacNeil T et al (1997) ART (protein product of agouti-related transcript) as an antagonist of MC-3 and MC-4 receptors. Biochem Biophys Res Commun 237:629–631
29. Cone RD, Lu D, Koppula S et al (1996) The melanocortin receptors: agonists, antagonists, and the hormonal control of pigmentation. Recent Prog Horm Res 51:287–317

30. Benoit SC, Schwartz MW, Lachey JL et al (2000) A novel selective melanocortin-4 receptor agonist reduces food intake in rats and mice without producing aversive consequences. J Neurosci 20:3442–3448
31. Yaswen L, Diehl N, Brennan MB et al (1999) Obesity in the mouse model of pro-opiomelanocortin deficiency responds to peripheral melanocortin. Nature Med 5:1066–1070
32. Huszar D, Lynch CA, Fairchild-Huntress V et al (1997) Targeted disruption of the melanocortin-4 receptor results in obesity in mice. Cell 88:131–141
33. Krude H, Biebermann H, Luck W et al (1998) Severe early-onset obesity, adrenal insufficiency and red hair pigmentation caused by POMC mutations in humans. Nature Gen 19:155–157
34. Koylu EO, Couceyro PR, Lambert PD, Ling NC et al (1997) Immunohistochemical localization of novel CART peptides in rat hypothalamus, pituitary and adrenal gland. J Neuroendocr 9:823–833
35. Kristensen P, Judge ME, Thim L et al (1998) Hypothalamic CART is a new anorectic peptide regulated by leptin. Nature 393:72–76
36. Sipols AJ, Baskin DG, Schwartz MW (1995) Effect of intracerebroventricular insulin infusion on diabetic hyperphagia and hypothalamic neuropeptide gene expression. Diabetes 44:147–151
37. Baskin DG, Wilcox BJ, Figlewicz DP et al (1988) Insulin and insulin-like growth factors in the CNS. Trends Neurosci 11:107–111
38. Schwartz MW, Seeley RJ, Woods SC et al (1997) Leptin increases hypothalamic pro-opiomelanocortin mRNA expression in the rostral arcuate nucleus. Diabetes 46:2119–2123
39. Spina M, Merlo-Pich E, Chan RK et al (1996) Appetite-suppressing effects of urocortin, a CRF-related neuropeptide. Science 273:1561–1564
40. Li C, Vaughan J, Sawchenko PE et al (2002) Urocortin III-immunoreactive projections in rat brain: partial overlap with sites of type 2 corticotrophin-releasing factor receptor expression. J Neurosci 22:991–1001
41. Inui A (2000) Transgenic approach to the study of body weight regulation. Pharmacol Rev 52:35–61
42. Härfstrand A, Fuxe K, Agnati LF et al (1986) Studies on neuropeptide Y-catecholamine interactions in the hypothalamus and in the forebrain of the male rat. Relationship to neuroendocrine function. Neurochem Int 8:355–1376
43. Sakurai T, Amemiya A, Ishii M et al (1998) Orexins and orexin receptors: a family of hypothalamic neuropeptides and G protein-coupled receptors that regulate feeding behavior. Cell 92:573–585
44. Yamanaka A, Sakurai T, Katsumoto T et al (1999) Chronic intracerebroventricular administration of orexin-A to rats increases food intake in daytime, but has no effect on body weight. Brain Res 849:248–252
45. Hara J, Beuckmann CT, Nambu T et al (2001) Genetic ablation of orexin neurons in mice results in narcolepsy, hypophagia, and obesity. Neuron 200130:345–354
46. Wang J, Osaka T, Inoue S (2001) Energy expenditure by intracerebroventricular administration of orexin to anesthetized rats. Neurosci Lett 315:49–52
47. Griffond B, Risold PY, Jacquemard C et al (1999) Insulin-induced hypoglycemia increases preprohypocretin (orexin) mRNA in the rat lateral hypothalamic area. Neurosci Lett 262:77–80
48. Cai XJ, Widdowson PS, Harold J et al (1999) Hypothalamic orexin expression: modulation by blood glucose and feeding. Diabetes 48:2132–2137
49. Stratford TR, Kelley AE (1997) GABA in the nucleus accumbens shell participates in the central regulation of feeding behavior. J Neurosci 19:121–131
50. Berridge KC, Pecina S (1999) Benzodiazepines, appetite, and taste palatability. Neurosci Biobehav Rev 37:735–740
51. Merali Z, McIntosh J, Anisman H (1999) Role of bombesin-related peptides in the control of food intake. Neuropeptides 33:376–386
52. Fathi Z, Corjay MH, Shapira H et al (1993) BRS-3: a novel bombesin receptor subtype selectively expressed in testis and lung carcinoma cells. J Biol Chem 268:5979–5984

53. Johansson JO, Jarbe TU, Henriksson BG (1975) Acute and subchronic influences of tetrahydrocannabinols on water and food intake, body weight and temperature in rats. Life Sci 5:17–27
54. Gonzalez S, Manzanares J, Berrendero F et al (1999) Identification of endocannabinoids and cannabinoid CB(1) receptor mRNA in the pituitary gland. Neuroendocrinology 70:137–145
55. Devane WA, Hanus L, Breuer A et al (1992) Isolation and structure of a brain constituent that binds to the cannabinoid receptor. Science 258:1946–1949
56. Williams CM, Kirkham TC (1999) Anandamide induces overeating: mediation by central cannabinoid (CB1) receptors. Psycopharmacol 143:315–317
57. Arnone M, Maruani J, Chaperone F et al (1997) Selective inhibition of sucrose and ethanol intake by SR141716, an antagonist of central cannabinoid (CB1) receptor. Psycopharmacol 132:104–106
58. Di Marzo V, Goparaju SK, Wang L et al (2001) Leptin-regulated endocannabinoids are involved in maintaining food intake. Nature 410:822–825
59. Gibbs J, Young RC, Smith GP (1973) Cholecystokinin decreases food intake in rats. J Comp Physiol Psychol 84:488–495
60. Moran TH, Ameglio PJ, Schwartz GJ, McHugh PR et al (1992) Blockade of type A, not type B, CCK receptors attenuates satiety actions of exogenous and endogenous CCK. Am J Physiol 262:R46–R50
61. Moran TH, McHugh PR (1988) Gastric and non-gastric mechanisms for satiety action of cholecystokinin. Am J Physiol 254:R628–R632
62. Howard AD, Feighner SD, Cully DF et al (1996) A receptor in pituitary and hypothalamus that functions in growth hormone release. Science 273:974–977
63. Ariyasu H, Takaya K, Tagami T et al (2001) Stomach is a major source of circulating ghrelin, and feeding state determines plasma ghrelin-like immunoreactivity levels in humans. J Clin Endocrinol Metab 86:4753–4758
64. Tschop M, Wawarta R, Riepl RL et al (2001) Post-prandial decrease of circulating human ghrelin levels. J Endocrinol Invest 24:RC19–21
65. Tschop M, Weyer C, Tataranni PA et al (2001) Circulating ghrelin levels are decreased in human obesity. Diabetes 50:707–709
66. Cummings DE, Weigle DS, Frayo RS et al (2002) Plasma ghrelin levels after diet-induced weight loss or gastric bypass surgery. N Engl J Med 346:1623–1630
67. Meeran K, O'Shea D, Edwards CM et al (1999) Repeated intracerebroventricular administration of glucagon-like peptide-1-(7-36) amide or exendin-(9-39) alters body weight in the rat. Endocrinology 140:244–250
68. Valassi E, Scacchi M, Cavagnini F (2008) Neuroendocrine control of food intake. Nutr Metab Cardiovasc Dis 18:158–168
69. Estall JL, Drucker DL (2006) Glucagon-like Peptide-2. Annu Rev Nutr 26:391–411
70. Lund A, Vilsboll T, Bagger JI et al (2011) The separate and combined impact of the intestinal secretion in type 2 diabetes hormones, GIP, GLP-1, and GLP-2, on glucagon. Am J Physiol Endocrinol Metab 300:E1038–E1046
71. Bremholm L, Hornum M, Henriksen BM et al (2009) Glucagon-like peptide-2 increases mesenteric blood flow in humans. Scand J Gastroenterol 44:314–319
72. Lovshin J, Estall J, Yusta B et al (2001) Glucagon-like peptide (GLP)-2 action in the murine central nervous system is enhanced by elimination of GLP-1 receptor signaling. J Biol Chem 276:21489–21499
73. Sorensen LB, Flint A, Raben A et al (2003) No effect of physiological concentrations of glucagon-like peptide-2 on appetite and energy intake in normal weight subjects. Int J Obes Relat Metab Disord 27:450–456
74. Zhang Y, Proenca R, Maffei M et al (1994) Positional cloning of the mouse obese gene and its human homologue. Nature 372:425–432
75. Ahima RS, Saper CB, Flier JS et al (2000) Leptin regulation of neuroendocrine systems. Front Neuroendocr 21:263–307

76. Tritos NA, Mantzoros CS (1997) Leptin: its role in obesity and beyond. Diabetologia 40:1371–1379
77. Grasso P (2011) Novel approaches to the treatment of obesity and type 2 diabetes mellitus: bioactive leptin-related synthetic peptide analogs. Recent Pat Endocr Metab Immune Drug Discov 5:163–175
78. Clement K, Garner C, Hager J et al (1996) Indication for linkage of the human OB gene region with extreme obesity. Diabetes 45:687–690
79. Schwartz MW, Peskind E, Raskind M et al (1996) Cerebrospinal fluid leptin levels: relationship to plasma levels and to adiposity in humans. Nature Med 2:589–593
80. Ahima RS, Osei SY (2001) Molecular regulation of eating behavior: new insights and prospects for therapeutic strategies. Trends Mol Med 7:205–213
81. Woods SC, Lotter EC, McKay LD et al (1979) Chronic intracerebroventricular infusion of insulin reduces food intake and body weight of baboons. Nature 282:503–505
82. Cusin I, Dryden S, Wang Q et al (1995) Effect of sustained physiological hyperinsulinaemia on hypothalamic neuropeptide Y and NPY mRNA levels in the rat. J Neuroendocrinol 7:193–197
83. Bruning JC, Gautam D, Burks DJ et al (2000) Role of brain insulin receptor in control of body weight and reproduction. Science 289:2122–2125
84. Bray GA, York DA (1979) Hypothalamic and genetic obesity in experimental animals: an autonomic and endocrine hypothesis. Physiol Rev 59:719–809
85. Dallman MF, Strack AM, Akana SF et al (1993) Feast and famine: critical role of glucocorticoids with insulin in daily energy flow. Front Neuroendocrinol 14:303–347
86. Bradley RL, Cheatham B (1999) Regulation of ob gene expression and leptin secretion by insulin and dexamethasone in rat adipocytes. Diabetes 48:272–278
87. Jeanrenaud B, Rohner-Jeanrenaud F (2000) CNS-periphery relationships and body weight homeostasis: influence of the glucocorticoid status. Int J Obes 24(Suppl 2):S74–S76
88. Malendowicz LK, Macchi C, Nussdorfer GG et al (1998) Acute effects of recombinant murine leptin on rat pituitary-adrenocortical function. Endocrinol Res 24:235–246
89. Ainslie DA, Morris MJ, Wittert G et al (2001) Estrogen deficiency causes central leptin insensitivity and increased hypothalamic neuropeptide Y. Int J Obes 25:1680–1688
90. Mystkowski P, Schwartz MW (2000) Gonadal steroids and energy homeostasis in the leptin era. Nutrition 16:937–946
91. Plata-Salaman CR (1998) Cytokine-induced anorexia. Behavioral, cellular, and molecular mechanisms. Ann N Y Acad Sci 856:160–170
92. Fawcett RL, Waechter AS, Williams LB et al (2000) Tumor necrosis factor-alpha inhibits leptin production in subcutaneous and omental adipocytes from morbidly obese humans. J Clin Endocrinol Metab 85:530–535
93. Langhans W, Hrupka B (1999) Interleukins and tumor necrosis factor as inhibitors of food intake. Neuropeptides 1999(33):415–524
94. Wallenius V, Wallenius K, Ahren B et al (2002) Interleukin-6-deficient mice develop mature-onset obesity. Nature Med 8:75–79
95. Gloaguen I, Costa P, Demartis A et al (1997) Ciliary neurotrophic factor corrects obesity and diabetes associated with leptin deficiency and resistance. Proc Natl Acad Sci U S A 94:6456–6461
96. Bjorbaek C, Elmquist JK, El-Haschimi K et al (1999) Activation of SOCS-3 messenger ribonucleic acid in the hypothalamus by ciliary neurotrophic factor. Endocrinology 140:2035–2043
97. Leibowitz SF, Roossin P, Rosenn M (1984) Chronic norepinephrine injection into the hypothalamic paraventricular nucleus produces hyperphagia and increased body weight in the rat. Pharmacol Biochem Behav 21:801–808
98. Oltmans GA (1983) Norepinephrine and dopamine levels in hypothalamic nuclei of the genetically obese mouse (ob/ob). Brain Res 273:369–373
99. Brunetti L, Michelotto B, Orlando G, Vacca M et al (1999) Leptin inhibits norepinephrine and dopamine release from rat hypothalamic neuronal endings. Eur J Pharmacol 372:237–240

100. Salamone JD, Mahan K, Rogers S (1993) Ventrolateral striatal dopamine depletions impair feeding and food handling in rats. Pharmacol Biochem Behav 44:605–610
101. Szczypka MS, Rainey MA, Kim DS et al (1999) Feeding behavior in dopamine-deficient mice. Proc Natl Acad Sci U S A 96:12138–12143
102. Pothos EN, Creese I, Hoebel BG (1995) Restricted eating with weight loss selectively decreases extracellular dopamine in the nucleus accumbens and alters dopamine response to amphetamine, morphine, and food intake. J Neurosci 15:6640–6650
103. Nonogaki K, Strack AM, Dallman MF et al (1998) Leptin-independent hyperphagia and type 2 diabetes in mice with a mutated serotonin 5-HT2C receptor gene. Nature Med 4:1152–1156
104. Oomura Y, Yoshimatsu H (1984) Neural network of glucose monitoring system. J Auton Nerv Syst 10:359–372
105. Levin BE (2006) Metabolic sensing neurons and the control of energy homeostasis. Physiol Behav 89:486–489
106. Oomura Y, Nakamura T, Sugimori M et al (1975) Effect of free fatty acid on the rat lateral hypothalamic neurons. Physiol Behav 14:483–486
107. Wang R, Cruciani-Guglielmacci C, Migrenne S et al (2006) Effects of oleic acid on distinct populations of neurons in the hypothalamic arcuate nucleus are dependent on extracellular glucose levels. J Neurophysiol 95:1491–1498
108. Ruge T, Hodson L, Cheeseman J et al (2009) Fasted to fed trafficking of fatty acids in human adipose tissue reveals a novel regulatory step for enhanced fat storage. J Clin Endocrinol Metab 94:1781–1788
109. Escartin C, Pierre K, Colin A et al (2007) Activation of astrocytes by CNTF induces metabolic plasticity and increases resistance to metabolic insults. J Neurosci 27:7094–7104
110. Pellerin L (2003) Lactate as a pivotal element in neuron-glia metabolic cooperation. Neurochem Int 43:331–338
111. Lam CK, Chari M, Wang PY et al (2008) Central lactate metabolism regulates food intake. Am J Physiol Endocrinol Metab 295:E491–E496
112. Blouet C, Jo YH, Li X et al (2009) Mediobasal hypothalamic leucine sensing regulates food intake through activation of a hypothalamus-brainstem circuit. J Neurosci 29:8302–8311
113. Cota D, Proulx K, Smith KA et al (2006) Hypothalamic mTOR signaling regulates food intake. Science 312:927–930
114. Minokoshi Y, Alquier T, Furukawa N et al (2004) AMP-kinase regulates food intake by responding to hormonal and nutrient signals in the hypothalamus. Nature 428:569–574

Obesity: Definition and Epidemiology

Stefania Maggi, Luca Busetto, Marianna Noale,
Federica Limongi, and Gaetano Crepaldi

3.1 Introduction

In the recent years, obesity has received considerable attention as a major health risk, to the point that some scientists have predicted that it could become responsible for reversing the current trend of increasing life expectancy [1]. Indeed, obesity is the most prevalent form of malnutrition in the industrialized countries, and it is rapidly becoming highly prevalent also in the developing world. It is considered a multifactorial condition, caused by a complex interaction between the environment, genetic predisposition, and human behavior.

The relevance of obesity as a risk factor for medical conditions is very well appreciated; it is now considered as a major contributor to the global burden of disease and disability, because it is linked to various disabling conditions, such as heart disease, diabetes, hypertension, stroke, certain cancers, osteoarthritis, and respiratory abnormalities, and to several digestive diseases, including gastro-esophageal reflux disease (GERD) and its complications, colorectal polyps and cancer, and liver disease (e.g., nonalcoholic fatty liver disease, cirrhosis, and hepatocellular carcinoma) [2]. Moreover, it has been reported that obesity is associated with an increased risk of death, although the relation of BMI categories with mortality has been the subject of much controversy, because epidemiologic studies have found linear, U-shaped, or J-shaped relationship between BMI and total mortality [3].

S. Maggi (✉) • M. Noale • F. Limongi • G. Crepaldi
CNR-Neuroscience Institute, Aging Branch-Padova,
Via Giustiniani 2, 35128 Padova, Italy
e-mail: Stefania.maggi@in.cnr.it; Marianna.noale@in.cnr.it

L. Busetto
Department of Medicine, University of Padova,
Via Giustiniani 2, 35128 Padova, Italy
e-mail: Luca.busetto@unipd.it

3.2 Definition

Many definitions of overweight and obesity have been proposed over time for adults. According to the World Health Organization, overweight and obesity are defined as abnormal or excessive fat accumulation that presents a risk to health. A crude population measure of overweight and obesity is the body mass index (BMI), a person's weight (in kilograms) divided by the square of his height (in meters). BMI (kg/m^2) is used in epidemiology and in clinical practice to define underweight, normal weight, overweight (pre-obesity), and obesity [4]. However, BMI is not a biological trait, but a calculated value based on body weight. The use of BMI as a proxy for adiposity, the true determinant of the obese state, may be misleading, given that body weight is the sum of individual organs and tissues and therefore it includes adipose tissue, skeletal muscle mass, and organs mass. Moreover, BMI does not convey any information on fat distribution (e.g., visceral fat accumulation and fatty infiltrations in individual organs) that is now considered an important determinant of metabolic and cardiovascular risk [5]. On the other hand, current reference methods for the direct measurement of fat mass (underwater weighing, total body densitometry) or total and regional adipose tissue volumes (CT or MRI) are costly and not applicable in large epidemiologic investigations or in routine clinical practice.

On a population level, a strong positive correlation between BMI and overall body fat content has been extensively reported [6]. However, this can mask significant variations in the relationship between BMI and adiposity on an individual level. For instance, the body fat content of a healthy subject with a normal BMI value (24 kg/m^2) has been demonstrated to vary from 8 % to 38 % in men and from 30 to 44 % in women [7]. This large variability implies that an individual subject may have a BMI corresponding to an obese state having both a low fat-free mass and a substantial fat accumulation or having a large skeletal muscle mass and normal fat mass. This latter condition typically occurs in athletes, in which high BMI may simply reflect increased muscle mass, which does not have anything to do with obesity and associated diseases. Even at an epidemiologic level, the poor performance of BMI as a marker of adiposity is emphasized by the large differences in percentage body fat observed between men and women having the same BMI level. In particular, women are characterized by a higher percentage of body fat than men, and by a different distribution, with higher subcutaneous rather than visceral adipose tissue [8]. Ethnic factors should also be taken into consideration. A BMI of 20–25 kg/m^2, which would be considered normal and healthy within a Caucasian population, corresponds to an elevated body fat content and is associated with an increased disease risk in other ethnic groups, and particularly in Asian populations. This observation prompted the WHO to adopt different cutoff points for overweight and obesity in people of Asian origin (Table 3.1) [9].

Table 3.1 The classification of weight category by BMI

Classification	BMI (kg/m^2) general cutoff points	BMI (kg/m^2) cutoff points for Asian populations
Underweight	<18.5	<18.5
Normal range	18.5–24.9	18.5–22.9
Pre-obese	25.0–29.9	23.0–27.4
Obese class I	30.0–34.9	27.5–32.4
Obese class II	35.0–39.9	32.5–37.4
Obese class III	≥40.0	≥37.5

Source: Adapted from WHO [4, 9]

3.3 Prevalence Rates and Trends

The prevalence of obesity around the world is monitored by the WHO through the Global Database on BMI that gathered data from surveys or population studies, where weight and height are measured or self-reported [10].

In 2008, 35 % of adults aged 20+ were overweight and 11 % were obese (meaning that 205 million men and 300 million women were obese). The worldwide prevalence of obesity had nearly doubled since 1980 (10 % of men and 14 % of women were obese in 2008, compared with 5 % for men and 8 % for women in 1980). The prevalence of overweight and obesity was highest in the WHO Regions of the Americas (62 % for overweight in both sexes and 26 % for obesity) and lowest in the WHO Region for Southeast Asia (14 % overweight in both sexes and 3 % for obesity). In the WHO Region for Europe, for the Eastern Mediterranean, and for the Americas, over 50 % of women were overweight; for all three of these regions, roughly half of overweight women are obese (23 % in Europe, 24 % in the Eastern Mediterranean, 29 % in the Americas). In all WHO regions, women were more likely to be obese than men, and in the WHO regions for Africa, Eastern Mediterranean, and Southeast Asia, women had roughly double the obesity prevalence of men (Fig. 3.1).

The prevalence rates of overweight and obesity increase with income level of countries up to upper middle income levels. The prevalence of overweight in high income and upper middle income countries was more than double that of low and lower middle income countries. For obesity, the difference more than triples from 7 % obesity in both sexes in lower middle income countries to 24 % in upper middle income countries. Women's obesity was significantly higher than men's, with the exception of high income countries where it was similar.

The current epidemic of obesity has been reported in most, but not all, regions of the world.

The more recent US data are from the National Health and Nutrition Examination Survey, 2011–2012. More than one-third (35 %) of adults were obese and the

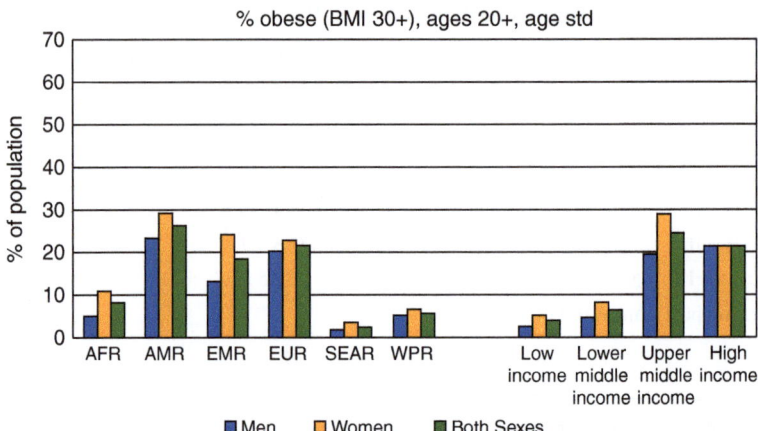

Fig. 3.1 Prevalence of obesity (BMI 30+) in the population aged 20+ in the WHO Regions (age standardized) [10]

prevalence of obesity was higher among middle-aged adults (40 %). The overall prevalence rates of obesity did not differ by gender, but they differ within ethnic groups: for example, among non-Hispanic black adults 57 % of women were obese, compared to 37 % of men. The highest prevalence rate of obesity was among non-Hispanic black adults (48 %), the lowest among non-Hispanic Asian adults (10.8 %). The prevalence of obesity among adults did not change between 2009–2010 and 2011–2012. In the early 1960s, the prevalence of obesity was 11 % among men and 16 % among women, and it changed relatively little until 1980. Data from NHANES II (between 1976 and 1980) and NHANES III (between 1988 and 1994) demonstrate that the prevalence rates of obesity increased considerably, to about 21 % in men and to about 26 % in women. By 2003–2004 the prevalence had increased to almost 32 % in men and 34 % in women [11].

Overall, most countries have rising trends of obesity. Only 2 of the 28 countries in the Global Database on BMI showed a falling trend in the prevalence of obesity in men (Denmark and Saudi Arabia), and 5 of the 28 countries showed a falling trend in the prevalence of obesity in women (Denmark, Ireland, Saudi Arabia, Finland, and Spain) [10].

However, the secular trend on the prevalence of obesity must be considered with caution: a continuous variable, such as body weight, is used to classify dichotomous variables, such as obesity and overweight. This could imply that an average modest weight gain might lead to a relevant increase in the incidence of overweight and obesity. However, in the USA it has been reported that the average increase of BMI has been very relevant, changing from 25.6 in 1976–1980 to 27.9 in 1999–2004 in men and from 25.3 to 28.7 in women, respectively (this corresponds to an increase of more than 7 kg in weight for men and women of average heights) [12].

Overweight and obesity lead to adverse metabolic effects on blood pressure, cholesterol, triglycerides, and insulin resistance. Risks of coronary heart disease, ischemic stroke, and type 2 diabetes mellitus increase steadily with increasing body mass index (BMI). Raised body mass index also increases the risk of sleep apnea, musculoskeletal disease, infertility, dementia, and cancer of the breast, colon, prostate, kidney, endometrium, and gall bladder. Recent analyses show that, in spite of advances in cardiovascular prevention and treatment, it is likely that the overall health burden associated with excess body weight will increase over time, particularly through an increasing prevalence of all other more disabling conditions associated with it [2].

Many epidemiologic studies report a U-shaped relationship between total mortality and BMI, with significant increased mortality at either extremes of BMI, but lower mortality in the overweight category [13]. The relation between overweight and total mortality is controversial, because some studies report an inverse relationship, but methodological issues might be responsible for this "obesity paradox," for example, reverse causality, given that elevated mortality rates at low BMI might be due to weight loss associated with occult or preexisting diseases, to smoking, or, in older population, to the development of frailty. Moreover, potential over-controlling by adjustment for weight-related conditions (such as diabetes and hypertension) might mislead and decrease the association of BMI and mortality [14, 15]. A recent long-term prospective study of older men indicates that a good overall health prognosis is associated with maintaining normal weight over the life course. It also demonstrates that age is an effect modifier in the association between overweight and risk of death and disability: midlife overweight is associated with a higher mortality rate, whereas in late life, the associations become more complex. Those who lose weight after being overweight in midlife not only have a higher risk of death but also have a higher risk of developing frailty and incident mobility-related disability in late life [16]. One important consideration is that higher BMI values may also be due to higher lean body mass, and a further indication comes from the Cardiovascular Health Study, where in men and women 65+, higher waist circumference was related to higher mortality risk, after controlling for BMI, while high BMI was associated with lower mortality, when controlling for waist circumference, probably because it represented the protective effect of lean mass [17]. During recent years, the obesity paradox has been a popular topic in the research of chronic diseases, such as cardiovascular disease, diabetes, and cancer. The suggestion that overweight or obesity could have beneficial effects may even have raised questions about the need for weight control programs. However, as reported in recent studies, the apparent paradox may be due to relatively short follow-up times and, especially, the inability of most studies to account for weight trend during the life course.

Weight should be rigorously controlled since birth. A study comparing data from large nationwide surveys has shown that the combined prevalence of obesity and overweight in children was high in the USA (25 %), moderate in Russia (16 %), and low in China (7 %) [18]. Previous studies indicate that in many developed countries children obesity has reached levels similar to those in the USA and that it is increasing in developing countries (e.g., in Brazil it has tripled from 1970 (4 %) to 1990 (14 %)). To the contrary, recent trend seems to stabilize in US children, and this might be due to the aggressive campaign against obesity and unhealthy dietary patterns. Data from other countries have shown a decline or stabilization of obesity levels, especially in children. For example, in Germany a study found a significant decline in overweight or obesity in children aged 4–7 years and a stabilization in children from 8 to 16 years of age, between 2004 and 2008 [19]. An Italian survey (Okkio alla salute) shows that 22.2 % of children aged <14 years are overweight, while 10.6 % are obese, with higher percentages in the southern regions. However, in Italy, as well as in the USA, prevalence seems to be stabilized in the very recent years [20].

In conclusion, we believe that the high prevalence rate of overweight and obesity, in spite of stabilized trends observed in the recent past in some developed countries, has to be considered with great concern, particularly in children. A high percentage of obese children and adolescents nowadays present complications which, until a decade ago, characterized only adulthood: insulin resistance, type 2 diabetes, dyslipidemia, hepatic steatosis, hypertension, that sometimes cluster in the metabolic syndrome, and all of them are associated to cardiovascular events, cancer and premature death as an adult. [21]. Obese children are also at higher risk of precocious puberty, polycystic ovary syndrome, nighttime sleep apnea, orthopedic complications, and psychological and social disturbances [22]. Nor should it be forgotten that obese children have a higher probability of becoming obese adults [23].

3.4 Determinants of Obesity

Environmental factors are likely to be major contributors to the obesity epidemic, together with biological predisposition. It is certain that obesity develops when there is a positive imbalance between energy intake and energy expenditure, but the relative contribution of these factors is poorly understood. Evidence supports the contribution of both excess energy intake and decreased energy expenditure in determining obesity:

1. Dietary data from four consecutive NHANES studies, consisting of 39,094 adults in the USA, have shown that the temporal trends in the increase of the quantity and energy density of foods consumed by adults parallel the increasing prevalence of obesity in the US population [24].
2. Data from the Central Statistical Office show that car ownership and television viewing, proxy measures of physical inactivity, closely parallel the rising trends in obesity in England [25].
3. Using data from NHANES, Dietz et al. demonstrated that the prevalence of obesity increased by 2 % for each additional hour of television viewed [26].
4. There is also evidence that the relative availability and price of different food products affect food consumption [27] and that the built environment, such as quality of local parks, affects the level of physical activities in a community [28].

These findings not only emphasize the impact of environmental factors on the obesity epidemic but also indicate that policies affecting the availability of high-caloric-density food, the cost of fruits and vegetables, and the built environment may contribute to the alarming prevalence rates of overweight and obesity.

In addition to environmental factors, there is genetic predisposition to obesity, and there is growing evidence that common genetic variants or single-nucleotide polymorphisms (SNP) may play an important role in the obesity epidemic. These SNPs have modest effects on an individual susceptibility to common forms of obesity, but due to their high frequency, they can have a large contribution to obesity on the population level [29].

Body size often is associated with socioeconomic status. However, the magnitude and the direction of the association tend to differ by level of economic development, sex, and race/ethnicity. In less-developed countries, higher weight may be associated with wealth and high income, and there may be a positive association between socioeconomic status and body size for both men and women. Historically, in many contexts, greater body size, including tallness, increased muscularity, and increased fatness, has symbolized power, dominance, wealth, or high social standing. For men in developed countries, height is associated positively with socioeconomic status, but weight and BMI tend to be weakly, if at all, associated with socioeconomic status. For women in developed countries, however, weight and BMI have a strong inverse association with socioeconomic status [18].

3.5   Summary and Conclusions

The prevalence of obesity has increased dramatically in the last decades in both adults and children, with evidence of possible recent stabilization, according to data from the USA and also from Italy [19, 20]. Nevertheless, the prevalence rates continue to be greater than one-third of the population, and, therefore, the Healthy People 2020 goal is not met yet [30]. The reduction of the prevalence rate of obesity is a public health priority. The epidemic of obesity is not limited to developed countries but has been documented in several regions worldwide, with the prevalence of obesity rising in most countries. Obesity is affected by a complex interaction between the environment, genetic predisposition, and human behavior. It is associated with an increased risk of numerous chronic diseases, from diabetes and cancers to many digestive diseases and to disability and death. In addition, the obesity epidemic represents a heavy burden on the economy with its massive healthcare costs. The problem of overweight and obesity has therefore emerged as one of the most pressing global issues that we will continue to face during the next several decades and demands attention from the healthcare community, researchers, and policy makers.

To fight the global obesity epidemic is a public health priority, and population-based, social, and environmental approaches should be developed.

References

1. Olshansky SJ, Passaro DJ, Hershow RC et al (2005) A potential decline in life expectancy in the United States in the 21st century. N Engl J Med 352(11):1138–1145
2. Peeters A, Backholer K (2012) Is the health burden associated with obesity changing? Am J Epidemiol 176(10):840–845

3. Campos P, Saguy A, Ernsberger P et al (2006) The epidemiology of overweight and obesity: public health crisis or moral panic? Int J Epidemiol 35(1):55–60
4. WHO (2000) Obesity: preventing and managing the global epidemic. Report of a WHO consultation. World Health Organ Tech Rep Ser 894:1–253
5. Müller MJ, Lagerpusch M, Enderle J et al (2012) Beyond the body mass index: tracking body composition in the pathogenesis of obesity and the metabolic syndrome. Obes Rev 13:6–13
6. Okorodudu DO, Jumean MF, Montori VM et al (2010) Diagnostic performance of body mass index to identify obesity as defined by body adiposity: a systematic review and meta-analysis. Int J Obes 34:791–799
7. Thomas EL, Frost G, Taylor-Robinson SD, Bell JD (2012) Excess body fat in obese and normal-weight subjects. Nutr Res Rev 25:150–161
8. Karastergiou K, Smith SR, Greenberg A (2012) Sex differences in human adipose tissues – the biology of pear shape. Biol Sex Differ 3:13
9. WHO (2004) Appropriate body-mass index for Asian populations and its implications for policy and intervention strategies. Lancet 363:157–163
10. World Health Organization (2008) Obesity. Available at: http://www.who.int/topics/obesity/en/. Accessed 7 Mar 2014
11. Ogden CL, Carroll BK, Flegal KM (2013) Prevalence of obesity among adults: United States, 2011–2012. NCHS Data Brief 131
12. Finucane MM, Stevens GA, Cowan MJ, Danaei G et al (2011) National, regional, and global trends in body-mass index since 1980: systematic analysis of health examination surveys and epidemiological studies with 960 country-years and 9·1 million participants. Lancet 377(9765):557–567
13. Flegal KM, Kit BK, Orpana H, Graubard BI (2013) Association of all-cause mortality with overweight and obesity using standard body mass index categories: a systematic review and meta-analysis. JAMA 309(1):71–82
14. Ferreira I, Stehouwer CDA (2012) Obesity paradox or inappropriate study designs? Time for life-course epidemiology. J Hypertens 30(12):2271–2275
15. Adams KF, Schatzkin A, Harris TB et al (2006) Overweight, obesity, and mortality in large prospective cohort of persons 50 to 71 years old. N Engl J Med 355(8):763–778
16. Strandberg TE, Stenholm S, Strandberg AY et al (2013) The "obesity paradox," frailty, disability, and mortality in older men: a prospective, longitudinal cohort study. Am J Epidemiol 178(9):1452–1460
17. Janssen I, Katzmarzyk PT, Ross R (2005) Body mass index is inversely related to mortality in older people after adjustment for waist circumference. J Am Geriatr Soc 53(12): 2112–2118
18. Wang Y (2001) Cross-national comparison of childhood obesity: the epidemic and the relationship between obesity and socioeconomic status. Int J Epidemiol 30(5):1129–1136
19. Ogden CL, Carroll MD, Kit BK, Flegal KM (2014) Prevalence of childhood and adult obesity in the United States, 2011–2012. JAMA 311(8):806–814
20. Dati Nazionali 2012. Okkio alla Salute, www.okkioallasalute.it (2012)
21. Weiss R, Dziura J, Burgert TS et al (2004) Obesity and the metabolic syndrome in children and adolescents. N Engl J Med 350:2362–2374
22. Han JC, Lawlor DA, Kimm SYS (2010) Childhood obesity. Lancet 375:1737–1748
23. Franks PW, Hanson RL, Knowler WC et al (2010) Childhood obesity, other cardiovascular risk factors, and premature death. N Engl J Med 362:485–493
24. Kant AK, Graubard BI (2006) Secular trends in patterns of self-reported food consumption of adult Americans: NHANES 1971–1975 to NHANES 1999–2002. Am J Clin Nutr 84(5): 1215–1223
25. Prentice AM, Jebb SA (1995) Obesity in Britain: gluttony or sloth? BMJ 311(7002):437–439
26. Dietz WH Jr, Gortmaker SL (1985) Do we fatten our children at the television set? Obesity and television viewing in children and adolescents. Pediatrics 75(5):807–812

27. Holsten JE (2008) Obesity and the community food environment: a systematic review. Public Health Nutr 14:1–9
28. Kipke MD, Iverson E, Moore D et al (2007) Food and park environments: neighborhood-level risks for childhood obesity in east Los Angeles. J Adolesc Health 40(4):325–333
29. Andreasen CH, Andersen G (2009) Gene-environment interactions and obesity-further aspects of genomewide association studies. Nutrition 25(10):998–1003
30. Wang YC, Orleans CT, Gortmaker SL (2012) Reaching the healthy people goals for reducing childhood obesity: closing the energy gap. Am J Prev Med 42(5):437–444

Part II

Metabolism and Endocrinology

Obesity and Thyroid Function

4

Giovanni Ceccarini, Alessio Basolo, and Ferruccio Santini

4.1 Introduction

The prevalence of both obesity and thyroid disorders is fairly elevated among the general population. This fact, together with the well-known action of thyroid hormone on energy expenditure, has contributed to generate the belief that there is a pathogenic link between fat accumulation and undetected thyroid function deficiency. The relationships between serum thyroid hormones, body weight, and feeding have been intensively investigated over the last decades. The aim of this chapter is to review relevant studies on the reciprocal interaction between the hypothalamo-pituitary-thyroid axis and adipose tissue, to verify scientific evidence over implausible beliefs.

4.2 Thyroid Hormone and Adipose Tissue

Thyroxine (T4) is the major secretory product of the thyroid gland and may be considered a precursor of the active form of the hormone *3,5,3'-triiodothyronine* (*T3*) that is mainly produced in peripheral tissues by 5'-deiodination of T4 [1]. Thyroid hormone synthesis and release are controlled by the thyroid-stimulating hormone (TSH), secreted by the anterior pituitary gland. T3 acts directly on the pituitary and hypothalamus to regulate TSH production through a classical negative feedback loop [2].

Thyroid hormone significantly contributes to the phenotype of mature adipocytes, by regulating important transcription factors and genes involved in the

---

G. Ceccarini • A. Basolo • F. Santini (✉)
Obesity Center at the Endocrinology Unit, University Hospital of Pisa,
Via Paradisa 2, Pisa 56100, Italy
e-mail: ceccarg@gmail.com; ale-bax@hotmail.it; ferruccio.santini@med.unipi.it

process of adipocyte differentiation. In vitro studies on cell cultures often require the presence of T3 in the milieu, as a factor that promotes the transformation of preadipocyte into mature adipocyte. T3 has a permissive effect on lipogenesis, by inducing the activity of genes involved in the triglyceride synthesis, thus displaying a trophic effect on the white adipocytes. Furthermore, T3 stimulates the lipolytic action induced by catecholamines, by increasing the sensitivity and the expression of the β-adrenergic receptor [3]. Thyroid hormone also exerts a relevant function in *brown adipocytes (BA)*, by enhancing the mitochondrial biogenesis and the *uncoupling protein 1 (UCP-1)* activity. Within BA, T3 produced from T4 by *type 2 deiodinase* (D2) increases the expression of UCP-1 both directly and by potentiating the effect of the adrenergic system [1]. The adrenergic system, on this hand, acts with a positive feedback by stimulating D2 activity and therefore increasing T3 intracellular levels. UCP-1 is localized in the inner membrane of mitochondria and uncouples proton transport across the membrane, thus dissipating the electrochemical gradient under the form of heat. In homoeothermic species, T3 has acquired a critical role in temperature homeostasis, sustaining approximately 30 % of the resting energy expenditure [4] and regulating the so-called adaptive (facultative) thermogenesis. During cold exposure or overfeeding, the thyroid hormone-activating D2 increases the generation of T3 in BA and promotes heat production [5]. Mice lacking thyroid hormone receptors exhibit decreased basal metabolic rate, decreased body temperature, and cold intolerance [6]. The impact of facultative thermogenesis on body weight regulation in humans remains an intriguing area of investigation that has received a great deal of attention after the demonstration that BA activity is impaired in obese subjects and significantly enhanced by cold exposure [7–9]. It is worth mentioning that human fat depots previously classified as "brown" were recently shown to be mainly composed of "beige adipocytes," a newly described cell lineage characterized by a phenotype that is intermediate between white and brown fat [10]. The physiological relevance of this findings remains to be fully elucidated.

4.3 The Interaction Between Nutrition and Thyroid Hormones

The nutritional status has to be carefully considered when interpreting the results of thyroid function tests in obese or overweight subjects [11]. A caloric deficit is characterized by a reduction of T3 and a concomitant increase of *reverse (r) T3* in the bloodstream. By converse, the production rate of T3, but not that of T4, is significantly increased during overfeeding and may explain the increased serum levels of T3 in some obese cohorts compared to controls. Thus, examination of patients at different caloric intakes, either while overeating or when on a *hypocaloric diet*, could account for discrepant results of serum thyroid hormones. Consistent evidence has been provided that thyroid hormone and deiodinases regulate feeding by acting at the central nervous level. In rodents, T3 administration in the hypothalamus increases appetite and may favor body weight gain in the long term. At this site T3 exerts a negative feedback on the expression of type 4 melanocortin receptor [12], a critical mediator of the anorectic effects of leptin [13]. Furthermore, fasting increases glial D2 activity and local T3 production in the arcuate nucleus. This favors excitability of NPY/AgRP orexigenic neurons [14] and promotes hyperphagia following food deprivation.

4.4 Leptin Regulation of the Hypothalamo-Pituitary-Thyroid Axis

Several endocrine factors produced and secreted by the white adipocytes are involved in fuel homeostasis. Among them, *leptin*, a 16 kd proteic hormone, is one of the most important long-term regulators of body weight, acting through the inhibition of food intake and promotion of energy expenditure and locomotor activity [15, 16]. The principal site of leptin action is the central nervous system and particularly the *arcuate nucleus* (ARC) of the hypothalamus. Besides the ARC, leptin receptors have been found both in the pituitary and in the TRH-secreting neurons of the paraventricular nucleus (PVN) [17].

Reduction of serum leptin, which occurs after prolonged fasting, plays a main role in the neuroendocrine adaptation to reduced caloric intake (amenorrhea, altered sympathetic tone, etc.), and it is associated with a downregulation of the hypothalamo-pituitary-thyroid axis.

Direct and indirect evidence suggests that leptin has a regulatory action on TSH secretion: (1) circadian rhythms of TSH and leptin are superimposable [18]; (2) subcutaneous administration of leptin to normal-weight subjects significantly blunts the fall of TSH secretion induced by fasting [19]; and (3) leptin administration to obese patients at physiological doses can partially reverse the fall of circulating thyroid hormones, which occurs during chronic caloric restriction [20]. A number of studies have investigated the effect of thyroid hormones on serum leptin [21], but evidence supporting a regulatory action of thyroxine or triiodothyronine on leptin is overall modest.

TSH receptors are expressed on the adipocytes [22], and the administration of recombinant human TSH can induce the release of leptin [23]. These findings suggest an in vivo activity of the TSH receptor in white adipocytes, although the related pathophysiological implications remain to be established. Interestingly enough, TSH receptors are also expressed also on brown adipocytes. This suggests that in hypothyroid subjects TSH might stimulate thermogenesis and counteract the drop of body temperature [24].

In summary, the decrease of serum leptin due to fat mass reduction is a signal capable of inhibiting the hypothalamo-pituitary-thyroid axis, by acting at the hypothalamic (PVN) level through inhibition of both *TRH* expression and secretion. This is likely an ancestral mechanism aimed at saving energy during periods of food shortage.

4.5 Thyroid Function Assessment in Obese Subjects

A recent review has assessed the relationship between serum TSH and *body mass index* (BMI) in euthyroid subjects [25], by analyzing the abundant literature accumulated on this topic over the last decade. Among the 29 selected studies, 18 reported a positive correlation between measures of adiposity and serum *TSH*. Some of these are large population studies including unselected obese and normal-weight individuals; other studies are focused on obese cohorts compared to control groups. It is important to underline that the described association between BMI and TSH is for TSH values that are within the normal reference range. Still, this observation raises the question if minimal thyroid function alterations may predispose to weight gain.

It is our opinion that this is not the case, as suggested by several lines of evidence. Firstly, the results of longitudinal studies showing a parallel increase of both TSH and BMI do not necessarily indicate that individuals with higher TSH levels do gain weight over time [26, 27], but TSH values might simply follow body weight changes [27]. Secondly, epidemiological studies have shown that women affected by undiagnosed subclinical hypothyroidism did not present with increased BMI if compared to euthyroid controls [28]. Thirdly, TSH serum levels tend to normalize after weight loss (obtained either through hypocaloric diet or bariatric surgery) [29, 30]. These observations taken together suggest that the slight increase of TSH observed in obese patients (*isolated hyper-thyrotropinemia*) may be an adaptive response of the hypothalamo-pituitary-thyroid axis to weight gain. Experimental evidence in the rodent model, showing a 3.7-fold increase of serum TSH after feeding with a high-fat diet, is in line with this view [31]. Data regarding the circulating concentrations of thyroid hormones in obese subjects are less univocal because of the serum levels of T3, which are reported increased, unchanged, or decreased, while T4 is generally reported low/normal [32–35]. These inconsistencies may be ascribed to the heterogeneity of the study populations that include people with variable caloric intakes, various degrees of obesity, and different distribution of body fat.

Overall, the causes responsible for the increased levels of serum TSH in obese patients are still a matter of debate. To offer a valid explanation, we have to consider that an expansion of the fat mass is usually associated with an increase of the lean mass that, in turn, would produce an accelerated turnover of thyroid hormone. The increased rate of thyroid hormone disposal would be the primary event promoting an activation of the hypothalamo-pituitary-thyroid axis, aimed at maintaining serum thyroid hormones within the euthyroid range. This succession of events would eventually produce low to normal serum T4 and slightly increased TSH, while serum T3 will remain mainly related to the current nutritional status of the individual.

4.6 Thyroid Structure in Obesity

Ultrasound studies indicate that in obese patients, the *thyroid volume* is larger than in nonobese subjects and it positively correlates to the amount of lean body mass rather than to body weight [32]. After weight loss, a reduction of the thyroid volume can also be observed [33]. Studies in obese children or adults showed a prevalent hypo-echogenic pattern at *thyroid ultrasound*, which was not related to thyroid autoimmunity [36, 37]. A clear association between obesity and autoimmune thyroid diseases has not been demonstrated to date, and ultrasound, a useful aid for diagnosing thyroid autoimmune diseases, shows unfortunately poor diagnostic accuracy in patients with morbid obesity.

Obesity has been reported as a risk factor for the development of *multinodular goiter* [38]. However, several limitations apply to the available studies, such as the small number of the population samples as well as biases in the selection of patients and controls. Similarly, systematic reviews of prospective observational studies showed a positive association between BMI at diagnosis and the risk of developing *differentiated thyroid cancer* [39]. A recent cross-sectional study indicates that BMI is a significant predictor of thyroid cancer in women but not in men [40] although this observation needs to be confirmed. The mechanisms theoretically responsible for the increased susceptibility to the development of goiter or thyroid cancer may be identified in the increased serum level of TSH (a growth factor for thyroid cells and a predictor of malignancy in thyroid nodules [41]), insulin, or additional growth factors.

4.7 Thyroid Function Alterations and Energetic Metabolism

Hyperthyroidism is usually (85 % of the cases) associated with a variable decrease of body weight [42]. During long-lasting hyperthyroidism, a decline of lean and fat mass associated with an increase in total energy expenditure is observed [43–45]. The extent of these phenomena depends upon the severity of the thyrotoxic state, the length of exposure to the excess of thyroid hormone, and possibly the age of the patient. The magnitude of weight loss is also related to the degree of compensatory hyperphagia; when the increased caloric intake exceeds the augmented energy expenditure, a paradoxical weight gain in thyrotoxic patients may be observed. The correction of hyperthyroidism is usually associated with an increase of body weight, but the changes of body composition during the recovery phase may differ among various patients. The putative risk predictors for the development of obesity after correction of hyperthyroidism are listed in Table 4.1. It is worth noting that the excessive body weight gain after treatment of hyperthyroidism is independent of the treatment modality: surgery, radioiodine, or antithyroid drugs [46].

Weight gain associated with overt *hypothyroidism* is a frequent complaint, being reported in over 50 % of patients [47], although of moderate extent [48]. Hypothyroidism and the related weight gain are frequently a theme of conversation between patient and physician who should be able to offer precise notions while dismissing myths. In overt hypothyroidism, the alterations in body weight reflect both the accumulation of body fat [49, 50], due to decreased resting energy expenditure and reduced physical activity, and the increase of body water [51], consequent to diminished capacity of excreting free-water [52] and increased tissue content of glycosaminoglycans [51]. Hypothyroidism is also associated with a worsening of the metabolic profile: increased total and LDL cholesterol and lipoprotein(a),

Table 4.1 Possible conditions predisposing to excessive weight gain after treatment of hyperthyroidism

Preexisting overweight or obesity
Familiar predisposition to obesity
Duration of hyperthyroidism
Extent of weight loss during hyperthyroidism
Inadequate or late correction of hypothyroidism following treatment of hyperthyroidism
Concurrent therapies (steroids, beta-blockers, etc.)
Prolonged physical inactivity

arterial medio-intimal thickness, and reduced HDL levels. Thus, thyroid function screening in obese and overweight subjects is recommended because, although hypothyroidism is unlikely to be the cause of the weight excess, correction of concurrent hypothyroidism is a prerequisite to restore the metabolic efficiency, to warrant an adequate compliance to lifestyle changes, and to improve the cardiovascular risk. Indeed, in spite of adequate substitution with L-thyroxine, hypothyroid patients experience only a modest weight loss following thyroid hormone administration [43, 53], and the excretion of excess body water, rather than reduction of the fat mass, accounts for most of the weight reduction [54]. When calculating the appropriate L-thyroxine needs, ideal body weight (not actual body weight) should be considered. Our experience gained by employing dual-energy x-ray absorptiometry to assess body composition in normal-weight, overweight, and obese subjects provided evidence that lean body mass is the best predictor of the daily requirements for L-thyroxine in hypothyroid patients [54]. In that study, the L-thyroxine daily dose necessary to suppress TSH levels reflected the different proportions of lean mass over the total body weight, and it was approximately 2.1 mcg/kg of body weight in normal-weight subjects, while it was only 1.63 mcg/kg in obese subjects. From these observations, the concept originates that thyroid hormones are mainly degraded in the lean compartment (including the muscles, liver, and skin), whereas fat is poorly involved in their metabolism.

It is our opinion that when no primary cause of hypothyroidism is found, the isolated elevation of serum TSH, which is likely secondary to obesity itself, should not be treated with L-thyroxine since the positive repercussions (if any) of this therapy on the patient's health have never been demonstrated.

4.8 Thyroid Hormone in the Treatment of Obesity

The history of the pharmacological treatment of obesity is constellated by disappointment. Thyroid hormone has been largely employed in the past years with the purpose to increase the energy expenditure and reduce the fat mass. An exhaustive meta-analysis of the literature has evaluated the effectiveness of T3 and/or T4 administration in euthyroid obese patients under caloric deprivation regimens [55]. Results of this work showed poor efficacy in terms of weight loss during most of T3 or T4 regimens. Furthermore, subclinical thyrotoxicosis and increased urinary nitrogen excretion were reported when T3 was employed at pharmacological doses. *Thyroid hormone derivatives* are potential candidates in the search for new aids capable of selectively increasing energy expenditure and promoting stable weight loss, without relevant side effects. A modulation of different isoforms of thyroid receptor-mediated pathways is a promising strategy for treating lipid disorders, hepatic steatosis, atherosclerosis, type 2 diabetes, and possibly obesity itself [56]. Selective agonists of thyroid hormone receptors have been recently employed, but clinical trials are required to evaluate their risk-to-benefit profile.

As a general concept, the search for a weight-lowering agent that generates a negative energy balance by increasing the caloric output should take into careful consideration that any stimulatory effect on resting energy expenditure may be counteracted by simultaneous effects at various sites (e.g., increased appetite, accelerated lipogenesis, and/or increased protein wasting), which could minimize or even neutralize the postulated beneficial outcome.

References

1. Marsili A, Zavacki AM, Harney JW, Larsen PR (2011) Physiological role and regulation of iodothyronine deiodinases: a 2011 update. J Endocrinol Invest 34:395–407
2. Costa-e-Sousa RH, Hollenberg AN (2012) Minireview: the neural regulation of the hypothalamic-pituitary-thyroid axis. Endocrinology 153:4128–4135
3. Viguerie N, Millet L, Avizou S, Vidal H, Larrouy D, Langin D (2002) Regulation of human adipocyte gene expression by thyroid hormone. J Clin Endocrinol Metab 87:630–634
4. Silva JE (2006) Thermogenic mechanisms and their hormonal regulation. Physiol Rev 86:435–464
5. Arrojo E, Drigo R, Fonseca TL, Werneck-de-Castro JP, Bianco AC (2013) Role of the type 2 iodothyronine deiodinase (D2) in the control of thyroid hormone signaling. Biochim Biophys Acta 1830:3956–3964
6. Golozoubova V, Gullberg H, Matthias A, Cannon B, Vennström B, Nedergaard J (2004) Depressed thermogenesis but competent brown adipose tissue recruitment in mice devoid of all hormone-binding thyroid hormone receptors. Mol Endocrinol 18:384–401
7. Cypess AM, Lehman S, Williams G, Tal I, Rodman D, Goldfine AB, Kuo FC, Palmer EL, Tseng YH, Doria A, Kolodny GM, Kahn CR (2009) Identification and importance of brown adipose tissue in adult humans. N Engl J Med 360:1509–1517
8. van der Lans AA, Hoeks J, Brans B, Vijgen GH, Visser MG, Vosselman MJ, Hansen J, Jörgensen JA, Wu J, Mottaghy FM, Schrauwen P, van Marken Lichtenbelt WD (2013) Cold acclimation recruits human brown fat and increases nonshivering thermogenesis. J Clin Invest 123:3395–3403
9. Yoneshiro T, Aita S, Matsushita M, Kayahara T, Kameya T, Kawai Y, Iwanaga T, Saito M (2013) Recruited brown adipose tissue as an antiobesity agent in humans. J Clin Invest 123:3404–3408
10. Wu J, Boström P, Sparks LM, Ye L, Choi JH, Giang AH, Khandekar M, Virtanen KA, Nuutila P, Schaart G, Huang K, Tu H, van Marken Lichtenbelt WD, Hoeks J, Enerbäck S, Schrauwen P, Spiegelman BM (2012) Beige adipocytes are a distinct type of thermogenic fat cell in mouse and human. Cell 150:366–376
11. Bray GA, Fisher DA, Chopra IJ (1976) Relation of thyroid hormones to body-weight. Lancet 1:1206–1208
12. Decherf S, Seugnet I, Kouidhi S, Lopez-Juarez A, Clerget-Froidevaux MS, Demeneix BA (2010) Thyroid hormone exerts negative feedback on hypothalamic type 4 melanocortin receptor expression. Proc Natl Acad Sci U S A 107:4471–4476

13. Santini F, Maffei M, Pelosini C, Salvetti G, Scartabelli G, Pinchera A (2009) Melanocortin-4 receptor mutations in obesity. Adv Clin Chem 48:95–109
14. Coppola A, Liu ZW, Andrews ZB, Paradis E, Roy MC, Friedman JM, Ricquier D, Richard D, Horvath TL, Gao XB, Diano S (2007) A central thermogenic-like mechanism in feeding regulation: an interplay between arcuate nucleus T3 and UCP2. Cell Metab 5:21–33
15. Friedman JM, Halaas JL (1998) Leptin and the regulation of body weight in mammals. Nature 395:763–770
16. Ribeiro AC, Ceccarini G, Dupré C, Friedman JM, Pfaff DW, Mark AL (2011) Contrasting effects of leptin on food anticipatory and total locomotor activity. PLoS One. doi:10.1371/journal.pone.0023364
17. Nillni EA (2010) Regulation of the hypothalamic thyrotropin releasing hormone (TRH) neuron by neuronal and peripheral inputs. Front Neuroendocrinol 31:134–156
18. Mantzoros CS, Ozata M, Negrao AB, Suchard MA, Ziotopoulou M, Caglayan S, Elashoff RM, Cogswell RJ, Negro P, Liberty V, Wong ML, Veldhuis J, Ozdemir IC, Gold PW, Flier JS, Licinio J (2001) Synchronicity of frequently sampled thyrotropin (TSH) and leptin concentrations in healthy adults and leptin-deficient subjects: evidence for possible partial TSH regulation by leptin in humans. J Clin Endocrinol Metab 86:3284–3291
19. Chan JL, Heist K, DePaoli AM, Veldhuis JD, Mantzoros CS (2003) The role of falling leptin levels in the neuroendocrine and metabolic adaptation to short-term starvation in healthy men. J Clin Invest 111:1409–1421
20. Rosenbaum M, Goldsmith R, Bloomfield D, Magnano A, Weimer L, Heymsfield S, Gallagher D, Mayer L, Murphy E, Leibel RL (2005) Low-dose leptin reverses skeletal muscle, autonomic, and neuroendocrine adaptations to maintenance of reduced weight. J Clin Invest 115:3579–3586
21. Feldt-Rasmussen U (2007) Thyroid and leptin. Thyroid 17:413–419
22. Sorisky A, Bell A, Gagnon A (2000) TSH receptor in adipose cells. Horm Metab Res 32:468–474
23. Santini F, Galli G, Maffei M, Fierabracci P, Pelosini C, Marsili A, Giannetti M, Castagna MG, Checchi S, Molinaro E, Piaggi P, Pacini F, Elisei R, Vitti P, Pinchera A (2010) Acute exogenous TSH administration stimulates leptin secretion in vivo. Eur J Endocrinol 163:63–67
24. Doniach D (1975) Possible stimulation of thermogenesis in brown adipose tissue by thyroid-stimulating hormone. Lancet 2:160–161
25. de Moura SA, Sichieri R (2011) Association between serum TSH concentration within the normal range and adiposity. Eur J Endocrinol 165:11–15
26. Fox CS, Pencina MJ, D'Agostino RB, Murabito JM, Seely EW, Pearce EN, Vasan RS (2008) Relations of thyroid function to body weight: cross-sectional and longitudinal observations in a community-based sample. Arch Intern Med 168:587–592
27. Svare A, Nilsen TI, Bjøro T, Asvold BO, Langhammer A (2011) Serum TSH related to measures of body mass: longitudinal data from the HUNT Study, Norway. Clin Endocrinol (Oxf) 74:769–775
28. Hak AE, Pols HA, Visser TJ, Drexhage HA, Hofman A, Witteman JC (2000) Subclinical hypothyroidism is an independent risk factor for atherosclerosis and myocardial infarction in elderly women: the Rotterdam Study. Ann Intern Med 15(132):270–278
29. Kok P, Roelfsema F, Langendonk JG, Frolich M, Burggraaf J, Meinders AE, Pijl H (2005) High circulating thyrotropin levels in obese women are reduced after body weight loss induced by caloric restriction. J Clin Endocrinol Metab 90:4659–4663
30. Moulin de Moraes CM, Mancini MC, de Melo ME, Figueiredo DA, Villares SM, Rascovski A, Zilberstein B, Halpern A (2005) Prevalence of subclinical hypothyroidism in a morbidly obese population and improvement after weight loss induced by Roux-en-Y gastric bypass. Obes Surg 15:1287–1291
31. Araujo RL, Andrade BM, Padrón AS, Gaidhu MP, Perry RL, Carvalho DP, Ceddia RB (2010) High-fat diet increases thyrotropin and oxygen consumption without altering circulating 3,5,3'-triiodothyronine (T3) and thyroxine in rats: the role of iodothyronine deiodinases, reverse T3 production, and whole-body fat oxidation. Endocrinology 151:3460–3469

32. Wesche MF, Wiersinga WM, Smits NJ (1998) Lean body mass as a determinant of thyroid size. Clin Endocrinol (Oxf) 48:701–706
33. Sari R, Balci MK, Altunbas H, Karayalcin U (2003) The effect of body weight and weight loss on thyroid volume and function in obese women. Clin Endocrinol (Oxf) 59:258–262
34. Knudsen N, Laurberg P, Rasmussen LB, Bülow I, Perrild H, Ovesen L, Jørgensen T (2005) Small differences in thyroid function may be important for body mass index and the occurrence of obesity in the population. J Clin Endocrinol Metab 90:4019–4024
35. Makepeace AE, Bremner AP, O'Leary P, Leedman PJ, Feddema P, Michelangeli V, Walsh JP (2008) Significant inverse relationship between serum free T4 concentration and body mass index in euthyroid subjects: differences between smokers and nonsmokers. Clin Endocrinol (Oxf) 69:648–652
36. Radetti G, Kleon W, Buzi F, Crivellaro C, Pappalardo L, di Iorgi N, Maghnie M (2008) Thyroid function and structure are affected in childhood obesity. J Clin Endocrinol Metab 93:4749–4754
37. Rotondi M, Cappelli C, Leporati P, Chytiris S, Zerbini F, Fonte R, Magri F, Castellano M, Chiovato L (2010) A hypoechoic pattern of the thyroid at ultrasound does not indicate autoimmune thyroid diseases in patients with morbid obesity. Eur J Endocrinol 163:105–109
38. Ayturk S, Gursoy A, Kut A, Anil C, Nar A, Tutuncu NB (2009) Metabolic syndrome and its components are associated with increased thyroid volume and nodule prevalence in a mild-to-moderate iodine deficient area. Eur J Endocrinol 161:599–605
39. Kitahara CM, Platz EA, Freeman LE, Hsing AW, Linet MS, Park Y, Schairer C, Schatzkin A, Shikany JM, Berrington de González A (2011) Obesity and thyroid cancer risk among U.S. men and women: a pooled analysis of five prospective studies. Cancer Epidemiol Biomarkers Prev 20:464–472
40. Han JM, Kim TY, Jeon MJ, Yim JH, Kim WG, Song DE, Hong SJ, BaeSJ KHK, Shin MH, ShongYK KWB (2013) Obesity is a risk factor for thyroid cancer risk in a large, ultrasonographically screened population. Eur J Endocrinol 168:879–886
41. Fiore E, Rago T, Provenzale MA, Scutari M, Ugolini C, Basolo F et al (2009) Lower levels of TSH are associated with a lower risk of papillary thyroid cancer in patients with thyroid nodular disease: thyroid autonomy may play a protective role. Endocr Relat Cancer 16:1251–1260
42. Ingbar SH (1985) The thyroid gland. in: J.D. Wilson, D.W. Foster (Eds.) Williams Textbook of Endocrinology. W.B. Saunders Company, Philadelphia, PA, USA; 1985: 975–1170
43. Hoogwerf BJ, Nuttall FQ (1984) Long-term weight regulation in treated hyperthyroid and hypothyroid subjects. Am J Med 76:963–970
44. Lovejoy JC, Smith SR, Bray GA, DeLany JP, Rood JC, Gouvier D, Windhauser M, Ryan DH, Macchiavelli R, Tulley R (1997) A paradigm of experimentally induced mild hyperthyroidism: effects on nitrogen balance, body composition, and energy expenditure in healthy young men. J Clin Endocrinol Metab 82:765–770
45. Riis AL, Jørgensen JO, Gjedde S, Nørrelund H, Jurik AG, Nair KS, Ivarsen P, Weeke J, Møller N (2005) Whole body and forearm substrate metabolism in hyperthyroidism: evidence of increased basal muscle protein breakdown. Am J Physiol Endocrinol Metab 288E:1067–1073
46. Dale J, Daykin J, Holder R, Sheppard MC, Franklyn JA (2001) Weight gain following treatment of hyperthyroidism. Clin Endocrinol (Oxf) 55:233–239
47. Zulewski H, Müller B, Exer P, Miserez AR, Staub JJ (1997) Estimation of tissue hypothyroidism by a new clinical score: evaluation of patients with various grades of hypothyroidism and controls. J Clin Endocrinol Metab 82:771–776
48. Baron DN (1956) Hypothyroidism; its aetiology and relation to hypometabolism, hypercholesterolaemia, and increase in body-weight. Lancet 271:277–281
49. Seppel T, Kosel A, Schlaghecke R (1997) Bioelectrical impedance assessment of body composition in thyroid disease. Eur J Endocrinol 136:493–498
50. Wolf M, Weigert A, Kreymann G (1996) Body composition and energy expenditure in thyroidectomized patients during short-term hypothyroidism and thyrotropin-suppressive thyroxine therapy. Eur J Endocrinol 134:168–173

51. Smith TJ, Bahn RS, Gorman CA (1989) Connective tissue, glycosaminoglycans, and diseases of the thyroid. Endocr Rev 10:366–391
52. Skowsky WR, Kikuchi TA (1978) The role of vasopressin in the impaired water excretion of myxedema. Am J Med 64:613–621
53. Karmisholt J, Andersen S, Laurberg P (2011) Weight loss after therapy of hypothyroidism is mainly caused by excretion of excess body water associated with myxoedema. J Clin Endocrinol Metab 96E:99–103
54. Santini F, Pinchera A, Marsili A, Ceccarini G, Castagna MG, Valeriano R, Giannetti M, Taddei D, Centoni R, Scartabelli G, Rago T, Mammoli C, Elisei R, Vitti P (2005) Lean body mass is a major determinant of levothyroxine dosage in the treatment of thyroid diseases. J Clin Endocrinol Metab 90:124–127
55. Kaptein EM, Beale E, Chan LS (2009) Thyroid hormone therapy for obesity and nonthyroidal illnesses: a systematic review. J Clin Endocrinol Metab 94:3663–3675
56. Baxter JD, Webb P (2009) Thyroid hormone mimetics: potential applications in atherosclerosis, obesity and type 2 diabetes. Nat Rev Drug Discov 8:308–320

Hypothalamic Growth Hormone/IGF-1 Axis

Annamaria Colao, Silvia Savastano, and Carolina Di Somma

5.1 Introduction

In the past years, a growing body of evidence showed that obese subjects with visceral adiposity have decreased growth hormone (GH) secretion [1], in analogy with adult patients with organic GH deficiency (GHD), a well-recognized acquired clinical entity commonly due to hypothalamic pituitary disorders and/or their treatments, such as surgery and radiotherapy. Of interest, GH replacement therapy in adult GHD can reduce visceral adipose tissue, with minimal alterations in total body weight. This evidence supports the hypothesis that regulation of the GH/insulin-like growth factor (IGF)-1 axis and the state of the adipose tissue depots are closely related [2].

Although generally reversible after sustained weight loss, the low GH status in obesity is associated with increased prevalence of cardiometabolic risk factors [1] and detrimental alterations of body composition [3]. Thus, the low GH status in obese subjects might be included in the maladaptive endocrine-metabolic changes accounting for heterogeneity in metabolic phenotype among equally obese subjects.

A. Colao (✉) • S. Savastano
Dipartimento di Medicina Clinica e Chirurgia – Unità di Endocrinologia,
Università degli Studi di Napoli Federico II, Via S. Pansini, 5,
Naples 80131, Italy
e-mail: colao@unina.it; sisavast@unina.it

C. Di Somma
IRCCS SDN Napoli, Via Gianturco, 113,
Naples 80143, Italy
e-mail: cdisomma@unina.it

This chapter aims at investigating the complex relationships between obesity and GH/IGF-1 axis and at discussing the main benefits of GH treatment in the management of obesity.

5.2   Effects of the GH/IGF-1 Axis on Adipose Tissue

GH is secreted in a pulsatile manner reflecting the integrated regulation by GH-releasing hormone (GHRH), somatostatin (SS), and GH-releasing peptides. A number of central and peripheral peptides involved in the control of food intake and energy expenditure, including adiponectin, ghrelin, and leptin, participate to the regulation of GH secretion. GH and IGF-1 have major anabolic action on muscle and lipolytic effects on adipose tissue [4]. Some of the GH effects on adipose tissue are exerted directly, via its receptor. Other effects, such as the stimulation of preadipocyte proliferation, differentiation, and survival, are produced by upregulation of IGF-1 secretion, the anabolic GH mediator mainly produced by the liver in response to GH stimulation. GH affects directly adipocyte metabolism by inhibiting the lipoprotein lipase and by increasing the hormone-sensitive lipase activity through the activation of the β-adrenergic receptor. By these effects, GH stimulates the preferential oxidation of lipids, directing the energy from metabolic processes towards the synthesis of proteins. In addition, GH downregulates the expression of 11βHSD1 (11β-hydroxysteroid dehydrogenase type 1), the enzyme that amplifies the action of glucocorticoid in visceral adipose tissue by stimulating the conversion of inactive dehydrocorticosterone to active corticosterone. Moreover, GH modulates the expression of lipid droplet proteins, such as CIDE-A (cell-death-inducing DFF45-like effector), and the secretion of adiponectin, thus promoting a more favorable peripheral adipose tissue distribution. More recently, the evidence that GH differentially regulates the NF-kB activity in adipocytes and macrophages suggests a modulating role for GH on chronic inflammation involved in obesity-associated insulin resistance [5]. IGF-1 is integrated in the IGF regulatory system consisting of IGFs (IGF-1 and IGF-2); type I and type II IGF receptors; regulatory proteins, including IGF-binding proteins (IGFBP-1–6); and the acid-labile subunit (ALS) [6]. IGF-1 circulates within the intravascular space as part of a ternary complex with ALS and IGFBP-3, the predominant plasma-binding globulin regulated by GH concentration, constituting both a reservoir and a carrier system for IGF-1. Free IGF-1, which accounts for less than 1 % of the total circulating IGF-1, is responsible for the bioactivity on target tissues. IGF-1 also has metabolic actions on its own in regulating lipolysis, proteolysis, and insulin resistance as part of the IGF-1/insulin system. In particular, a "fine-tuning" of IGF-1 signaling cascade, especially the IRS-1/PI3K/Akt pathway, is critical for proper adipogenesis [7]. Besides GH, many other different factors, primarily age, gender, body composition, nutritional-driven components, and glucose homeostasis, have been reported to affect IGF-1 metabolism [8]. The interaction between GH/IGF-1 axis and adipose tissue can be viewed as part of the overall regulation of feeding and fasting in order to maintain an adequate body weight and body composition.

5.3 Effects of Adipose Tissue on Somatotropic Axis

Despite a normal pituitary function, in obese individuals the endogenous GH secretion is markedly reduced compared to age-matched controls [1]. In particular, the reduction in the half-life of GH is associated with the reduction in both frequency and amplitude of GH secretory bursts and the increase in metabolic clearance rate; moreover, the severity of the secretory defects is proportional to the degree of obesity. The pathophysiological mechanism responsible for the low GH secretion in obesity is probably multifactorial. The inhibitory role of high circulating free fatty acid (FFA), as commonly seen in obese individuals, is supported by the restoration of GH release after the administration of the antilipolytic agent acipimox [9]. This evidence indicates that high circulating FFA might be responsible for a low GH status via the derangement of a classical endocrine feedback loop between GH and FFA released by GH-induced lipolysis. Similarly, orlistat, a gastrointestinal lipase inhibitor, is effective in inducing a weight-independent increase in GH peak, IGF-I levels, and IGF-I/IGFBP-3 ratio along with reduction in postprandial FFA [10]. Of interest, the acute reduction in circulating FFA induced by acipimox significantly increases the stimulated GH secretion only in obese individuals without organic GHD [11]. Besides FFA, a chronic state of SS or insulin excess, increased leptin levels, as well as overeating per se and a deficient ghrelin secretion, probably contribute to the impaired GH secretion.

Total IGF-1 concentrations could be normal or low in obesity [12], with reduced circulating levels of IGFBP-3 and ALS [13]. Differences in the assay methods across the studies might be responsible for this variability, but different peripheral mechanisms might contribute to reduce IGF-1 levels in obesity, such as hyperinsulinemia and chronic inflammation associated with obesity [14]. In particular, adipose tissue, as source of proinflammatory mediators, might directly affect the IGF-1/IGF-binding protein system by reducing IGF-1 bioactivity [15]. On the other side, increased free IGF-1 levels, namely, bioactive IGF-1, linked to blunted IGFBP-1 and IGFBP-2 levels due to the hyperinsulinemia and high IGFBP proteolysis activity, might be responsible for the negative feedback on somatotroph cells [16]. Actually, about 10 % obese individuals present with an overlap in the association of both reductions in peak-stimulated GH and low IGF-1 levels [17], where this concordance depicts the poorest condition of GH secretion. Of interest, IGF-1 levels commonly increase along with the normalization of GH secretion in obese individuals after weight loss [12]. The hypothetical maladaptive mechanisms likely involved in the etiopathogenesis of obesity-related alterations in GH/IGF-1 axis are shown in Fig. 5.1.

5.4 The Challenge to Diagnose Low GH Status in Obesity

It is of great practical importance to differentiate organic GHD versus obesity-related decrease in GH secretion as body fat and nutritional status are the main confounding factors in the interpretation of biochemical tests commonly used in the

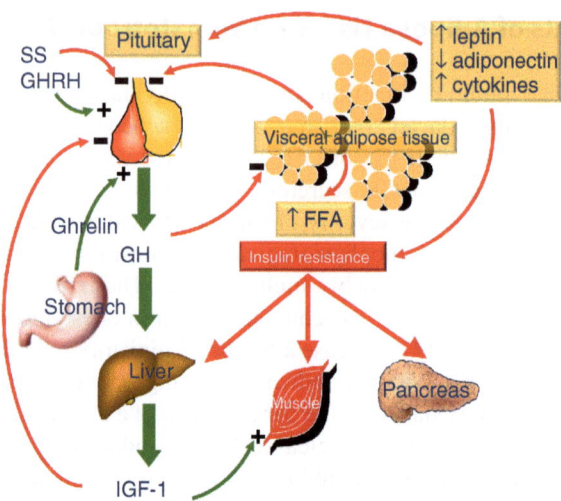

Fig. 5.1 The hypothetical maladaptive mechanisms likely involved in the etiopathogenesis of obesity-related alterations in GH/IGF-1 axis. The elevation of circulating FFA, adipokines, and cytokines induced by increased visceral adipose tissue depot responsible for insulin resistance at the liver, skeletal muscle, and pancreatic levels is also able to markedly affect the normal feedback control system operating in GH/IGF-1 axis. The "functional" low GH/IGF-1 axis, in turn, might act on body composition by inducing unfavorable changes in body composition similarly to those observed in GHD, thus contributing to worsen the insulin resistance state and the associated metabolic sequelae. *SS* somatostatin, *GHRH* growth hormone-releasing hormone, *GH* growth hormone, *IGF-1* insulin-like growth factor-1, *FFA* free fatty acids

diagnosis of GHD [18]. Considering the pulsatile nature of GH secretion, the diagnosis of GHD would require multiple sampling to obtain a 24-h integrated GH profile. IGF-1 and IGFBP-3 are nonpulsatile GH target hormones, and IGF-1 levels <2 standard deviation below the age-matched mean, in a well-nourished adult with pituitary disease, are a strong evidence for significant GHD. However, a provocative test of GH reserve is required for many adult patients with suspected GHD. The assessment of the GH secretion is commonly performed using pharmacological challenges such as the insulin tolerance test (ITT) or the GHRH+arginine. The latter, using the effect of arginine in potentiating the response to GHRH via inhibition of hypothalamic release of somatostatin, is currently considered the favorite diagnostic tool due to its high specificity and sensitivity, as well as tolerability. While BMI specific cutoff points for the diagnosis of severe GHD has not yet been available for ITT, GHRH+arginine is the only test for which BMI-dependent variability of GH responsiveness has been investigated [19]. In particular, appropriate GH cutoff in adults with BMI >30 kg/m^2 is considered 4.2 μg/L [20]. Using this new cutoff value of the GHRH+arginine test, about one third morbidly obese individuals presented with a low peak GH [2]. In addition, waist circumference adds per se predictive information to the determination of GH response, independent of BMI [21]. The adipose tissue effects on GH secretion have also been confirmed in healthy adolescents with normal stature during transition period [22], although appropriate cutoff

Table 5.1 Cutoff values of peak GH after GHRH +arginine according to BMI

First author (Ref.)	Age	BMI	Cutoff values (µg/L)
Corneli et al. [20][a]	Adults	<25 kg/m^2	<11.5
		25–30 kg/m^2	<8.0
		>30 kg/m^2	<4.2
Colao et al. [19][a]	Adults	<25 kg/m^2	11.8
		25–30 kg/m^2	8.1
		>30 kg/m^2	5.5
Perotti et al. [22]	Transition period	>85th percentile	<19

[a]Accepted by The Endocrine Society Clinical Practice Guideline on Evaluation and Treatment of Adult Growth Hormone Deficiency (GHD) [18]

values for overweight/obese adolescents are still missing. In Table 5.1 are reported cutoff values of peak GH after different stimulation tests according to BMI. The main criticism to GH stimulation testing in obesity is that this functional hyposomatotropism is fully reversed by weight loss and might cause misleading diagnosis of GHD [23], especially in view of a possible expensive unjustified treatment with GH. Whatever might be the central and peripheral mechanisms linking adipose tissue and low GH status, this condition, albeit functional, serves as a vicious circle that is reinforced with further accumulation of visceral adipose tissue. Thus, beyond the issue to erroneously classify obese individuals' low peak GH as really GH deficient, a low status of GH/IGF-1 axis, especially when the low GH secretion is paralleled by low IGF-1 levels, is however responsible for unfavorable changes in body composition and increased cardiovascular risk profile, similarly to those observed in organic GHD [24]. This hypothesis is in line with recent reports suggesting that low IGF-1 levels are linked to the pathogenesis of type 2 diabetes, metabolic syndrome, cardiovascular disease, and chronic inflammation [25, 26].

5.5 Metabolic Consequences of Low GH/IGF-1 Status in Obesity

The low GH/IGF-1 axis status is associated with a different obesity phenotype. In particular, obese individuals with blunted peak GH showed a significantly different body composition compared with normal responder counterpart, with the highest values of BMI, waist circumference, waist-to-hip ratio, and fat mass, and the lowest fat-free mass [1, 2, 12]. A similar association is found in patients with Prader-Willi syndrome (PWS), the most common known genetic cause of marked obesity characterized by multiple endocrine dysfunctions, including a reduced GH secretory capacity, who presented with changes in body composition that are worse than those observed in obese subjects with comparable BMI. In this respect, it is conceivable that the unfavorable changes in body composition associated with the low GH/IGF-1 status contribute to worsen the obesity-related metabolic sequelae, amplifying the cardiometabolic risk profile in the subset of obese individuals with low GH status. Accordingly, obese individuals with reduced GH secretion have increased cardiovascular disease risk factors, including dyslipidemia, chronic inflammation, and increased carotid intima-media thickness, and increased prevalence of metabolic syndrome [1, 27]. In addition, low peak GH has also been reported to be associated with increased intramyocellular and intrahepatic lipid content in premenopausal obese women, further suggesting the contribution of low GH status in the development of insulin resistance and other complications of the metabolic syndrome [28]. The cardiovascular risk profile increases when there is concordance between reductions in peak-stimulated GH and low IGF-1 levels in the same patient [17]. Thus, there may be different degrees of impairment of GH/IGF-1 axis in obesity. Further evidence on the effect of the low GH status in obesity is provided by the studies evaluating the effectiveness of GH treatment in obese individuals.

5.6 Effectiveness of GH Treatment in Obesity

A number of clinical trials have assessed the efficacy of recombinant human (rh) GH as adjuvant therapy in association with a standard weight loss program for unselected obese adults [1]. The major issues in evaluating rhGH treatment in obesity are the limited number of participants, the lack of placebo control, the short duration of the treatments, and the doses used. A recent comprehensive meta-analysis by Mekala et al. [29] has evidenced that rhGH treatment leads to decrease in total fat mass, visceral adiposity, and increase in lean body mass, even if without resulting in significant weight loss. Along with these little, albeit significant, changes in body composition, plasma lipid profile is improved, with decreases in total cholesterol and LDL cholesterol. In addition, no significant changes in markers of adiposity, such as leptin or adiponectin, are reported. In short-term studies, fasting plasma glucose and insulin increase transiently during the first few weeks of GH treatment, whereas improvements in glucose metabolism are observed only in long-term studies. In particular, significant beneficial effects on fat mass and glucose metabolism are observed in the studies reporting a longer mean duration of treatment (>12 weeks) compared to the short-term studies. This evidence is likely due to the longer lap of time required to evidence the insulin-sensitizing effects due to the reduction in visceral adipose tissue and the increase in IGF-1 levels. Accordingly, similar beneficial effects of GH treatment have been reported in obese type 2 diabetic patients with poor glycemic control [30]. Alternatively, GH treatment might act through decreased 11βHSD1 activity in visceral adipose tissue, increased glucose transport in the skeletal muscle, the major site of glucose disposal mediated via the IGF-1 receptor, increased proportion of insulin-sensitive type I muscle fibers, or increased capillarization in the skeletal muscle. There is no general agreement on the effective dose of rhGH in obese individuals. Many trials used relatively higher doses of rhGH compared with those recommended for adult GHD. Indeed, low doses that normalize age-related IGF-1 levels are more likely to minimize the number of dose-related side effects and the unfavorable effects on glucose metabolism, such as GH-induced hyperinsulinemia, which may oppose the lipolytic effect of

GH. This observation suggests that a careful investigation of GH/IGF-1 axis might be mandatory in the evaluation of obese individuals to be assigned to rhGH treatment. In this respect, it should be conceivable to limit the therapy to only subjects with reduced GH secretory capacity, in relation to their worse cardiometabolic risk profile, and for a period of time sufficient to obtain the spontaneous recovery of GH/IGF-1 axis, if any, along with weight loss. The adverse events most commonly reported are hypertension, arthralgia, paresthesia, and peripheral edema; more recently, an increased severity of obstructive sleep apnea in abdominally obese men during GH treatment likely due to the GH-induced increase of measures of neck volume has been reported [31]. Of interest, either the beneficial effects on body composition and cardiovascular risk or the side effect of altered glucose tolerance returns to pretreatment levels after GH withdrawal. Finally, GHRH analogues increasing endogenous GH secretion, such as tesamorelin [32], have recently evidenced to be efficacious in improving body composition without adversely affecting glucose metabolism, while studies on GH fragments with predominant antilipolytic activity have not yet yielded convincing results.

5.7   GH/IGF-I Axis and Bariatric Surgery

Bariatric surgery currently provides the only long-term control of obesity, resulting in major weight loss and weight maintenance. Up to now, very few well-designed clinical trials have been performed to scientifically investigate the GH/IGF-1 axis following bariatric procedures. Bariatric surgical techniques can be separated in malabsorptive procedures, such as biliopancreatic diversion (BPD), and restrictive procedures, such as laparoscopic adjustable gastric banding (LAGB) or sleeve gastrectomy, with a growing variety of procedures using one or both of these techniques over the years, such as the Roux-en-Y gastric bypass (RYGB). Among the postsurgical endocrine changes, those related to the GH/IGF-I axis have been poorly investigated. Stimulated GH secretion significantly increases after BPD [33]. Partial recovery of GH secretion is also observed after RYGB [34]. Although with some discrepancy [35, 36], postoperative IGF-1 secretion shows a long-lasting impairment, similarly to that showed after nonsurgical weight loss, presumably linked to the catabolic state induced by BPD [37] and RYGB [38]. Yet, in a prospective study 6 months after LAGB, when the initial catabolic state should have already been overcome, about 20 % obese women are found to be both GH and IGF-1 deficient and another fifth have IGF-1 levels still below the normal range calculated according with age normative ranges [13]. Interestingly, excess of weight loss (EWL) and fat mass loss are higher in patients who normalize their GH/IGF-1 axis after surgery than in those who do not [39]. Thus, the question arises as whether persistent failures of the GH/IGF-1 axis might negatively influence the outcome of bariatric surgery. Indeed, percent decrease of waist circumference, EWL, and fat mass is greater in obese individuals with normal preoperative GH secretion and IGF-1 levels, suggesting that the evaluation of GH/IGF-1 axis might be useful to predict the individual postoperative outcome [39].

Considering the effectiveness GH therapy to preserve fat-free mass in catabolic conditions, such as hypocaloric diets and wasting conditions, the possible favorable influence of the rhGH replacement treatment in preventing loss of fat-free mass during the early postoperative period in morbidly obese females with persistent low GH/IGF-1 status after LAGB has been investigated [40]. Indeed, patients treated with rhGH present with the same amount of EWL as those who do not, but in the former the weight loss is mainly due to fat mass loss, with a significant sparing of lean body mass. The beneficial effects of GH treatment are also accompanied by improvements of lipid profile and insulin sensitivity.

Conclusions

Obesity and GH/IGF-1 axis exhibit multiple and bidirectional relationships. The low GH status in obese adults, albeit functional and almost reversed by weight loss, is responsible for anthropometric and metabolic alterations favoring visceral obesity and increasing cardiometabolic risk profile. In this respect, the functional low GH status in obese individuals might be part of the multiple maladaptive endocrine changes involved in the pathogenesis of their obesity. This hypothesis generates the following considerations. Firstly, the different GH/IGF-1 axis status might be one of the mechanisms responsible for the heterogeneity in the obese phenotype. Secondly, preoperatively testing the GH/IGF-1 axis in obese patients might be useful to predict the individual postoperative outcome. Thirdly, the impairment of the GH/IGF-1 axis might be the rationale to consider GH as an adjunctive treatment in the subset of obese individuals with reduced GH secretory capacity and low circulating levels of IGF-1, in relation to their worst cardiometabolic risk profile, with particular regard to those patients who are candidates for bariatric surgery. This evidence might be of particular relevance in obese patients considering the protective effect of IGF-1 against cardiovascular disease, atherosclerosis, and diabetes.

Acknowledgments We are very grateful to Prof. P. Forestieri (Department of Clinical Medicine and Surgery, University Federico II, Naples, Italy), Prof. L. Angrisani (General and Laparoscopic Surgery Unit, San Giovanni Bosco Hospital, Naples, Italy), Prof. L. Docimo (Division of General and Bariatric Surgery, Second University of Naples, Naples, Italy), Prof. M. Musella (Department of General Surgery, Advanced Biomedical Sciences, University Federico II, Naples, Italy), and Dr. C. Giardiello (Mininvasive and Metabolic Surgery Unit, University, Pineta Grande Hospital, Castel Volturno (CE), Italy) for their long-lasting enthusiastic cooperation in sharing with us the difficult task to investigate the GH/IGF-1 axis in obese patients eligible for surgery.

References

1. Berryman DE, Glad CA, List EO, Johannsson G (2013) The GH/IGF-1 axis in obesity: pathophysiology and therapeutic considerations. Nat Rev Endocrinol 9:346–356
2. Savastano S, Di Somma C, Belfiore A et al (2006) Growth hormone status in morbidly obese subjects and correlation with body composition. J Endocrinol Invest 29:536–543
3. Savastano S, Di Somma C, Mentone A et al (2006) GH insufficiency in obese patients. J Endocrinol Invest 29(Suppl 5):42–53

4. Vijayakumar A, Yakar S, Leroith D (2011) The intricate role of growth hormone in metabolism. Front Endocrinol (Lausanne) 2:1–11
5. Kumar PA, Chitra PS, Lu C et al (2014) Growth hormone (GH) differentially regulates NF-kB activity in preadipocytes and macrophages: implications for GH's role in adipose tissue homeostasis in obesity. J Physiol Biochem 70:433–440
6. Vottero A, Guzzetti C, Loche S (2013) New aspects of the physiology of the GH-IGF-1 axis. Endocr Dev 24:96–105
7. Kawai M, Rosen CJ (2010) The IGF-I regulatory system and its impact on skeletal and energy homeostasis. J Cell Biochem 111:14–19
8. Frystyk J (2004) Free insulin-like growth factors: measurements and relationships to growth hormone secretion and glucose homeostasis. Growth Horm IGF Res 14:337–375
9. Cordido F, Peino R, Peñalva A et al (1996) Impaired growth hormone secretion in obese subjects is partially reversed by acipimox-mediated plasma free fatty acid depression. J Clin Endocrinol Metab 81:914–918
10. Di Somma C, Rivellese A, Pizza G et al (2011) Effects of short-term treatment with orlistat on growth hormone/insulin-like growth factor-I axis in obese post-menopausal women. J Endocrinol Invest 34:90–96
11. Scacchi M, Orsini F, Cattaneo A et al (2010) The diagnosis of GH deficiency in obese patients: a reappraisal with GHRH plus arginine testing after pharmacological blockade of lipolysis. Eur J Endocrinol 163:201–206
12. Rasmussen MH (2010) Obesity, growth hormone and weight loss. Mol Cell Endocrinol 316:147–153
13. Di Somma C, Angrisani L, Rota F et al (2008) GH and IGF-I deficiency are associated with reduced loss of fat mass after laparoscopic-adjustable silicone gastric banding. Clin Endocrinol (Oxf) 69:393–399
14. Savastano S, Di Somma C, Pizza G et al (2011) Liver-spleen axis, insulin-like growth factor-(IGF)-I axis and fat mass in overweight/obese females. J Transl Med 9:136
15. Fuentes E, Fuentes F, Vilahur G et al (2013) Mechanisms of chronic state of inflammation as mediators that link obese adipose tissue and metabolic syndrome. Mediators Inflamm 2013:1–11
16. Frystyk J, Brick DJ, Gerweck AV et al (2009) Bioactive insulin-like growth factor-I in obesity. J Clin Endocrinol Metab 94:3093–3097
17. Stanley TL, Feldpausch MN, Murphy CA et al (2014) Discordance of IGF-1 and GH stimulation testing for altered GH secretion in obesity. Growth Horm IGF Res 24:10–15
18. Molitch ME, Clemmons DR, Malozowski S et al (2011) Evaluation and treatment of adult growth hormone deficiency: an Endocrine Society clinical practice guideline. J Clin Endocrinol Metab 96:1587–1609
19. Colao A, Di Somma C, Savastano S et al (2009) A reappraisal of diagnosing GH deficiency in adults: role of gender, age, waist circumference, and body mass index. J Clin Endocrinol Metab 94:4414–4422
20. Corneli G, Di Somma C, Baldelli R et al (2005) The cut-off limits of the GH response to GH-releasing hormone-arginine test related to body mass index. Eur J Endocrinol 153:257–264
21. Bredella MA, Utz AL, Torriani M et al (2009) Anthropometry, CT, and DXA as predictors of GH deficiency in premenopausal women: ROC curve analysis. J Appl Physiol 106:418–422
22. Perotti M, Perra S, Saluzzi A et al (2013) Body fat mass is a strong and negative predictor of peak stimulated growth hormone and bone mineral density in healthy adolescents during transition period. Horm Metab Res 45:748–753
23. Popovic V (2013) Approach to testing growth hormone (GH) secretion in obese subjects. J Clin Endocrinol Metab 98:1789–1796
24. Colao A, Di Somma C, Cuocolo A et al (2004) The severity of growth hormone deficiency correlates with the severity of cardiac impairment in 100 adult patients with hypopituitarism: an observational, case-control study. J Clin Endocrinol Metab 89:5998–6004
25. Colao A, Di Somma C, Cascella T et al (2008) Relationships between serum IGF1 levels, blood pressure, and glucose tolerance: an observational, exploratory study in 404 subjects. Eur J Endocrinol 159:389–397

26. Akanji AO, Smith RJ (2012) The insulin-like growth factor system, metabolic syndrome, and cardiovascular disease risk. Metab Syndr Relat Disord 10:3–13
27. Di Somma C, Pivonello R, Pizza G et al (2010) Prevalence of the metabolic syndrome in moderately-severely obese subjects with and without growth hormone deficiency. J Endocrinol Invest 33:171–177
28. Bredella MA, Torriani M, Thomas BJ et al (2009) Peak growth hormone-releasing hormone-arginine-stimulated growth hormone is inversely associated with intramyocellular and intrahepatic lipid content in premenopausal women with obesity. J Clin Endocrinol Metab 94: 3995–4002
29. Mekala KC, Tritos NA (2009) Effects of recombinant human growth hormone therapy in obesity in adults: a meta analysis. J Clin Endocrinol Metab 94:130–137
30. Ahn CW, Kim CS, Nam JH et al (2006) Effects of growth hormone on insulin resistance and atherosclerotic risk factors in obese type 2 diabetic patients with poor glycaemic control. Clin Endocrinol (Oxf) 64:444–449
31. Karimi M, Koranyi J, Franco C et al (2010) Increased neck soft tissue mass and worsening of obstructive sleep apnea after growth hormone treatment in men with abdominal obesity. J Clin Sleep Med 6:256–263
32. Makimura H, Feldpausch MH, Rope AM et al (2012) Metabolic effects of a growth hormone-releasing factor in obese subjects with reduced growth hormone secretion: a randomized controlled trial. J Clin Endocrinol Metab 97:4769–4779
33. Camastra S, Manco M, Frascerra S et al (2009) Daylong pituitary hormones in morbid obesity: effects of bariatric surgery. Int J Obes (Lond) 33:166–172
34. Mancini MC, Costa AP, de Melo ME et al (2006) Effect of gastric bypass on spontaneous growth hormone and ghrelin release profiles. Obesity (Silver Spring) 14:383–387
35. Galli G, Pinchera A, Piaggi P et al (2012) Serum insulin-like growth factor-1 concentrations are reduced in severely obese women and raise after weight loss induced by laparoscopic adjustable gastric banding. Obes Surg 22:1276–1280
36. Mittempergher F, Pata G, Crea N et al (2013) Preoperative prediction of growth hormone (GH)/insulin-like growth factor-1 (IGF-1) axis modification and postoperative changes in candidates for bariatric surgery. Obes Surg 23:594–601
37. De Marinis L, Bianchi A, Mancini A et al (2004) Growth hormone secretion and leptin in morbid obesity before and after biliopancreatic diversion: relationships with insulin and body composition. J Clin Endocrinol Metab 89:174–180
38. Edén Engström B, Burman P, Holdstock C et al (2006) Effects of gastric bypass on the GH/IGF-I axis in severe obesity–and a comparison with GH deficiency. Eur J Endocrinol 154:53–59
39. Savastano S, Angrisani L, Di Somma C et al (2010) Relationship between growth hormone/insulin-like growth factor-1 axis integrity and voluntary weight loss after gastric banding surgery for severe obesity. Obes Surg 20:211–220
40. Savastano S, Di Somma C, Angrisani L et al (2009) Growth hormone treatment prevents loss of lean mass after bariatric surgery in morbidly obese patients: results of a pilot, open, prospective, randomized, controlled study. J Clin Endocrinol Metab 94:817–826

Adrenal Function and Obesity

6

Laura Proietti Pannunzi, Cecilia Motta, and Vincenzo Toscano

6.1 Hypothalamus–Pineal–Adrenal Axis and Glucocorticoid Functions

Cortisol production by the adrenal cortex (zona fasciculata and zona reticularis) is stimulated and controlled by adrenocorticotropic hormone (ACTH), itself subject to the action of pituitary secretagogues; among these, the most powerful are corticotrophin-releasing hormone (CRH) and antidiuretic hormone (ADH). Cortisol inhibits ACTH secretion by a negative feedback that acts on pituitary and hypothalamic levels [1].

In their turn, hypothalamic centers receive stimulatory signals from the central nervous system; the whole is regulated by a complex interaction of several systemic and paracrine factors, such as adrenergic, serotoninergic, and dopaminergic systems, cells in the vascular wall, and immune system, in a way that is not completely understood [2].

All these settings lead to ACTH and cortisol secretion, which occurs in a pulsatile manner and with a circadian rhythm, resulting in a diurnal profile characterized by high cortisol activity in early morning hours and low cortisol activity in the afternoon and evening [3]. The hypothalamic–pituitary–adrenal (HPA) axis has a central role in maintaining homeostasis in several regulatory systems, by the integration through hypothalamic centers of numerous environmental factors.

The HPA axis is regulated by a feedback system that controls the cortisol secretion in order to avoid its excessive production, which might cause, especially in the long term, severe damage; this setting takes place through glucocorticoid receptors (GRs), which are located in different areas of the central nervous system, particularly in the hippocampus.

Cortisol secreted into the circulation is then metabolized in the peripheral target tissues by two different enzymes: 11-β-hydroxysteroid dehydrogenase (11-β-HSD)

L. Proietti Pannunzi • C. Motta • V. Toscano (✉)
UOC Endocrinologia – Azienda Ospedaliera Sant'Andrea,
Università di Roma Sapienza, Via di Grottarossa 1035-1039, Rome 00189, Italy
e-mail: l.pannunzi@yahoo.it; dott.cecilia.motta@gmail.com; vincenzo.toscano@uniroma1.it

© Springer International Publishing Switzerland 2015
A. Lenzi et al. (eds.), *Multidisciplinary Approach to Obesity: From Assessment to Treatment*, DOI 10.1007/978-3-319-09045-0_6

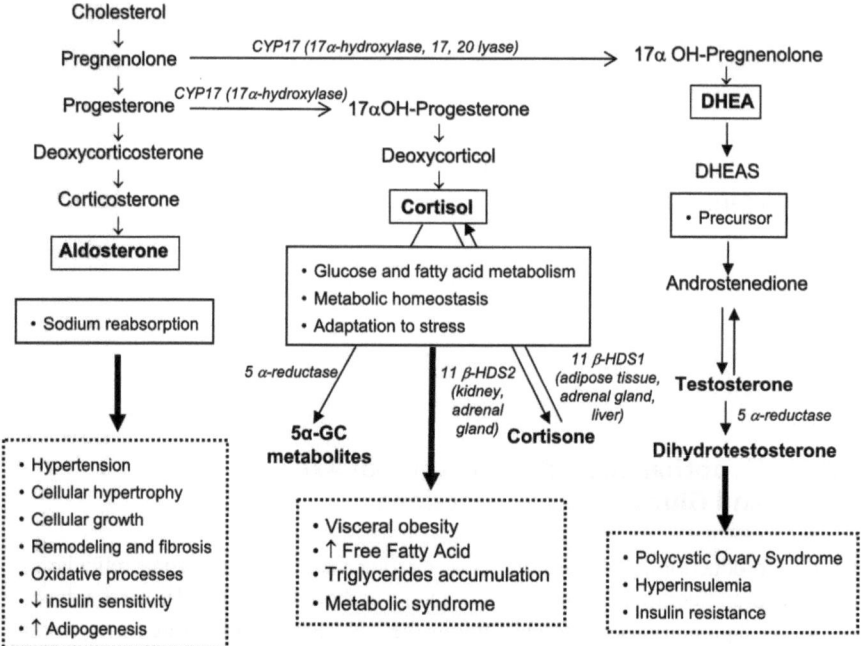

Fig. 6.1 Actions of adrenal hormones from Roberge [6]

type 1, which transforms cortisone into cortisol, and 11-β-hydroxysteroid dehydrogenase type 2, which transforms cortisol into the less active cortisone. 11-β-HSD2, which is thought to protect tissues from a cortisol excess, has been described to be found in the kidney, adipose tissue, liver, and muscle [3].

The effects of cortisol are exerted through the GR–hormone complex that interacts with some genes. The effect obviously depends on both the amount of active cortisol and on the receptor density; the concentration of active cortisol depends on which type of 11-β-HSD is present in the tissue. The transformation of cortisol to cortisone and back leads both to the modification of the locally active hormone concentrations and to changes in circulating levels of cortisol [3].

Cortisol is also irreversibly inactivated by 5-α and 5-β reductases, enzymes that convert ring A of the hormone, which is then excreted through the bile [3].

Glucocorticoids, insulin, growth hormone, cytokines, and stress seem to be all involved in the regulation of these enzymes [4].

Glucocorticoids play an important role in the regulation of metabolic homeostasis, initiating a broad range of actions on various organs [5, 6]. Metabolic effects of glucocorticoids are well known and can be summarized as:

- Inhibition of glucose uptake in peripheral tissues
- Stimulation of gluconeogenesis
- Increase of blood glucose and insulin in the postabsorptive phase
- Altered post-receptor insulin function, reducing insulin signaling via stimulation of oxygen species production and oxidative stress [1] (Fig. 6.1)

6.2 Effects of Glucocorticoids on Adipose Tissue

Glucocorticoids have a number of very important functions. Their involvement to contrast stressor agents or situations is known for many years, although not completely elucidated.

Recent studies showed that obesity cannot be explained just as a mechanism of cause–effect, but many factors and conditions can contribute to its pathophysiology. In this regard, physiological and pathophysiological stresses have a significant long-term impact. In fact, in a stressful situation, GCs are secreted through the CRH pathway, and these elevated levels of CGs seem to stimulate appetite, increasing feeding and consequently producing obesity [7]. GCs play an important role in lipid uptake. It has been demonstrated that GC receptor is expressed in adipose tissue and its density in visceral adipose tissue is higher than in other adipose deposits [8]. Visceral adipose tissue has been associated to cardiovascular disease [9]. Veilleux et al. showed an increased accumulation of visceral adipose tissue in humans with a higher 11-β-HSD1 activity, increased lipolysis, and increased levels of lipoprotein lipase (LPL) activity [10]. Moreover, Morton et al. demonstrated that 11-β-HSD1-deficient mice were resistant to diet-induced visceral obesity [11]. Taken together, all these data can suggest that there is an irrefutable correlation between GCs and visceral adipose tissue; anyway, the underlying mechanisms are not completely elucidated.

The action of GCs on fatty acid metabolism is very complicated and can be explicated through the beta-adrenergic pathway, where cAMP is usually the first target of investigation. The action of GCs can be shared in the short term and long term. At short term, GC infusion enhances the release of non-esterified fatty acids from the adipocytes through the activation of a particular type of LPL, hormone-sensitive lipase [12]. Long-term effects, instead, were mediated by the regulation of the transcription of specific gene target including HSL, ATGL, and perilipin (cf. Table 6.1).

Bjorntorp has demonstrated that GCs determine the activation of LPL with consequent increase of visceral adipose deposit [3].

However, in literature there are many different evidences about the pathway of GCs on lipolysis, but often they are in contrast with each other; a summary of the previous studies is reported in Table 6.1.

6.3 Effects of Glucocorticoids on the Differentiation of Adipose Tissue

Since several years, it is known that glucocorticoids stimulate lipolysis; people with glucocorticoid excess usually present increased fat deposits. The increased appetite sense and the lipogenic effect of the associated hyperinsulinemia caused by the high levels of GCs may explain this contradiction. Anyway, the relationship between adipogenesis and glucocorticoid hormones is very complex.

In the last 15 years, many new knowledge about the adipose tissue have been discovered. In fact, adipose tissue is discerned in visceral and subcutaneous fat. The

Table 6.1 Summary of previous studies investigating the effects of GCs on lipolysis

Article	Adipose model	Dose/type of GC	Duration	Lipolysis	Suggested mechanisms
Fain et al.	Isolated parametrial adipocytes; high-fat–fed rats	Dexamethasone 0.016 µg/mL (0.04 µmol/L)	4 h	↑ FFA release	Altered transcription
–	–	–	–	↔ glycerol release	–
Fain et al.	Isolated parametrial adipocytes; rat	Dexamethasone 0.1 µg/mL (2.5 µmol/L)	4 h	↔ glycerol	↔ cAMP
Lamberts et al.	Isolated epididymal adipocytes; rat	Dexamethasone 0.1 µg/mL (2.5 µmol/L)	4 h	↔ glycerol	↔ cAMP
Samra et al.	In vivo human	Hydrocortisone 1.5 µmol/L	Acute IV infusion	↑ overall NEFA release	↑ LPL activity
–	–	–	–	↓ NEFA venoarterial difference in abdominal	↑ peripheral lipase activity
–	–	–	–	–	↓ visceral lipase activity
Ottosson et al.	Isolated subcutaneous human	Hydrocortisone 1 µmol/L	3 days	↓ basal lipolysis	↓ Production or
–	–	–	–	–	↑ elimination of cAMP
–	–	–	–	–	↓ β-adrenergic–stimulated lipolysis
Campbell et al.	3T3-L1 adipocytes	Corticosterone 1–100 µmol/L	48 h	↑ glycerol release	↑ HSL and ATGL transcription
–	–	–	48 h	↓ glycerol release	↓ cAMP activity

Adapted from [31]

relationship between human fat topography and metabolic syndrome was investigated at molecular level, and an important role of glucocorticoid hormones was found.

In vitro studies were performed to explain the pathway of differentiation from stem cell to adipose tissue. Significant differences of adipocyte differentiation were found between human and rodent culture cells [13].

In rodent preadipocyte cell lines, the addition of glucocorticoid in the first 48 h (expansion clonal phase) to the calf serum showed a stimulatory effect. This effect

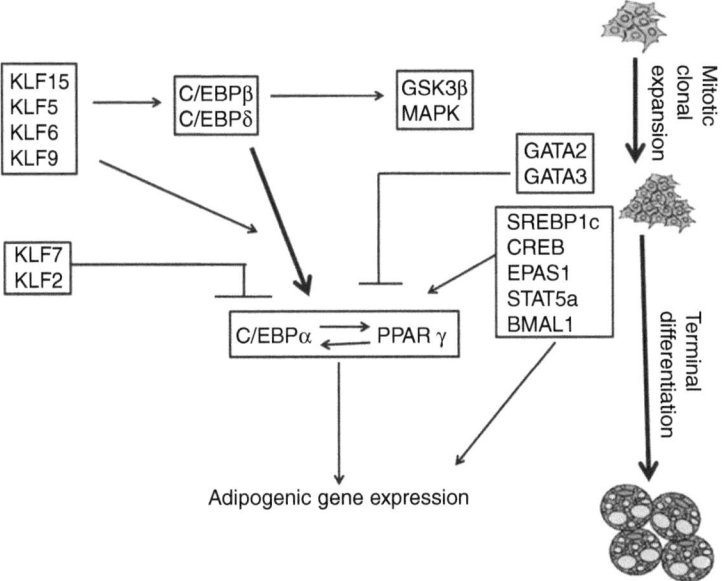

Fig. 6.2 Transcriptional regulation of adipocyte differentiation from [14]

has been attributed to a direct stimulation of C/EBPδ transcription, repression of the pref-1, an antiadipogenic preadipocite factor and to the depletion of a specific subcellular pool of histone deacetylase 1 (HDAC1) [13, 14].

In human primary preadipocyte differentiation, the action of GCs is limited to the first 48 h and determines an increased level of transcription factors and adipogenic markers such as C/EBPα that is not present in rodent cells [15] (Fig. 6.2).

This early elevation does not reflect an increase in mRNA levels; in a second moment, elevated levels of C/EBPα and PPARγ are observed, and at this time, they are correlated to the mRNA levels. At day 2–4, mRNA levels of both molecules remain elevated, but protein expression of the only C/EBPα starts to decline despite the high mRNA levels. These observations could explain a different role in adipocyte maturation of PPARγ vs. C/EBPα, with a predominant role for PPARγ in mature adipocyte [13].

In vivo studies were also performed. Part of literature indicates that cortisol in humans and corticosterone in mice stimulate the adipogenesis; in fact, in obese mice, adrenalectomy decreases the rate of body weight gain, but this effect is completely reversed when the animals are treated with corticosterone [16].

Many theories have been hypothesized to explain the mechanisms at the basis of visceral obesity.

Of course, increased secretion of glucocorticoid is associated to obesity; anyway, cortisol levels are not elevated in idiopathic obesity suggesting an increased metabolism of glucocorticoid hormones.

Some authors suppose that in obesity there is an increased local active glucocorticoid concentration and that this determines a peripheral amplified activation of its receptors.

Other authors presume a pivotal role of 11-β-HSD type 1.

Disorders of this enzyme were found in obese models. In fact, 11β-HSD is impaired in obese rats and an increased local activity in visceral fat was found. The consequence of this hyperactivity is a higher concentration of active glucocorticoid responsible for visceral fat increase [17]. In the same manner, it could be speculated that in human an increased activity of 11-β-HSD plays a role in visceral obesity and metabolic syndrome.

GCs may contribute to obesity in many ways. It has been demonstrated that GCs regulate the appetite center through direct and indirect actions. Although an acute stress condition seems to suppress appetite sense, the GCs released in the hours and days after the event play a feeding role. However, recent studies have also demonstrated that, in humans, high levels of cortisol are related to the amount of ingested food 1 h after the injection of CRH and the amount of food is directly correlated to the cortisol peak.

Several studies have examined the possible interactions of GC target molecules and their mechanism on the appetite center. Various molecules have been invoked:

1. Neuropeptide Y (NPY) and agouti-related peptide (AgRP) [the gene expression of these molecules is upregulated in the arcuate nucleus by an increase of AMP-activated protein kinase signaling through GC stimulus] [18].
2. Leptin, whose sensitivity to the brain is reduced in the presence of high levels of GCs [18], can also act through the pancreatic stimulation of insulin, which has an intricate role in the regulation of the sense of hunger [19].
3. Ghrelin, whose levels increase during stress, resulting in increased release of CRH. The CRH therefore could act both in a direct way and in an indirect way through the stimulation of noradrenergic fibers at the level of the paraventricular nucleus (PVN). However, this theory has yet to be validated. Lastly, it has been hypothesized that a chronic stress could determine a rise of the ghrelin signaling with subsequent increase of food intake.

6.4 Glucocorticoid Hormone Variations in Obesity

The well-known metabolic effects of glucocorticoids have stimulated interest in the possible role of alterations of the HPA axis in primitive obesity [1].

Ever since 1963, Schteingart et al. showed an increased production of cortisol in obese subjects; later it became clear that alterations of cortisol in obesity were mostly characterized by an increased production of this hormone associated with a parallel increase in its metabolic clearance, therefore with normal or even low levels of serum cortisol concentrations [1, 3, 20]. These alterations are significantly more evident with visceral distribution of fat. Some studies have measured salivary

Table 6.2 Modifications of the HPA axis in the obese subject

Hormone	Obesity
Basal cortisol	Normal
Metabolic clearance of GCs	Increased
Synthesis and production of GCs	Increased
GC production in adipose tissue	Increased activity of 11β-HSD type 1
Free urinary cortisol	Normal/increased
Basal ACTH	Normal
Number of ACTH secretory pulses	Increased
Amplitude of ACTH secretory pulses	Decreased
17-OH corticosteroids	Increased

Table 6.3 Modification to adrenal stimulation test in obese subject

Hormone	Obesity
Cortisol after CRH (and AVP)	Increased
ACTH after CRH (and AVP)	Increased
Cortisol after ACTH	Increased
Cortisol after hypoglycemia	Increased
ACTH and cortisol after stress	Increased
Cortisol after meal	Increased
HPA axis sensitivity to an increase in the noradrenergic tone	Increased
Cortisol suppression after dexamethasone	Normal/decreased

cortisol in obese subjects finding both increased and reduced basal concentrations: these discrepancies are probably due to a different degree of activation of the HPA axis, which in turn could depend on environmental stress [1, 3] (Tables 6.2 and 6.3).

It is well known that cortisol secretion or production and urinary cortisol excretion are regularly increased in obesity; the reasons for this elevated turnover are only partially understood: the increased cortisol secretion may be influenced by lean body mass, by an HPA axis hyperactivity, and by alterations in the hormone's metabolism [22].

Numerous studies have examined the urinary output of urinary free cortisol and cortisol metabolites (17-ketogenic steroids), and their excretion rates are frequently elevated in obese subjects, particularly in those with visceral obesity [3].

Pasquali et al. showed that daily urinary free cortisol excretion rates were one- to sixfold higher in women with abdominal body fat distribution than in women with peripheral body fat distribution and in controls [21]. Many of these studies, however, do not consider the fact that obese subjects have an increased body mass and surface area; some studies have therefore applied a correction factor (for body surface or to calculate lean mass, estimated by using creatinine's output values), and cortisol excretion has been found to be elevated by some authors but not by all [3, 20, 23].

ACTH and cortisol response to physiological and pharmacological stimuli is thought to be impaired in subjects with visceral obesity: it has been described that the percentage increase in ACTH and cortisol after administration of CRH alone or in combination with vasopressin is significantly greater compared to that of subjects with peripheral obesity and lean controls [1, 23, 24]. However, not all studies are in agreement: in some of these, plasma cortisol and ACTH response to CRH did not differ from obese and lean subjects [25]. In addition a normal cortisol suppression after dexamethasone administration is supported by numerous studies, with only few exceptions [20, 22, 25–27].

Several studies provided direct evidence of an increased cortisol metabolism rate in obesity. As discussed above, 11-β-HSD2 has been found in the kidney and also in adipose tissue; hence, if there is a large cortisol inactivation systemically, due to the elevated body fat mass in obesity, the HPA axis is expected to increase the hormone secretion, to compensate for the higher cortisol degradation and to maintain normal free cortisol blood levels; there is a realistic possibility that the increased cortisol secretion described in obese subjects would be a consequence of its elevated peripheral inactivation. However, this mechanism of parallel changes in metabolic clearance and HPA axis activity has not been observed in all obese subjects [3, 22].

11-β-HSD1 activity, which reactivates cortisone to active cortisol, also appears to be altered in obesity; numerous studies found an increase in 11-β-HSD1 mRNA and activity in subcutaneous and omental adipose tissue in human obesity, and this has been associated with BMI, body fat percentage, waist circumference, and insulin resistance [22, 25, 28]. Furthermore, in studies conducted on animals, it has been reported that mice overexpressing 11-β-HSD1 selectively in adipose tissue develop visceral obesity, insulin resistance, and hyperlipidemia [29]. 11-β-HSD1 activity could thus result in the development of a local hypercortisolism; this alteration potentially leads to an increased adipocyte differentiation and increased secretion of free fatty acids [1].

Some authors found that the activity of 5-α and 5-β reductases, enzymes that irreversibly inactivate cortisol, is associated with obesity, in particular with BMI, waist circumference and waist–hip ratio, and fat mass-related insulin resistance [22, 30].

References

1. Chiovato L, Magri F (2006) Modificazioni del sistema endocrino nei soggetti obesi. In: Pinchera A, Bosello O, Carruba MO (eds) Obesità e sistema endocrino. Mediserve, Milano, pp 189–205
2. Chrousos GP, Gold PW (1992) The concept of stress and stress system disorders. Overview of physical and behavioral homeostasis. JAMA 267:1244–1252
3. Bjorntorp P, Rosmond R (2000) Obesity and cortisol. Nutrition 16:924–936
4. Andrews RC, Walker BR (1999) Glucocorticoids and insulin resistance: old hormones, new targets. Clin Sci 96(5):513–523
5. Schoneveld OJ, Gaemers IC, Lamers WH (2004) Mechanisms of glucocorticoid signalling. Biochim Biophys Acta 1680:114–128
6. Roberge C, Carpentier AC, Langlois MF et al (2007) Adrenocortical dysregulation as a major player in insulin resistance and onset of obesity. Am J Physiol Endocrinol Metab 29:E1465–E1478
7. De Vriendt T, Moreno LA, De Henauw S (2009) Chronic stress and obesity in adolescent: scientific evidence and methodological issue for epidemiological research. Nutr Metab Cardiovasc Dis 19:511–519

8. Rebuffè-Scrive M, Brönnegard M, Nilsson A et al (1990) Steroid hormone receptors in human adipose tissue. J Clin Endocrinol Metab 71:1215–1219
9. Bjorntorp P (2001) Do stress reactions cause abdominal obesity and comorbidities? Obes Rev 2:73–76
10. Veilleux A, Rhéaume C, Daris M et al (2009) Omental adipose tissue type 1 11 beta-hydroxysteroid dehydrogenase oxoreductase activity, body fat distribution, and metabolic alterations in women. J Clin Endocrinol Metab 94:3550–3557
11. Morton NM, Paterson JM, Masuzaki H et al (2004) Novel adipose tissue-mediated resistance to diet-induced visceral obesity in 11 beta-hydroxysteroid dehydrogenase type 1-deficient mice. Diabetes 53:931–938
12. Slavin BG, Ong JM, Kern PA (1994) Hormonal regulation of hormone-sensitive lipase activity and mRNA levels in isolated rat adipocytes. J Lipid Res 35:1535–1541
13. Tomlinson JJ, Boudreau A, Dongmei W et al (2006) Modulation of early human preadipocyte differentiation by glucocorticoids. Endocrinology 174:5284–5293
14. Moreno-Navarrete JM, Fernandez-Real JM (2012) Adipocyte differentiation. In: Symonds ME (ed) Adipose tissue biology. Springer, New York, pp 17–38
15. Cao Z, Umek RM, McKnight SL (1991) Regulated expression of three C/eBP isoforms during adipose conversion of 3 T3-L1 cells. J Biol Chem 253:7570–7578
16. Shimomura Y, Bray GA, Lee M (1987) Adrenalectomy and steroid treatment in obese (ob/ob) and diabetic (db/db) mice. Horm Metab Res 19:295–299
17. Livingstone DE, Kenyon CJ, Walker BR (2000) Mechanism of dysregulation of 11 beta-hydroxysteroid dehydrogenase type 1in obese Zucker rats. J Endocrinol 167:533–539
18. Strack AM, Sebastian RJ, Schwartz MW et al (1995) Glucocorticoids and insulin: reciprocal signals for energy balance. Am J Physiol 268:R142–R149
19. Spencer SJ, Tilbrook A (2011) The glucocorticoid contribution to obesity. Stress 14:233–246
20. Schteingart DE, Gregerman RI, Conn JW (1963) A comparison of the characteristics of increased adrenocortical function in obesity and Cushing's syndrome. Metabolism 12:484–497
21. Pasquali R, Cantobelli S, Casimirri F et al (1993) The hypothalamic-pituitary-adrenal axis in obese women with different patterns of body fat distribution. J Clin Endocrinol Metab 77(2):341–346
22. Mussig K, Remer T, Maser-Gluth (2010) Brief review: glucocorticoid excretion in obesity. J Steroid Biochem Mol Biol 121:589–593
23. Murphy BPE (1968) Clinical evaluation of urinary cortisol determinations by competitive protein-binding radioassay. J Clin Endocrinol Metab 28:343–348
24. Simkim-Silverman LR, Wing RR (2000) Weight gain during menopause. Is it inevitable or can it be prevented? Postgrad Med 108(47–50):53–56
25. Rask E, Olsson T, Soderberg S et al (2001) Tissue-specific dysregulation of cortisol metabolism in human obesity. J Clin Endocrinol Metab 86(3):1418–1421
26. Duclos M, Gatta B, Corcuff JB et al (2001) Fat distribution in obese women is associated with subtle alterations of the hypothalamic-pituitary-adrenal axis activity and sensitivity to glucocorticoids. Clin Endocrinol 55(4):447–454
27. Jessop DS, Dallman MF, Fleming D, Lightman SL (2001) Resistance to glucocorticoid feedback in obesity. J Clin Endocrinol Metab 86(9):4109–4114
28. Desbriere R, Vuaroqueaux V, Achard V et al (2006) 11 beta-hydroxysteroid dehydrogenase type 1 mRNA is increased in both visceral and subcutaneous adipose tissue of obese patients. Obesity 14(5):794–798
29. Masuzaki H, Paterson J, Shinyama H et al (2001) A transgenic model of visceral obesity and the metabolic syndrome. Science 294(5549):2166–2170
30. Fraser R, Ingram MC, Anderson NH et al (1999) Cortisol effects on body mass, blood pressure, and cholesterol in the general population. Hypertension 33(6):1364–1368
31. Peckett AJ, Wright D, Riddell MC (2011) The effects of glucocorticoids on adipose tissue lipid metabolism. Metabolism 60:1500–1510

Ovarian Function and Obesity: PCOS, Menopause

Carla Lubrano, Lucio Gnessi, and Silvia Migliaccio

7.1 Ovarian Function and Energy Metabolism

Energy metabolism and fertility in women are tightly connected and reciprocally regulated to meet the need to feed a developing embryo, forcing metabolic pathways to adapt to this reproductive request [1]. The female body composition, characterized by higher fat mass, and the propensity to weight gain might be the consequence of evolutionary adaptations that enable reproduction in food-scarce environments [2]. The regulatory mechanisms linking food availability and reproductive function take into account the variable energy demands at each stage of the reproductive cycle (menstrual cycles, pregnancy, and lactation). Reproductive disorders can lead to changes in metabolic function, and similarly, metabolic disorders can underlie changes in reproductive function. All the signals about nutritional status are integrated at hypothalamic levels in the arcuate nucleus which regulates both ovulation and energy homeostasis; in fact, sensors of energy status in this nucleus direct the synthesis of gonadotropins in the pituitary by regulating, through kisspeptin neurons, the activity of gonadotropin-releasing hormone (GnRH) neurons located in the preoptic area, in relation to individual's metabolic status [3–5]. Moreover, estrogen signaling potentiates leptin sensitivity [6]. The overall effects of increased estrogen signaling are induction of an anorexigenic response and fat redistribution to subcutaneous rather than to visceral depots.

C. Lubrano (✉) • L. Gnessi
Department of Experimental Medicine, Section of Medical Pathophysiology,
Food Science and Endocrinology, Sapienza University of Rome,
Viale del Policlinico 155, Rome 00161, Italy
e-mail: carla.lubrano@uniroma1.it; Lucio.gnessi@uniroma1.it

S. Migliaccio
Department of Movement, Human and Health Sciences, Unit of Endocrinology,
Foro Italico University, Largo Lauro De Bosis 15, Rome 00195, Italy
e-mail: silvia.migliaccio@uniroma4.it

The concentration of various circulating estrogen metabolites such as estradiol, estrone, estriol, and their ratio varies and depends on fertility status [7]. The high degree of reciprocal control of energy sensing and reproduction is implemented through estrogen receptor (ER) α and ERβ as the nexus between these two functions [8]. Accordingly, the set of genes controlled by ERα and ERβ might substantially change in response to different concentrations and ratios of estrogens. Hence, in the same target tissue, the intracellular activity of ERs might vary at each reproductive stage or during the menstrual cycle, leading to an alternate activation of pathways that control energy metabolism. Indeed, liver ERs can be activated by nutritional signaling molecules (such as amino acids and IGF-1), as well as gonadal hormones, and can regulate liver production of both apoB and IGF-1. Moreover, dietary intakes of amino acids can also regulate fertility [9]. ERα and ERβ are expressed in all tissues relevant to glucose metabolism, including the adipose tissue [10], skeletal muscle, and pancreas [11]. In pancreatic β cells, estrogens have an antiapoptotic action; repress both lipid biosynthesis and the accumulation of fat, preventing lipotoxicity; and directly stimulate insulin biosynthesis [12], but sex hormones counteract the effects of insulin in the periphery [13]. Insulin resistance (IR) is related to abdominal obesity, and in women, it is often inextricably linked with ovarian dysfunctions, leading to clinical manifestations across the entire female reproductive life. Specifically, obesity in women manifests as early menarche, subfertility, polycystic ovary syndrome (PCOS), and symptomatic menopause and increases the risk of breast cancer. In fact, the cessation of ovarian function is linked with obesity as menopause precipitates abdominal weight gain and the associated adverse metabolic derangements. Overall, obese women with superimposed reproductive alterations may be considered to be at high risk for further progression to metabolic syndrome (MetS), type 2 diabetes mellitus (T2DM), and potentially cardiovascular diseases (CVD). These patients can then be targeted for early screening, lifestyle optimization, and the prevention of the subsequent metabolic derangement [14] (Fig. 7.1).

7.2 Subfertility and Obesity

Adipose tissue is an endocrine organ and has a role in the metabolism of sex steroids. Central obesity in women appears to impair reproduction even in the absence of PCOS. Potential mechanisms of subfertility in obese women include IR with hyperinsulinemia, which stimulates ovarian androgen production, as well as increased peripheral aromatization of androgens. Altogether, these events may modify gonadotropin secretion pattern altering follicular development [15]. In subfertile couples, it has been shown that the probability of spontaneous pregnancy declined linearly with the women's body mass index (BMI) [16]. These data suggest that obesity per se may impair reproduction in women.

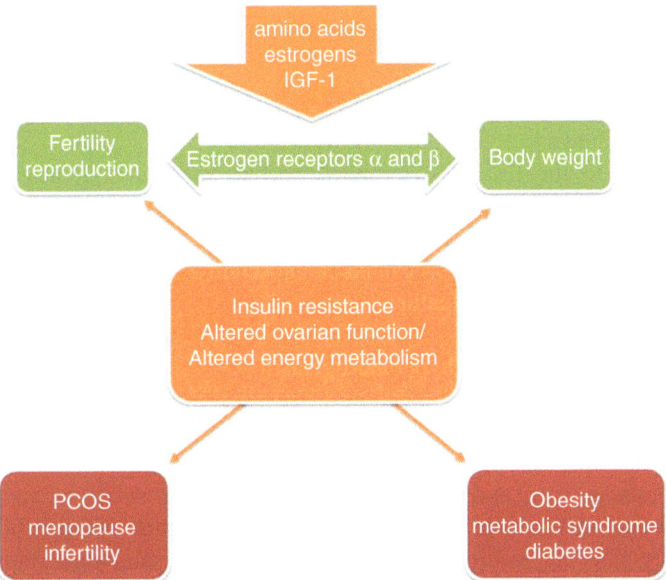

Fig. 7.1 Reciprocal regulation of energy metabolism and ovarian function in order to guarantee a metabolic status tuned to reproductive needs. The alteration of one or both of these compartments may lead to metabolic and/or reproductive diseases

7.3 Age of Menarche and Obesity

It is well known that sexual maturation depends on total body fat and tends to occur earlier in overweight and obese girls. Women who experienced early menarche have higher BMI in adult life compared to the late-maturing girls; data from animal and human studies suggest that leptin may be the link between total body fat and the onset of menarche [17]. This association between earlier menarche and adult obesity may be considered as the beginning of the interaction between body weight, metabolism, and reproduction which persists throughout the female reproductive life; earlier age of menarche, in fact, increases the risk of adult T2DM, and this appears to be mediated by greater adult adiposity [18].

7.4 PCOS and Obesity in Adult Women

PCOS is the most frequent ovarian disorder in premenopausal women (6–10 %), and obesity is a common feature of this endocrinopathy (present in 20–69 % of patients) [19]. PCOS is a heterogeneous disorder characterized by multiple endocrine disturbances, and its underlying causes are likely to be both genetic and environmental. It is possible that this condition begins prenatally, and the consequences extend past in the reproductive years, with multigenerational impact [20]. The fundamental pathophysiologic defect in PCOS is not known, but changes in insulin action, gonadotropin dynamics, as well as ovarian and steroidogenic defects have all been shown to contribute to the disorder.

According to the ESHRE (European Society of Human Reproduction and Embryology)/ASRM (American Society for Reproductive Medicine) consensus and to the evidence-based clinical practice guidelines of an Endocrine Society-appointed task force [21], PCOS can be diagnosed in a woman presenting with two out of three of the following features:

1. Clinical and/or biological hyperandrogenism
2. Chronic anovulation
3. Presence of polycystic ovaries (PCO) on ultrasound [22]

During the physical examination, it is important to assess the cutaneous manifestations (hirsutism, acne, alopecia, acanthosis nigricans, and skin tags), using grading systems that minimize the subjectivity of the evaluations, and to record BMI and waist circumference, as visceral obesity worsens the severity of the PCOS phenotype and increases the incidence of PCOS-related metabolic risk factors. A 2-h oral glucose tolerance test using a 75-g oral glucose load is also recommended to screen for impaired glucose tolerance (IGT) andT2M, and rescreening within 5 years is suggested. Different phenotypes such as "ovulatory PCOS" and "nonhyperandrogenic PCOS" have received much criticism and probably represent less severe forms. Women with PCOS face a lifetime of reproductive and metabolic risk, but the focus of attention has been on fertility, which remains a challenge for many women with this condition. Reduced fertility, however, seems to be present only in the presence of oligo-ovulation or anovulation, but there is no clear data of the fertility of patients with PCOS who have normal ovulatory function. IR is recognized to be the key pathophysiological element of PCOS and a significant contributor to its reproductive and metabolic complications [23, 24]. PCOS patients often display other indices of cardiovascular risk such as dyslipidemia, high serum homocysteine, and inflammatory markers (serum TNF and IL-6) [1]. They also present clinical features of premature atherosclerosis such as impaired pulse wave velocity, increased carotid intima-media wall thickness, presence of carotid plaque, and increased coronary artery calcification [25, 26]. Despite the prevalence and health implications of PCOS, clinical gaps exist including delayed diagnosis, inconsistent management, inadequate support for lifestyle change, and limited attention to psychological and metabolic features. Intervention was needed to improve awareness, patient experience, early diagnosis, self-management, complication screening, and treatment across reproductive, metabolic, and psychological features [27].

7.5 Insulin Resistance, Androgens, and Abdominal Obesity

Increased serum insulin stimulates ovarian androgen production and also reduces sex hormone-binding globulin (SHBG) production in the liver further increasing serum levels of free bioavailable androgens. Apart from reproductive (anovulation) and cosmetic (acne, alopecia, and hirsutism) consequences of elevated serum androgens in women, hyperandrogenemia can increase abdominal obesity, which in turn further aggravates existing IR. Preadipocytes are known to have androgen receptors, and high androgen levels have been shown to induce selective IR in cultured adipocytes. Conversely, adipokines secreted by the intra-abdominal adipose tissue may also promote ovarian androgen production. TNF may directly stimulate proliferation and steroidogenesis in the rat theca cells and is involved in the apoptosis and anovulation in the rat's ovary. Additionally, intra-abdominal fat tissue has been shown to express several enzymes involved in the metabolism of androgens which may further contribute to the hyperandrogenism in women with PCOS [28].

7.6 Endocrine-Disrupting Chemicals (EDCs), PCOS, and Obesity

Recently, there has been interest in whether EDCs in the environment, particularly bisphenol A (BPA), may contribute to the disorder. A growing body of research documents the effects of EDCs on the differentiation of adipocytes and the central nervous system circuits that control food intake and energy expenditure [29]. In parallel, interest has grown in epigenetic influences, including maternal programming, the process by which the mother's experience has permanent effects on energy-balancing traits in the offspring [30]. In animal models, exposure to BPA during the perinatal period dramatically disrupts ovarian and reproductive function in females. BPA also appears to have obesogenic properties, disrupting normal metabolic activity and making the body prone to overweight. In humans, cross-sectional data suggest that BPA concentrations are higher in women with PCOS than in reproductively healthy women, but the link of causality has not been established, and additional work is needed to understand the mechanisms by which EDCs may contribute to PCOS as well as the critical periods of exposure, which may even be transgenerational [31].

7.7 PCOS and Obesity in Adolescents

The use of diagnostic criteria established during the consensus conference held in Rotterdam in 2003 is recommended in adults, whereas in adolescent and perimenopausal and postmenopausal women, the diagnostic criteria for PCOS have not been validated [32]. Of particular concern is that many of the features considered to be diagnostic for PCOS may evolve over time and change during the first few years after menarche. Nonetheless, attempts to define young women who may be at risk for development of PCOS are pertinent since associated morbidity such as obesity, IR, and dyslipidemia may benefit from early intervention. Some suggest that even using the strictest criteria, the diagnosis of PCOS may not be valid in adolescents younger than 18 years. In addition, evidence does not necessarily support that lack of treatment of PCOS in younger adolescents will result in untoward outcomes since features consistent with PCOS often resolve with time [33].

7.8 Menopause and Obesity

Age-dependent cessation of ovarian functions is associated with a disruption of metabolic homeostasis and consequent inflammatory reactions that trigger the onset of metabolic, cardiovascular, skeletal, and neurologic pathologies. Recent data show that obese menopausal patients are not protected from osteoporosis [34, 35]. With menopause, estradiol levels decrease markedly, although estrone levels remain at reproductive level. In adipose tissue, estrogens increase subcutaneous fat deposition in lower body areas and decrease lipolytic activity, and when estrogen signaling decreases, the subcutaneous fat redistributes to visceral areas and increases hepatic fat deposition [36, 37]. These phenomena can be reversed by the administration of hormone replacement therapy (HRT) that might aid the restoration of metabolic homeostasis and highlight the pathogenic mechanisms underlying the disordered energy metabolism associated with human ovarian dysfunction. Furthermore, PCOS is common among reproductive-aged women (8–10 %). Although the medical and metabolic consequences of PCOS are well described in young women, its impact on female reproductive senescence and the menopausal transition is poorly understood [38]. Randomized controlled clinical trials should be carried out to better evaluate the long-term effects of oral contraceptives or HRT in women. The use of contraceptives can deteriorate glucose tolerance; however, low estrogen doses when administered orally can improve tolerance. Recent evidences suggest that genistein aglycone and phytoestrogens may act beneficially on surrogate cardiovascular risk markers in postmenopausal women and on bone loss [39–41].

7.9 Non-pharmacological Treatment of PCOS-Related Obesity

Lifestyle modification studies to reduce IR in obese women with PCOS are limited by small numbers, lack of controls, and variable methodologies used to evaluate IR. Small reductions in weight (~5 % body weight) have led to positive clinical improvements, but long-term dietary restriction is generally difficult to maintain, while specific dietary recommendations lack evidences. Beneficial effects of exercise in women with PCOS have been proved: a 3-month structured exercise training program caused significant improvement in cardiopulmonary functional capacity, IR, and BMI and after 6 months even restored ovulation [42]. Young patients show very good compliance to lifestyle modifications (unlike adult women), and loss of body weight can result in a spontaneous resumption of menstrual cycles. There are very few data on different kinds of diets (Mediterranean, hyperproteic) and on the role of physical exercise alone in not obese PCOS patients.

7.10 Pharmacological Treatment of PCOS-Related Obesity

Considering the reciprocal interactions between pathways that control fertility and energy metabolism and the key roles of molecules such as estrogens and IGF-1 in these pathways, these new data could challenge current therapeutic strategies—amelioration of metabolic disorders, for example, might become an important goal of hormone replacement therapy (HRT) in menopausal obese women. Women with PCOS, however, frequently present a number of risk factors that could be absolute or relative contraindications to the use of a contraceptive pill. Insulin sensitizers have been used to control body weight gain in patients with PCOS, and most of the data demonstrate that metformin surely improves insulin sensitivity and show evidences of benefit on parameters of MetS (reduction of blood pressure and low-density lipoprotein cholesterol) [43]. The effects of other insulin sensitizers such as glitazones have also been evaluated in patients with PCOS [44]. Treatment with orlistat, a potent inhibitor of gastric and pancreatic lipase which impairs digestion of dietary fats, combined with hypocaloric diet apart from decreasing body weight also led to a reduction of serum insulin and androgen levels in obese PCOS patients [45]. The new guidelines [31] do not recommend the use of inositols, thiazolidinediones, or statins, considering that the latter may improve chronic inflammation and lipid profile but impair insulin sensitivity in women with PCOS [46], and suggest the use of metformin only in women with glucose intolerance. Metformin is well known to improve the ovarian response to clomiphene citrate, improve the likelihood of mono-ovulatory cycles and lower the risk of ovarian hyperstimulation syndrome [47]. Common sense also suggests using metformin in young patients with PCOS who do not require immediate infertility treatment [48].

7.11 Bariatric Surgery in the Treatment of PCOS-Related Obesity

Bariatric surgery should only be advocated to morbidly obese individuals after careful evaluation of the risk-to-benefit ratio. According to the current National Institute of Health clinical recommendations, surgical treatment of obesity should be considered when BMI is greater than 40 or greater than 35 in patients with a high-risk obesity-related condition following failure of other treatments for weight control [49, 50]. Results from uncontrolled studies assessing the effect of bariatric surgery in morbidly obese women with PCOS reported sustained weight loss and complete resolution of all features defining PCOS, including hirsutism, hyperandrogenism, menstrual irregularity, anovulation, and improved menstrual cyclicity as well as natural conception [51].

7.12 Breast Cancer and Obesity

The main risk factors for breast cancer are associated with reproductive status, genetic, lifestyle, ethnicity, and anthropometric characteristics [52, 53]. In particular, overweight and obesity have been clearly associated with an increased overall risk of breast cancer. These associations appeared to be extremely consistent for postmenopausal breast cancer, but there is still controversy on their impact on the risk of premenopausal breast cancer. An inverse association between BMI and the risk of premenopausal breast cancer, with a 50 % reduction in risk among obese women and an 8 % reduction in risk per 5 kg m^{-2} increase in BMI, has been reported. A recent meta-analysis shows that obesity (BMI) is predictive of an adverse clinical outcome in both premenopausal and postmenopausal breast cancer and that (Waist to Hip Ratio) WHR and height are associated with a small increase of this risk. Overall, this analysis suggests that WHR as a marker of the intra-abdominal (central) fat has a positive impact on the risk of breast cancer [54].

References

1. Della Torre S, Benedusi V, Fontana R et al (2014) Energy metabolism and fertility—a balance preserved for female health. Nat Rev Endocrinol 10:13–23
2. Shapira N (2013) Women's higher health risks in the obesogenic environment: a gender nutrition approach to metabolic dimorphism with predictive, preventive, and personalized medicine. EPMA J 4:1
3. Davis LK, Hiramatsu N, Hiramatsu K et al (2007) Induction of three vitellogenins by 17β-estradiol with concurrent inhibition of the growth hormone-insulin-like growth factor 1 axis in a euryhaline teleost, the tilapia (Oreochromis mossambicus). Biol Reprod 77:614–625
4. Olofsson LE, Pierce AA, Xu AW (2009) Functional requirement of AgRP and NPY neurons in ovarian cycle-dependent regulation of food intake. Proc Natl Acad Sci U S A 106:15932–15937
5. Oakley AE, Clifton DK, Steiner RA (2009) Kisspeptin signaling in the brain. Endocr Rev 30:713–743
6. Clegg DJ, Brown LM, Woods SC et al (2006) Gonadal hormones determine sensitivity to central leptin and insulin. Diabetes 55:978–987
7. Chervenak J (2009) Bioidentical hormones for maturing women. Maturitas 64:86–89
8. Villa A, Della Torre S, Stell A et al (2012) Tetradian oscillation of estrogen receptor α is necessary to prevent liver lipid deposition. Proc Natl Acad Sci U S A 109:11806–11811
9. Della Torre S, Rando G, Meda C et al (2011) Amino acid-dependent activation of liver estrogen receptor α integrates metabolic and reproductive functions via IGF-1. Cell Metab 13:205–214
10. D'Eon TM, Souza SC, Aronovitz M et al (2005) Estrogen regulation of adiposity and fuel partitioning. Evidence of genomic and non-genomic regulation of lipogenic and oxidative pathways. J Biol Chem 280:35983–35991
11. Couse JF, Korach KS (1999) Estrogen receptor null mice: what have we learned and where will they lead us? Endocr Rev 20:358–417

12. Tiano JP, Delghingaro-Augusto V, Le May C et al (2011) Estrogen receptor activation reduces lipid synthesis in pancreatic islets and prevents β cell failure in rodent models of type 2 diabetes. J Clin Invest 121:3331–3342
13. Jovanovic L (2004) Advances in diabetes for the millennium: diabetes in women. MedGenMed 6:3
14. Racho'n D, Teede H (2010) Ovarian function and obesity—interrelationship, impact on women's reproductive lifespan and treatment options. Mol Cell Endocrinol 316:172–179
15. Diamanti-Kandarakis E, Bergiele A (2001) The influence of obesity on hyperandrogenism and infertility in the female. Obes Rev 2:231–238
16. Van der Steeg JW, Steures P, Eijkemans MJ et al (2008) Obesity affects spontaneous pregnancy chances in subfertile, ovulatory women. Hum Reprod 23:324–328
17. Shalitin S, Phillip M (2003) Role of obesity and leptin in the pubertal process and pubertal growth – a review. Int J Obes Relat Metab Disord 27:869–874
18. Lakshman R, Forouhi N, Luben R et al (2008) Association between age at menarche and risk of diabetes in adults: results from the EPIC-Norfolk cohort study. Diabetologia 51: 781–786
19. Carmina E, Bucchieri S, Esposito A et al (2007) Abdominal fat quantity and distribution in women with polycystic ovary syndrome and extent of its relation to insulin resistance. J Clin Endocrinol Metab 92:2500–2505
20. Hoeger KM (2014) Developmental origins and future fate in PCOS. Semin Reprod Med 32(03):157–158
21. Orio F, Palomba S (2014) New guidelines for the diagnosis and treatment of PCOS. Nat Rev Endocrinol 10:130–132
22. Moran LJ, Teede HJ (2009) Metabolic features of the reproductive phenotypes of polycystic ovary syndrome. Hum Reprod Update 15:477–488
23. Boudreaux MY, Talbott EO, Kip KE et al (2006) Risk of T2DM and impaired fasting glucose among PCOS subjects: results of an 8-year follow-up. Curr Diabetes Rep 6:77–83
24. Toscano V, Bianchi P, Balducci R et al (1992) Lack of linear relationship between hyperinsulinaemia and hyperandrogenism. Clin Endocrinol Oxford 36:197–207
25. Moran LJ, Hutchison SK, Meyer C et al (2009) A comprehensive assessment of endothelial function in overweight women with and without polycystic ovary syndrome. Clin Sci (Lond) 116(10):761–770
26. Orio F, Palomba S, Colao A (2006) Cardiovascular risk in women with polycystic ovary syndrome. Fertil Steril 86(Suppl 1):S20–S21
27. Misso M, Boyle J, Norman R, Teede H (2014) Development of evidenced-based guidelines for PCOS and implications for community health. Semin Reprod Med 32(3):230–240
28. Gambineri A, Patton L, Vaccina et al (2006) Treatment with flutamide, metformin, and their combination added to a hypocaloric diet in overweight-obese women with polycystic ovary syndrome: a randomized, 12-month, placebo-controlled study. J Clin Endocrinol Metab 91:3970–3980
29. Lubrano C, Genovesi G, Specchia P et al (2013) Obesity and metabolic comorbidities: environmental diseases? Oxid Med Cell Longev 2013:640673. doi:10.1155/2013/640673
30. Schneider JE, Brozek JM, Keen-Rhinehart E (2014) Our stolen figures: the interface of sexual differentiation, endocrine disruptors, maternal programming, and energy balance. Horm Behav, http://dx.doi.org/10.1016/j.yhbeh.2014.03.011
31. Barrett ES, Sobolewski M (2014) Polycystic ovary syndrome: do endocrine-disrupting chemicals play a role? Semin Reprod Med 32(03):166–176
32. Legro RS, Arslanian SA, Ehrmann DA et al (2013) Diagnosis and treatment of polycystic ovary syndrome: an Endocrine Society clinical practice guideline. J Clin Endocrinol Metab 98(12):4565–4592, http://dx.doi.org/10.1210/jc.2013-2350
33. Agapova SE, Cameo T, Sopher AB et al (2014) Diagnosis and challenges of polycystic ovary syndrome in adolescence. Semin Reprod Med 32(3):194–201
34. Greco EA, Fornari R, Rossi F et al (2010) Is obesity protective for osteoporosis? Evaluation of bone mineral density in individuals with high body mass index. Int J Clin Pract 64:817–820. doi:10.1111/j.1742-1241.2009.02301.x

35. Greco EA, Francomano D, Fornari R et al (2013) Negative association between trunk fat, insulin resistance and skeleton in obese women. World J Diabetes 4:31–39
36. Lovejoy JC, Champagne CM, de Jonge L et al (2008) Increased visceral fat and decreased energy expenditure during the menopausal transition. Int J Obes (Lond) 32:949–958
37. Wing RR, Matthews KA, Kuller LH et al (1991) Weight gain at the time of menopause. Arch Intern Med 151:97–102
38. Kudesia B, Neal-Perry G (2014) Menopausal implications of polycystic ovarian syndrome. Semin Reprod Med 32(03):222–229
39. Marini H, Bitto A, Altavilla D et al (2010) Efficacy of genistein aglycone on some cardiovascular risk factors and homocysteine levels: a follow-up study. Nutr Metab Cardiovasc Dis 20:332–340. doi:10.1016/j.numecd.2009.04.012
40. Marini H, Bitto A, Altavilla D, Burnett BP et al (2008) Breast safety and efficacy of genistein aglycone for postmenopausal bone loss: a follow-up study. J Clin Endocrinol Metab 93: 4787–4796. doi:10.1210/jc.2008-1087
41. Atteritano M, Marini H, Minutoli L et al (2007) Effects of the phytoestrogen genistein on some predictors of cardiovascular risk in osteopenic, postmenopausal women: a two-year randomized, double-blind, placebo-controlled study. J Clin Endocrinol Metab 92:3068–3075
42. Palomba S, Giallauria F, Falbo A et al (2008) Structured exercise training programme versus hypocaloric hyperproteic diet in obese polycystic ovary syndrome patients with anovulatory infertility: a 24-week pilot study. Hum Reprod 23:642–650
43. Meyer C, McGrath BP, Teede HJ (2007) Effects of medical therapy on insulin resistance and the cardiovascular system in polycystic ovary syndrome. Diabetes Care 30:471–478
44. Pi-Sunyer FX (2008) The effects of pharmacologic agents for type 2 diabetes mellitus on body weight. Postgrad Med 120:5–17
45. Panidis D, Farmakiotis D, Rousso D et al (2008) Obesity, weight loss, and the polycystic ovary syndrome: effect of treatment with diet and orlistat for 24 weeks on insulin resistance and androgen levels. Fertil Steril 89:899–906
46. Puurunen J, Piltonen T, Puukka K et al (2013) Statin therapy worsens insulin sensitivity in women with polycystic ovary syndrome (PCOS): a prospective, randomized, double-blind, placebo-controlled study. J Clin Endocrinol Metab 98(12):4798–4807, http://dx.doi.org/10.1210/jc.2013-2674
47. Palomba S, Falbo A, Zullo F et al (2009) Evidence-based and potential benefits of metformin in the polycystic ovary syndrome: a comprehensive review. Endocr Rev 30:1–50
48. Misso ML, Costello MF, Garrubba M et al (2013) Metformin versus clomiphene citrate for infertility in non-obese women with polycystic ovary syndrome: a systematic review and meta-analysis. Hum Reprod Update 19:2–11
49. Lubrano C, Cornoldi A, Pili M et al (2004) Reduction of risk factors for cardiovascular diseases in morbid-obese patients following biliary-intestinal bypass: 3 years' follow-up. Int J Obes Relat Metab Disord 28:1600–1606
50. Lubrano C, Mariani S, Badiali M et al (2010) Metabolic or bariatric surgery? Long-term effects of malabsorptive vs restrictive bariatric techniques on body composition and cardiometabolic risk factors. Int J Obes (Lond) 34:1404–1414. doi:10.1038/ijo.2010.54
51. Eid GM, Cottam DR, Velcu LM et al (2005) Effective treatment of polycystic ovarian syndrome with Roux-en-Y gastric bypass. Surg Obes Relat Dis 1:77–80
52. Petrangeli E, Lubrano C, Ortolani F et al (1994) Estrogen receptors: new perspectives in breast cancer management. J Steroid Biochem Mol Biol 49:327–331
53. Petrangeli E, Lubrano C, Ravenna L et al (1995) Gene methylation of oestrogen and epidermal growth factor receptors in neoplastic and perineoplastic breast tissues. Br J Cancer 72:973–975
54. Amadou A, Ferrari P, Muwonge R et al (2013) Overweight, obesity and risk of premenopausal breast cancer according to ethnicity: a systematic review. Obes Rev 14:665–678

Obesity and Osteoporosis

Emanuela A. Greco, Lorenzo M. Donini, Andrea Lenzi, and Silvia Migliaccio

8.1 Introduction

Obesity and osteoporosis are important widespread health problems which lead to high prevalence of both mortality and morbidity [1, 2]. Obesity has always been known and recognized as a risk factor for metabolic and cardiovascular diseases, however a protective factor for bone loss and osteoporosis. Age-related changes in body composition, metabolic factors, and hormonal levels, accompanied by a decline in physical activity, may all provide mechanisms for the propensity to lose muscle mass, gain fat mass and, also develop bone loss [3].

Obesity is due to an imbalance in which energy intake exceeds energy expenditure over a prolonged period. Several environmental, nutritional, and hormonal factors appear to influence body weight. For instance, postmenopausal women often show increased body weight, and are often affected by hypertension, dyslipidemia, diabetes, and cardiovascular disease, but they have always been considered protected against osteoporosis [4].

Osteoporosis is a bone metabolic disease characterized by a decrease in bone strength, due to a reduction in both bone quantity and quality, leading to an increased risk of developing spontaneous and traumatic fractures [5]. The rate of bone loss in adults reflects the interaction between genetic and environmental factors, which also influence the extent of bone acquisition during growth, known as peak bone mass [6]. Soon after menopause, a process of bone loss begins in women, due to increased bone resorption, exerted by osteoclasts, which overcomes bone formation

---

E.A. Greco • L.M. Donini • A. Lenzi
Department of Experimental Medicine, Section of Medical Pathophysiology, Endocrinology and Nutrition, Sapienza University, Rome, Italy

S. Migliaccio, MD, PhD (✉)
Department of Movement, Human and Health Sciences, Unit of Endocrinology, Foro Italico University, Largo Lauro De Bosis 15, 00135 Rome, Italy
e-mail: silvia.migliaccio@uniroma4.it

acted by osteoblasts [7, 8]. Moreover, osteoblast function declines with aging also in men [8]. Traditionally, osteoporosis has been regarded as a condition only associated with fracture and skeletal disability in old age, but recent studies demonstrate that bone mineral density (BMD) appears to be a better long-term predictor of death than blood pressure and cholesterol [9]. Further data published in the last decades indicated that low BMD is a strong and independent predictor of all-cause mortality including cardiovascular ones [10].

Body fat and lean mass are correlated with BMD, with obesity apparently exerting protection against bone loss [11]. The pathophysiological role of adipose tissue in skeletal homeostasis probably resides in the role that several adipokines play in bone remodeling through effects on either formation or resorption. Since the demonstration that bone cells expressed several specific hormone receptors, the skeleton has long been considered an endocrine target organ [12]. Additionally, more recent observations have shown that bone-derived factors such as osteocalcin and osteopontin might affect body weight control and glucose homeostasis suggesting a possible role of bone tissue as an endocrine organ itself with the presence of a potential feedback between the skeleton and other endocrine organs [13].

Thus, the cross talk between fat and bone likely constitutes a homeostatic feedback system in which adipokines and molecules secreted by bone cells represent the link of an active bone-adipose axis. However, the mechanism(s) by which all these events occur still remain(s) unclear.

8.2 Fat and Bone Correlation: Evidence-Based Observations

In the last decades, the association between obesity and osteoporosis has been actively investigated. Extensive data have shown that total body fat was positively related to BMD, an important and measurable determinant of fracture risk; that high body weight or body mass index (BMI) are correlated with high BMD; and that the decrease in body weight leads to bone loss in white women but not in white men [14].

Although these data indicate that obesity exerts a protective effect on bone tissue, some more recent studies have described an opposite event [15]. In particular, evidences suggest an inverse relationship between obesity and osteoporosis depending on how obesity is defined. In fact in the studies where obesity is defined on the basis of BMI or body weight, it appears to act as protective factor against bone loss and fractures; however, if obesity is considered as percentage of body fat and distribution, it becomes a risk factor for osteoporosis and fractures [16].

Our group has recently demonstrated that a population of obese subjects had significant skeletal alterations. In particular, the subdivision of the population into three different groups upon BMI status showed a slightly different BMD pattern among groups: overweight subjects (BMI > 25 < 30) did not show any modification in skeletal health, while obese and severely obese subjects (BMI > 30) had a significant alteration in their BMD levels [17]. Subsequently, we have demonstrated that in obese men and women, there is a significant inverse correlation between trunk fat and BMD [18, 19]. Moreover, data published by Blum et al. in a premenopausal women population demonstrated that high amount of fat mass is negatively associated with bone mass [20]. Thus, all these data suggest an important role of fat distribution as much as total fat mass itself, confirmed in a recent study on healthy postmenopausal women by Kim et al. in which body weight was positively related with BMD and low risk for vertebral fractures, whereas percent of body fat and waist circumference were related to a low BMD and to a higher risk for vertebral fractures [21].

Finally, several lines of evidence from environmental factors and medical interventions support an inverse correlation between fat and bone mass: physical exercise increases bone mass while reducing fat mass [22]; supplementation with calcium and vitamin D appears beneficial for the prevention of both osteoporosis and obesity [23]; estrogen replacement therapy in postmenopausal women improves both lean and bone mass and reverses menopause-related weight gain [24]; gonadotropin-releasing hormone agonists and glucocorticoids increase both osteoporosis and obesity [25]; some antidiabetic drugs, which interfere with PPARγ and thus with adipocytes differentiation, appear to influence significantly skeletal homeostasis and fracture risk [26].

8.3 Fat and Bone Correlation: From Basic Observations to Potential Mechanisms of Interaction

Several potential mechanisms have been proposed to explain the complex relationship between visceral white adipose tissue (VAT) and bone. VAT was long viewed as a passive energy reservoir, but since the discovery of leptin and following identification of other adipose tissue-derived hormones and serum mediators, fat has been considered an active endocrine organ which modulates energy homeostasis [27–29]. All these molecules affect human energy homeostasis and might as well be involved in bone metabolism, contributing to the complex relationship between adipose and bone tissues.

Leptin is the most important adipocyte-derived hormone and its effect on bone remodeling is complex: both negative and positive action on BMD have been reported in humans [27]. Adiponectin, in contrast to leptin, decreases in obese and diabetic subjects and increases after weight loss. Human osteoblasts express adiponectin and its receptors, and in vivo and in vitro studies show that adiponectin increases bone mass [28].

Resistin may play a role in bone remodeling, as it is expressed in bone marrow mesenchymal stem cells (MSCs), osteoblasts, and osteoclasts, but its effect on bone is still unclear [29].

VAT also secretes various inflammatory cytokines, such as interleukin-6 (IL-6) and tumor necrosis factor-α (TNF-α), well recognized as osteoclastogenesis and resorption-stimulating factors [30, 31].

Furthermore, adipocytes and osteoblasts originate from a common progenitor, a pluripotential MSC, which has an equal propensity for differentiation into either adipocytes or osteoblasts (or other lines) under the influence of several cell-derived transcription factors [32].

This process is complex, suggesting significant plasticity and multifaceted mechanism(s) of regulation within different cell lineages. One potential mechanism of regulation is the Wnt signaling pathway which inhibits adipogenesis and promotes osteogenesis [33, 34]. New experimental tools, such as gene microarrays, are being used to document the relationship of classical steroid hormones to bone and fat formation in marrow. One study has examined the skeletal phenotype of mice (SAM-P/6) deficient in both thyroid receptors α and β. These mice showed increased mRNA levels for adipocyte specific genes, increased bone marrow adipocyte numbers, and reduced trabecular and total bone mineral density [35]. Duque et al. found that vitamin D treatment inhibited adipogenesis and enhanced osteogenesis in the SAM-P/6 mice, demonstrating a coordinated induction of osteoblastogenic genes and a reduction of adipogenic genes after vitamin D treatment, which stimulates not only bone formation but also bone resorption [36].

Overall, these recent findings support the inverse relationship between adipogenic and osteogenic differentiation in the bone marrow microenvironment, which is mediated, in part, through cross talk between the pathways activated by steroid receptors, the PPARs, and other cytokines and paracrine factors [37].

Finally, other factors, such as total caloric intake, type of nutrients, alcohol consumption, oxygen tension, and cellular redox pathways influence bone marrow adipogenesis despite osteoblastogenesis, showing that the bone marrow MSC may consider multiple differentiation pathways during its lifetime and, indeed, may dedifferentiate and transdifferentiate in response to changes in the microenvironment [8].

Conclusions

Obesity and osteoporosis are major global health problems with an increasing prevalence and high impact on mortality and morbidity. Even though previous several data indicate that high body weight and BMI are protective factors against osteoporosis, an increasing number of evidence show conflicting results regarding this issue, suggesting that obesity might actually interfere with bone health. Thus, a specific and careful characterization of skeletal metabolism and further studies evaluating skeleton modifications might be useful in obese subjects.

References

1. Kado DM, Huang MH, Karlamangla AS et al (2004) Hyperkyphotic posture predicts mortality in older community-dwelling men and women: a prospective study. J Am Geriatr Soc 52:1662–1667
2. Rossner S (2002) Obesity: the disease of the twenty-first century. Int J Obes Relat Metab Disord 26(Suppl 4):S2–S4
3. Hu FB (2003) Overweight and obesity in women: health risks and consequences. J Women Health (Larchmt) 12(2):163–172
4. Reid IR (2002) Relationships among body mass, its components, and bone. Bone 31:547–555
5. NIH Consensus development panel on osteoporosis (2001) JAMA 285:785–795
6. Brown S, Rosen CJ (2003) Osteoporosis. Med Clin North Am 87:1039–1063

7. Cagnacci A, Zanin R et al (2007) Menopause, estrogens, progestins, or their combination on body weight and anthropometric measures. Fertil Steril 88(6):1603–1608
8. Migliaccio S, Greco EA et al (2011) Is obesity in women protective against osteoporosis? Diabetes Metab Syndr Obes 4:273–282
9. Johansson C, Black D et al (1998) Bone mineral density is a predictor of survival. Calcif Tissue Int 63:190–196
10. Von der Recke P, Hansen MA, Hassager C (1999) The association between low bone mass at the menopause and cardiovascular mortality. Am J Med 106:273–278
11. Reid IR, Plank LD et al (1992) Fat mass is an important determinant of whole body bone density in premenopausal women but not in men. J Clin Endoc Metab 75:779–782
12. Eriksen EF, Colvard DS et al (1988) Evidence of estrogen receptors in normal human osteoblast-like cells. Science 241(4861):84–86
13. Fukumoto S, Martrin TJ (2009) Bone as an endocrine organ. Trends Endocrinol Metab 20(5):230–236
14. Cummings SR, Black DM et al (1993) Bone density at various sites for prediction of hip fractures. The Study of Osteoporotic Fractures Research Group. Lancet 341:72–75
15. Compston JE, Watts NB, Investigators G et al (2011) Obesity is not protective against fracture in postmenopausal women: glow. Am J Med 124(11):1043–1050
16. Zhao LJ, Jiang H et al (2008) Correlation of obesity and osteoporosis: effect of fat mass on the determination of osteoporosis. J Bone Miner Res 23:17–29
17. Greco EA, Fornari R et al (2010) Is obesity protective for osteoporosis? Evaluation of bone mineral density in individuals with high body mass index. Int J Clin Pract 64(6):817–820
18. Greco EA, Francomano et al (2013) Negative association between trunk fat, insulin resistance and skeleton in obese women. World J Diabetes 4(2):31–39
19. Migliaccio S, Francomano D et al (2013) Trunk fat negatively influences skeletal and testicular functions in obese men: clinical implications for the aging male. Int J Endocrinol. doi:10.1155/2013/182753
20. Blum M, Harris SS et al (2003) Leptin, body composition and bone mineral density in premenopausal women. Calcif Tissue Int 73:27–32
21. Kim KC, Shin DH et al (2010) Relation between obesity and bone mineral density and vertebral fractures in Korean postmenopausal women. Yonsei Med J 51(6):857–863
22. Reid IR, Legge M et al (1995) Regular exercise dissociates fat mass and bone density in premenopausal women. J Clin Endocrinol Metab 80:1764–1768
23. Reid IR (1996) Therapy of osteoporosis: calcium, vitamin D, and exercise. Am J Med Sci 312:278–286
24. Manson JE, Martin KA (2001) Postmenopausal hormone replacement therapy. N Engl J Med 345:34–40
25. Steinbuch M, Youket TE et al (2004) Oral glucocorticoid use is associated with an increased risk of fracture. Osteoporos Int 15:323–328
26. Mieczkowska A, Baslé MF et al (2012) Thiazolidinediones induce osteocyte apoptosis by a G protein-coupled receptor 40-dependent mechanism. J Biol Chem 287(28):23517–23526
27. Steppan CM, Crawford DT et al (2000) Leptin is a potent stimulator of bone growth in ob/ob mice. Regul Pept 92:73–78
28. Kadowaki T, Yamauchi T (2005) Adiponectin and adiponectin receptors. Endocr Rev 26:439–451
29. Vendrell J, Broch M et al (2004) Resistin, adiponectin, ghrelin, leptin, and proinflammatory cytokines: relationships in obesity. Obes Res 12:962–971
30. Tilg H, Moschen AR (2008) Inflammatory mechanisms in the regulation of insulin resistance. Mol Med 14(3–4):222–231
31. Magni P, Dozio E et al (2010) Molecular aspects of adipokine-bone interactions. Curr Mol Med 10(6):522–532
32. Sekiya I, Larson BL et al (2004) Adipogenic differentiation of human adult stem cells from bone marrow stroma (MSCs). J Bone Miner Res 19:256–264
33. Bennett CN, Ross SE et al (2002) Regulation of Wnt signaling during adipogenesis. J Biol Chem 277:30998–31004

34. Zhou S, Eid K et al (2004) Cooperation between TGFbeta and Wnt pathways during chondrocyte and adipocyte differentiation of human marrow stromal cells. J Bone Miner Res 19:463–470
35. Uchiyama Y (1994) Adipose conversion is accelerated in bone marrow cells of congenitally osteoporotic SAMP6 mice [abstract]. J Bone Miner Res 9(Suppl 1):S321
36. Duque G, Macoritto M et al (2004) Vitamin D treatment of senescence accelerated mice (SAM-P/6) induces several regulators of stromal cell plasticity. Biogerontology 5:421–429
37. Moerman EJ, Teng K et al (2004) Aging activates adipogenic and suppresses osteogenic programs in mesenchymal marrow stroma/stem cells: the role of PPAR-gamma2 transcription factor and TGF-beta/BMP signaling pathways. Aging Cell 3:379–389

Sarcopenic Obesity

9

Lorenzo M. Donini, Stefan A. Czerwinski, Audry C. Choh,
Eleonora Poggiogalle, Silvia Migliaccio, and Andrea Lenzi

9.1 Introduction

Sarcopenic obesity is a condition that is characterized by age-related loss of muscle mass and function (i.e., sarcopenia) concomitant with increases in regional or total body adiposity (i.e., obesity). Sarcopenic obesity is a critical public health issue that underlies two important problems: the rising prevalence of obesity in Western and developing countries and the increasing life span of humans [1–4]. The changes in body composition that occur as a result of the aging process and with obesity represent a common ground where sarcopenic obesity develops [3]. Body composition progressively changes with age. These changes begin around the third decade of life and accelerate in later life. A number of studies have now demonstrated a progressive loss of lean body mass in the elderly that is simultaneously accompanied by an increase in fat mass. These changes typically occur while body weight and body mass index (BMI) remain relatively stable [5–10].

L.M. Donini (✉) • A. Lenzi
Department of Experimental Medicine, Section of Medical Pathophysiology,
Endocrinology and Nutrition, Sapienza University, Rome, Italy
e-mail: lorenzomaria.donini@uniroma1.it

E. Poggiogalle
Department of Experimental Medicine, Medical Physiopathology, Food Science
and Endocrinology Section, Food Science and Human Nutrition Research Unit,
Sapienza University of Rome, Ple Aldo Moro, 5, 00185 Rome, Italy

S.A. Czerwinski • A.C. Choh
Division of Epidemiology, Lifespan Health Research Center, Department of Community
Health, Boonshoft School of Medicine, Wright State University,
3171 Research Blvd., Dayton, OH 45420-4014, USA

S. Migliaccio
Department of Movement, Human and Health Sciences, Unit of Endocrinology,
Foro Italico University, Largo de Bosis 14, 00135 Rome, Italy

© Springer International Publishing Switzerland 2015
A. Lenzi et al. (eds.), *Multidisciplinary Approach to Obesity:
From Assessment to Treatment*, DOI 10.1007/978-3-319-09045-0_9

While sarcopenic obesity is often considered a condition of aging, there is substantial evidence now that suggests that this condition can manifest at earlier ages. One of the more significant findings emerging from the literature is that sarcopenia may be present in relatively young obese subjects [11]. In line with the hypothesis that obesity produces low-grade inflammation and hormonal changes affecting muscle function and metabolism, obese young people could have similar changes as the elderly and meet the criteria for the diagnosis of sarcopenic obesity [5–11]. Factors such as being sedentary and having an unhealthy diet may lead to the development of phenotypic aspects of sarcopenic obesity in these younger subjects [8–10]. Chronic inflammation induced by obesity is thought to be a pivotal element that may influence the additional depletion of muscle mass in the overweight/obese [3, 7].

Both sarcopenia and obesity are linked to functional impairment [12, 13]. Sarcopenia is independently associated with a reduction in muscle strength and impairment in physical performance [12, 14]. Likewise, a wealth of studies have also demonstrated that obesity detrimentally affects physical function and is connected with the onset of physical disabilities [5, 15]. When coupled with sarcopenia, the presence of obesity worsens functional status and exacerbates physical disability [5, 16]. Currently, although sarcopenic obesity represents a serious public health concern, evidence supporting effective strategies for its management is relatively scarce. Furthermore, a universal consensus for its diagnosis, as well as its treatment, does not yet exist [17, 18].

9.2 Definition of Sarcopenic Obesity

Diagnostic criteria for sarcopenic obesity are not universally established, and different definitions are currently available. Hence, the prevalence of sarcopenic obesity ranges from 2.75 % to over 20 %, depending on the criteria used for the diagnosis and the methods of body composition assessment used [9, 16].

In a recent systematic review summarizing the state of the science regarding the current literature about sarcopenic obesity [19], 26 studies examining more than 23,000 subjects were considered. In all of the studies examined, except one, the definition of sarcopenic obesity was based on the co-occurrence of obesity and sarcopenia. To define the obesity component, various obesity parameters were used including BMI, fat mass, and visceral fat area, either as single parameters or in association with other adiposity measures. To define sarcopenia, several different parameters were used including appendicular skeletal muscle mass standardized for height or weight, cross-sectional muscle area at the quadriceps level, muscle strength, and/or muscle/fat-free mass indices [13].

In our view, a definition of sarcopenia based on a reduction in muscle mass in "absolute" terms is limited in obese subjects and does not accurately describe the picture in terms of functional outcome. Initially, at least in younger obese subjects, increases in fat mass are accompanied by increases in muscle mass [20–23]. These increases in mass enable the body to maintain, for a relatively long time, reasonable metabolic control and a satisfactory physical efficiency. The ratio between real lean body mass and ideal lean body mass may represent an even more useful indicator of sarcopenia. According to existing literature concerning body composition in adults and healthy humans, the percentage of body weight that consists of lean mass is, respectively, 85 % for men and 75 % for women. A number of studies have also suggested that in obese subjects, excess body weight is not only made of fat mass but includes a certain amount of muscle mass that approximately corresponds to 25 % of the excess body weight [22–26]. In fact, a relative and not an absolute reduction of muscle mass is sufficient to trigger reduced functional performance.

The methods and tools used for the assessment of body composition, as well as the choice of functional indicators, represent another important issue in the identification of sarcopenic obese subjects. In research settings, computed tomography (CT scan) and magnetic resonance imaging (MRI) have been used for estimating muscle mass or fat mass. These techniques, and to a lesser extent, dual-energy X-ray absorptiometry (DXA), are considered to be very precise imaging systems able to separate fat from other soft tissues in the body. However, high cost and limited access to equipment in some facilities and concerns about radiation exposure limit the use of these whole-body imaging methods for routine clinical practice. Bioimpedance analysis (BIA) may represent a valid alternative to these methods in clinical practice as it is inexpensive, easy to use, and readily reproducible. BIA results, obtained under standard conditions, have been found to correlate well with gold standard techniques [27].

The choice of threshold values is also critical in properly identifying sarcopenic obese subjects. Cutoff points depend on the measurement technique chosen and on the availability of reference studies. Similarly to what happens for bone mineral density, a normative population (healthy young adults) needs to be used, with cut-off points at two standard deviations below the mean reference value. In the literature, the diverse threshold values and methods adopted by different authors makes it difficult to compare studies. This represents a significant limitation, given that different intervention procedures need to be compared in research fieldwork, as well as in clinical practice. Thus, it is important to verify the outcomes of these different intervention procedures. Further epidemiological data are needed in order to obtain good reference values for populations in different countries and for different ethnicities.

A final major obstacle in the creation of a reasonable definition for sarcopenic obesity is whether the definition of sarcopenic obesity should be based only on a criterion of body composition (i.e., reduced muscle mass or lean body mass and increased fat mass) or one that also includes functional criteria. Normally, obesity (one aspect of sarcopenic obesity) is defined using only fat mass or BMI. However, reduced fat-free mass along with muscle strength and functional impairment are used to define sarcopenia. In the case of sarcopenia, functional measurements are required for diagnosis. In the consensus by Cruz-Jentoft et al., the European Working Group on Sarcopenia in Older People (EWGSOP) [28] recommends considering the presence of both low muscle mass and low muscle function (strength or performance). Using this method, EWGSOP further classifies conceptual stages as "pre-sarcopenia," "sarcopenia," and "severe sarcopenia." In the case of sarcopenic obesity, it is likely that the same logical pathway should be followed, even if no study presently hypothesizes a diagnosis of sarcopenic obesity in this manner.

So far, only a simple evaluation of body composition has been used to define sarcopenic obesity. An implementation of this definition with muscle strength and functional parameters will probably be more useful in clinical practice. A wide range of tests is available for physical performance evaluation, particularly in the elderly population, including the Short Physical Performance Battery (SPPB), gait speed, the 6-min walk test, and the stair climb power test [29]. By including functional information, this definition will be more responsive to the patient's clinical status and to the severity of the disease. This is important as an increase in fat mass together with the deterioration of lean body mass (with possible fatty infiltration) may lead to a progressive worsening of functional parameters, such as aerobic capacity, muscle strength, walking speed, and ability to maintain balance. Moreover, using this definition will also make it easier to track the course of the nutritional and rehabilitation treatment and to identify outcomes to be achieved.

9.3 Biology of Sarcopenic Obesity

In the case of sarcopenic obesity, the augmentation of lean body mass in parallel with fat mass represents a protective mechanism allowing the obese individual to sustain increased fat mass. This avoids, at least in the early phases of the process, the onset of metabolic and functional impairment during fat accumulation and a reduction in lean body mass (due to the aging process, inflammation, poor diet leading to rapid weight loss, or inactivity) that may cause a precocious onset of disability in obese subjects [8, 9]. In obese adults, an imbalance between lean mass, excess body fat, and total body size occurs earlier than in normal-weight individuals [8, 9]. This imbalance results in disproportionate ratios between the remaining conserved lean mass and excess fat mass, thereby creating a situation where body weight exceeds that which the lean mass can support. The pathogenetic and functional role of sarcopenia in obese elderly subjects, as well as in younger obese adults, still remains to be fully clarified [11].

Weight cycling is also known to exert deleterious effects on body composition and sarcopenic obesity, particularly among elderly subjects. Weight cycling can result in a greater loss of lean body mass during the weight-loss phase. Often when weight is regained lean mass is not conserved [6]. Hunter et al. [30] found that after dieting and weight loss, premenopausal women regained limb body mass, while trunk lean mass was not restored. The researchers hypothesized that the mechanism explaining the reduction of resting energy expenditure, the basis of the potential adipose tissue increase after dieting, was a consequence of the mass depletion from highly metabolically active tissue. On the other hand, in a more recent paper [13], young overweight and obese men and women who regained weight did not see negative effects in terms of body fat distribution and composition of lean body mass. It is clear from the literature that further research is needed examining weight cycling and its effect on body composition, especially in younger obese subjects.

Inadequate dietary protein intake may also influence sarcopenic obesity. Current recommendations for protein intake [31] were determined based on studies performed in healthy individuals. These requirements may not be adequate when considering a complex condition such as sarcopenic obesity. Studies have shown that protein requirements in the elderly may not be adequate to maintain or prevent muscle loss [32]. Future studies are needed to address the question of what is a reasonable dietary protein intake to satisfy the nutritional requirements for sarcopenic obese subjects. Careful consideration should be made to increase protein intake while maintaining or reducing total calorie intake.

9.4 Sarcopenic Obesity, Physical Performance, Disability, and Quality of Life

Using a recently developed tool (TSD-OC) specifically designed to assess disability level in obese subjects [33], we investigated the relationship between sarcopenic obesity and performance. The TSD-OC test is composed of 36 items divided into seven sections (pain, stiffness, activities of daily living and indoor mobility, housework, outdoor activities, occupational activities, and social life), and in the validation study, the TSD-OC test was found to be significantly correlated to functional assessment (6MWT), handgrip strength and quality of life parameters (SF-36 questionnaire). Our results (not yet published) highlight that the presence of sarcopenia in obese subjects was associated with a worse TSD-OC test score. This finding is consistent with data presented in a recent study by Baumgartner, pointing out the coexistence of low physical capacity and sarcopenic obesity [5].

While evidence supports the synergistic pathological action exerted by obesity and sarcopenia, it is still a matter of debate which of the two components (increased fat mass or reduced lean body mass) in sarcopenic obesity is better correlated with disability. Some studies have concluded that excess body fat was a stronger contributor to physical function impairment than sarcopenia [30, 34]. However, Davison et al. [14] did not demonstrate any association between sarcopenia and functional limitations; instead, mobility impairment was related to percentage of body fat and BMI. Similarly, Cawthon et al. [35] found that adipose tissue and performance status were more closely related to disability than lean body mass. Some of this debate is depicted in the U-shaped relationship between BMI and physical limitations [36]. Our data suggest that the correlation is stronger for lean body mass and especially for the real lean body mass/ideal lean body mass ratio. In a recent paper [18], the authors hypothesized that disability caused by sarcopenia and sarcopenic obesity was related to the amount of adiposity or body weight bearing per unit of muscle mass (total body fat to lower limb muscle mass ratio). Our finding of increased disability in obese subjects with sarcopenia confirms that the sarcopenia, in the context of obesity, may be better defined as a "relative" sarcopenia. Despite the appearance that muscle mass is conserved, it probably is not enough in proportion to the total body mass to prevent the onset of functional impairment and disability. Moreover, fat infiltration of muscles, known as "myosteatosis" [11], could also be responsible for deteriorated muscle function in obese individuals.

9.5 Treatment of Sarcopenic Obesity

There are numerous potential approaches to consider in terms of treatment for sarcopenic obesity. Even though weight loss is beneficial in obese subjects in terms of reducing metabolic and cardiovascular risk [37], the concomitant changes in body composition that occur during caloric restriction create additional concerns for the maintenance of good functional status and physical performance. Especially in obese older adults, obesity-related disability tends to worsen because of the decline of lean mass with aging [5]. Even in younger subjects, a reduction in body weight consists of loss of both fat mass and lean body mass. The literature suggests that a decrease in lean body mass can range from 15 % of total body weight in the case of a mild energy restriction to as much as 50–70 % during semi-starvation [38]. Despite a reduction of body weight, diet combined with exercise has been shown to result in a minor decrease of fat-free mass when compared to diet alone. Intentional weight loss through diet alone was shown to deteriorate muscle mass particularly among the elderly [39, 40]. A number of other studies have shown that exercise has additional benefits in preserving or minimizing loss of lean mass during diet-induced weight loss [34]. In these studies, both aerobic and resistance activities, or their combination, appear to be effective in limiting muscle loss during dieting and preserving physical function. However, contrary to these findings, Hunter et al. demonstrated that resistance training, but not aerobic exercise, was able to conserve lean body mass and strength following weight loss [30]. Also, in a study by Hays et al. on sedentary older obese subjects [41], a dietary intervention based on fat restriction but not energy deficit resulted in beneficial effects on body weight and fat mass reduction that were greater than an ad libitum diet combined with exercise.

Evidence regarding macronutrient manipulation (e.g., fat restriction) and conventional caloric restriction in terms of weight loss and its effects on body composition in the context of sarcopenic obesity is lacking. To date, only one study on older overweight and obese men who underwent exercise training only reported significant weight loss as well as body fat percentage reduction without altering lean body mass. Interestingly, the positive body composition changes achieved in this study were also accompanied by an increase in resting salivary testosterone levels. Testosterone has been demonstrated to be related to increased levels of physical activity and greater aerobic capacity. Decreasing testosterone levels in aging men have been found to be associated with changes in body composition in late life [36]. Hence, further studies should be initiated in order to identify the type of exercise intervention that is most appropriate for the treatment of sarcopenic obesity.

Evidence concerning the effects of protein supplementation on body composition in sarcopenic obesity is scarce. In a study by Coker et al. [42], whey protein and essential amino acid supplementation promoted a greater body fat loss in sarcopenic obese elderly subjects during intentional weight loss. A higher skeletal muscle protein fractional synthetic rate, when compared to intact protein from sodium and calcium caseinate, may have accounted for this difference due to the energy cost of protein synthesis. The study also reported a sparing effect on lean mass. The high leucine content in whey protein may be responsible for increased fat loss and retained lean mass in younger, non-sarcopenic obese subjects [43]. The anabolic effect of whey protein, as a source of leucine, has consistently been demonstrated on muscle in healthy subjects and in older individuals [44–46].

As mentioned previously, in aging males, testosterone levels have been found to be associated with changes in body composition in late life [36]. Conversely, in women, hormonal changes (less estrogen activity) during menopause make women more prone to develop sarcopenia [47]. Isoflavone supplementation (phytoestrogens) in peri- and postmenopausal women appears to increase lean body mass, most likely by stimulating estrogen receptors ER-α and ER-β and increasing estrogen activity. The hormonal effect exerted by phytoestrogens may also be relevant on muscle tissue beyond the simple augmentation of dietary protein intake. Soy isoflavones may be responsible for changes in insulin, IGF-1, and IGFBP-3, and promoting increases in fat-free mass [48]. It should be noted, however, that in a study by Choquette et al. [49], as well as in a similar study carried out in normal-weight women [50], neither an interaction nor an additive effect was reported between isoflavones and exercise on body composition. Directly administering sex hormones has been shown to improve lean body mass [51]. This is likely due to the positive influence of sex hormones on muscle anabolism [47, 52]. In obese postmenopausal woman, the administration of sex hormones could represent a beneficial treatment for counteracting changes in lean and fat mass related to menopause. This avenue of treatment, however, should only be pursued after carefully evaluating the additional risks and benefits of such a treatment.

Understanding the nature of age-related changes in hormone levels may aid in the design of additional therapeutic targets for future interventions. However, pharmacological attempts, other than sex hormone replacement therapy, to reverse manifestations of sarcopenic obesity are sparse. In a study conducted by Shea et al. [53], it was demonstrated that in overweight and obese older nondiabetic men undergoing weight loss, pioglitazone (a diabetic medication) increased the loss of abdominal visceral fat and resistance training attenuated thigh muscle loss. This result was not observed in women, illustrating that gender differences should also be accounted for in future trials exploring potential benefits of PPAR-γ agonist on body composition in sarcopenic obese subjects [54, 55].

9.6 Summary

While sarcopenic obesity continues to be an important public health concern, there are numerous challenges that exist in its assessment and treatment. The biggest challenge continues to be the lack of a standard clinical definition. In spite of these challenges, research continues to provide insights into the disease process and its relationship to physical disability and frailty. Studies examining a variety of treatment options are being be conducted.

References

1. Baumgartner RN (2000) Body composition in healthy aging. Ann N Y Acad Sci 904:437–448
2. Flegal KM, Carroll MD, Ogden CL, Johnson CL (2002) Prevalence and trends in obesity among US adults, 1999–2000. JAMA 288:1723–1727
3. Roubenoff R (2004) Sarcopenic obesity: the confluence of two epidemics. Obes Res 12:887–888
4. Villareal D (2009) Obesity in older adults-a growing problem. Nutrition and health: handbook of clinical nutrition and aging. Humana Press, New York, pp 263–267
5. Baumgartner RN, Wayne SJ, Waters DL, Janssen I, Gallagher D, Morley JE (2004) Sarcopenic obesity predicts instrumental activities of daily living disability in the elderly. Obes Res 12:1995–2004
6. Dominguez LJ, Barbagallo M (2007) The cardiometabolic syndrome and sarcopenic obesity in older persons. J Cardiometab Syndr 2:183–189
7. Kim TN, Yang SJ, Yoo HJ, Lim KI, Kang HJ, Song W, Seo JA, Kim SG, Kim NH, Baik SH, Choi DS, Choi KM (2009) Prevalence of sarcopenia and sarcopenic obesity in Korean adults: the Korean sarcopenic obesity study. Int J Obes 33:885–892
8. Stenholm S, Harris TB, Rantanen T, Visser M, Kritchevsky SB, Ferrucci L (2008) Sarcopenic obesity: definition, cause and consequences. Curr Opin Clin Nutr Metab Care 11:693–700
9. Waters DL, Baumgartner RN (2011) Sarcopenia and obesity. Clin Geriatr Med 27:401–421
10. Zamboni M, Mazzali G, Fantin F, Rossi A, Di Francesco V (2008) Sarcopenic obesity: a new category of obesity in the elderly. Nutr Metab Cardiovasc Dis 18:388–395
11. Miljkovic I, Zmuda JM (2010) Epidemiology of myosteatosis. Curr Opin Clin Nutr Metab Care 13:260–264
12. Ritz P (2009) Editorial: obesity in the elderly: should we be using new diagnostic criteria? J Nutr Health Aging 13:168–169
13. Zamboni M, Mazzali G, Zoico E, Harris TB, Meigs JB, Di Francesco V, Fantin F, Bissoli L, Bosello O (2005) Health consequences of obesity in the elderly: a review of four unresolved questions. Int J Obes 29:1011–1029
14. Davison KK, Ford ES, Cogswell ME, Dietz WH (2002) Percentage of body fat and body mass index are associated with mobility limitations in people aged 70 and older from NHANES III. J Am Geriatr Soc 50:1802–1809
15. Zoico E, Di Francesco V, Guralnik JM, Mazzali G, Bortolani A, Guariento S, Sergi G, Bosello O, Zamboni M (2004) Physical disability and muscular strength in relation to obesity and different body composition indexes in a sample of healthy elderly women. Int J Obes Relat Metab Disord 28:234–241
16. Prado CM, Wells JC, Smith SR, Stephan BC, Siervo M (2012) Sarcopenic obesity: a critical appraisal of the current evidence. Clin Nutr 31:583–601
17. Aubertin-Leheudre M, Lord C, Goulet ED, Khalil A, Dionne IJ (2006) Effect of sarcopenia on cardiovascular disease risk factors in obese postmenopausal women. Obesity 14:2277–2283
18. Auyeung TW, Lee JS, Leung J, Kwok T, Woo J (2013) Adiposity to muscle ratio predicts incident physical limitation in a cohort of 3,153 older adults–an alternative measurement of sarcopenia and sarcopenic obesity. Age (Dordr) 35:1377–1385
19. Donini L, Poggiogalle E, Migliaccio S, Aversa A, Pinto A (2013) Body composition in sarcopenic obesity: systematic review of the literature. Mediterr J Metab 6:191–198
20. Elia M, Stubbs RJ, Henry CJ (1999) Differences in fat, carbohydrate, and protein metabolism between lean and obese subjects undergoing total starvation. Obes Res 7:597–604
21. Gallagher D, DeLegge M (2011) Body composition (sarcopenia) in obese patients: implications for care in the intensive care unit. J Parenter Enteral Nutr 35:21S–28S
22. Norgan NG, Durnin JV (1980) The effect of 6 weeks of overfeeding on the body weight, body composition, and energy metabolism of young men. Am J Clin Nutr 33:978–988
23. Passmore R, Meiklejohn AP, Dewar AD, Thow RK (1955) An analysis of the gain in weight of overfed thin young men. Br J Nutr 9:27–37

24. Deurenberg P, Deurenberg Yap M, Wang J, Lin FP, Schmidt G (1999) The impact of body build on the relationship between body mass index and percent body fat. Int J Obes Relat Metab Disord 23:537–542
25. Deurenberg P, Yap M, van Staveren WA (1998) Body mass index and percent body fat: a meta analysis among different ethnic groups. Int J Obes Relat Metab Disord 22:1164–1171
26. Gunther CM, Burger A, Rickert M, Crispin A, Schulz CU (2008) Grip strength in healthy Caucasian adults, reference values. J Hand Surg Am 33A:558–565
27. Kyle UG, Genton L, Karsegard L, Slosman DO, Pichard C (2001) Single prediction equation for bioelectrical impedance analysis in adults aged 20–94 years. Nutrition 17:248–253
28. Cruz-Jentoft AJ, Baeyens JP, Bauer JM, Boirie Y, Cederholm T, Landi F, Martin FC, Michel JP, Rolland Y, Schneider SM, Topinkova E, Vandewoude M, Zamboni M (2010) Sarcopenia: European consensus on definition and diagnosis: report of the European Working Group on Sarcopenia in Older People. Age Ageing 39:412–423
29. Working Group on Functional Outcome Measures (2008) Functional outcomes for clinical trials in frail older persons: time to be moving. J Gerontol A Biol Sci Med Sci 63:160–164
30. Hunter GR, Byrne NM, Sirikul B, Fernandez JR, Zuckerman PA, Darnell BE, Gower BA (2008) Resistance training conserves fat-free mass and resting energy expenditure following weight loss. Obesity 16:1045–1051
31. WHO Technical Report Series 935 (2011) Protein and amino acid requirements in human nature: report of a joint FAO/WHO/UNU expert consultation. Report of a joint FAO/WHO/UNU expert consultation
32. Campbell WW, Trappe TA, Wolfe RR, Evans WJ (2001) The recommended dietary allowance for protein may not be adequate for older people to maintain skeletal muscle. J Gerontol A Biol Sci Med Sci 56:M373–M380
33. Donini LM, Brunani A, Sirtori A, Savina C, Tempera S, Cuzzolaro M, Spera G, Cimolin V, Precilios H, Raggi A, Capodaglio P (2011) Assessing disability in morbidly obese individuals: the Italian Society of Obesity test for obesity-related disabilities. Disabil Rehabil 33:2509–2518
34. Garrow JS, Summerbell CD (1995) Metaanalysis – effect of exercise, with or without dieting, on the body-composition of overweight subjects. Eur J Clin Nutr 49:1–10
35. Cawthon PM, Fox KM, Gandra SR, Delmonico MJ, Chiou CF, Anthony MS, Caserotti P, Kritchevsky SB, Newman AB, Goodpaster BH, Satterfield S, Cummings SR, Harris TB (2011) Clustering of strength, physical function, muscle, and adiposity characteristics and risk of disability in older adults. J Am Geriatr Soc 59:781–787
36. Michalakis K, Goulis DG, Vazaiou A, Mintziori G, Polymeris A, Abrahamian-Michalakis A (2013) Obesity in the ageing man. Metab Clin Exp 62:1341–1349
37. Liebermeister H (2003) Effects of weight-reduction on obesity-related diseases. Ger Med Sci 1:Doc04
38. Ballor DL, Katch VL, Becque MD, Marks CR (1988) Resistance weight training during caloric restriction enhances lean body-weight maintenance. Am J Clin Nutr 47:19–25
39. Darmon P (2013) Intentional weight loss in older adults: useful or wasting disease generating strategy? Curr Opin Clin Nutr Metab Care 16:284–289
40. Miller SL, Wolfe RR (2008) The danger of weight loss in the elderly. J Nutr Health Aging 12:487–491
41. Hays NP, Starling RD, Liu XL, Sullivan DH, Trappe TA, Fluckey JD, Evans WJ (2004) Effects of an ad libitum low-fat, high-carbohydrate diet on body weight, body composition, and fat distribution in older men and women – a randomized controlled trial. Arch Intern Med 164:210–217
42. Coker RH, Miller S, Schutzler S, Deutz N, Wolfe RR (2012) Whey protein and essential amino acids promote the reduction of adipose tissue and increased muscle protein synthesis during caloric restriction-induced weight loss in elderly, obese individuals. Nutr J 11:105
43. Frestedt JL, Zenk JL, Kuskowski MA, Ward LS, Bastian ED (2008) A whey-protein supplement increases fat loss and spares lean muscle in obese subjects: a randomized human clinical study. Nutr Metab (Lond) 5:8. doi:10.1186/1743-7075-5-8

44. Burd NA, Yang YF, Moore DR, Tang JE, Tarnopolsky MA, Phillips SM (2012) Greater stimulation of myofibrillar protein synthesis with ingestion of whey protein isolate v. micellar casein at rest and after resistance exercise in elderly men. Br J Nutr 108:958–962
45. Churchward-Venne TA, Burd NA, Mitchell CJ, West DWD, Philp A, Marcotte GR, Baker SK, Baar K, Phillips SM (2012) Supplementation of a suboptimal protein dose with leucine or essential amino acids: effects on myofibrillar protein synthesis at rest and following resistance exercise in men. J Physiol 590:2751–2765
46. Murphy C, Miller BF (2010) Protein consumption following aerobic exercise increases whole-body protein turnover in older adults. Appl Physiol Nutr Metab 35:583–590
47. Messier V, Rabasa-Lhoret R, Barbat-Artigas S, Elisha B, Karelis AD, Aubertin-Leheudre M (2011) Menopause and sarcopenia: a potential role for sex hormones. Maturitas 68:331–336
48. Moeller LE, Peterson CT, Hanson KB, Dent SB, Lewis DS, King DS, Alekel DL (2003) Isoflavone-rich soy protein prevents loss of hip lean mass but does not prevent the shift in regional fat distribution in perimenopausal women. Menopause 10:322–331
49. Choquette S, Riesco E, Cormier E, Dion T, Aubertin-Leheudre M, Dionne IJ (2011) Effects of soya isoflavones and exercise on body composition and clinical risk factors of cardiovascular diseases in overweight postmenopausal women: a 6-month double-blind controlled trial. Br J Nutr 105:1199–1209
50. Wu J, Oka J, Tabata I, Higuchi M, Toda T, Fuku N, Ezaki J, Sugiyama F, Uchiyama S, Yamada K, Ishimi Y (2006) Effects of isoflavone and exercise on BMD and fat mass in postmenopausal Japanese women: a 1-year randomized placebo-controlled trial. J Bone Miner Res 21:780–789
51. Sorensen MB, Rosenfalck AM, Hojgaard L, Ottesen B (2001) Obesity and sarcopenia after menopause are reversed by sex hormone replacement therapy. Obes Res 9:622–626
52. Velders M, Diel P (2013) How sex hormones promote skeletal muscle regeneration. Sports Med 43:1089–1100
53. Shea MK, Nicklas BJ, Marsh AP, Houston DK, Miller GD, Isom S, Miller ME, Carr JJ, Lyles MF, Harris TB, Kritchevsky SB (2011) The effect of pioglitazone and resistance training on body composition in older men and women undergoing hypocaloric weight loss. Obesity 19:1636–1646
54. Gupta AK, Smith SR, Greenway FL, Bray GA (2009) Pioglitazone treatment in type 2 diabetes mellitus when combined with portion control diet modifies the metabolic syndrome. Diabetes Obes Metab 11:330–337
55. Shokouh P, Joharimoghadam A, Roohafza H, Sadeghi M, Golabchi A, Boshtam M, Sarrafzadegan N (2013) Effects of pioglitazone on asymmetric dimethylarginine and components of the metabolic syndrome in nondiabetic patients (EPICAMP Study): a double-blind, randomized clinical trial. PPAR Research 358074

Obesity and Testicular Function

Alessandro Ilacqua, Davide Francomano, and Antonio Aversa

10.1 Pathophysiology of Testicular Dysfunction with Relation to Adipose Tissue Excess

Testosterone deficiency syndrome (TDS) is becoming recognised as an increasingly common problem in the *ageing male* population. The European Male Ageing Study (EMAS) reports prevalence rates of 3.2 % in older men aged 60–69 and 5.1 % in those aged 70–79, based on a combination of a single morning testosterone after excluding those already diagnosed and treated for TDS or pituitary abnormalities [1]. *Erectile dysfunction* (ED), loss of morning erections and low sexual desire are the three most common symptoms likely to predict low *testosterone* (T) levels, but other important symptoms are often associated (Table 10.1). Low serum T is more common in men with *type 2 diabetes mellitus* (T2DM), *metabolic syndrome* (MetS) and *cardiovascular disease* (CVD) than in the general population, and this relationship is independent from the presence of obesity [2, 3]. Also, male *obesity* is associated with a reduction of testicular function mainly due to *secondary hypogonadism* (SH) [4, 5]. The prevalence of SH in T2DM was estimated to be 29 % (range 25–40 %), with a higher prevalence of 50 % when obesity and T2DM coexist [6, 7]. Several studies suggest that men who were obese at baseline and at follow-up, either if measured by body mass index (BMI) or by central obesity (waist–hip ratio or waist circumference), exhibit a greater decline of total and free T compared to men who were never classified as obese [8], mainly because of higher amounts of *visceral fat* [9]. Visceral adiposity is associated with elevated concentrations of insulin (hyperinsulinaemia), C peptide and glucose intolerance, which are negatively correlated to total and free T levels [10, 11]. The link between obesity and (decreased)

A. Ilacqua, MD, PhD • D. Francomano, MD • A. Aversa, MD, PhD (✉)
Department Experimental Medicine, Endocrinology and Food and Science Section,
Sapienza University of Rome, Viale Regina Elena 324, 00161 Rome, Italy
e-mail: alessandro_ilacqua@alice.it; davide.francomano@uniroma1.it;
antonio.aversa@uniroma1.it

Table 10.1 Signs and symptoms associated with testosterone deficiency syndrome

Loss of libido
Erectile dysfunction
Sarcopenia
Low bone mass
Depressive thoughts
Fatigue
Loss of body hair
Hot flushes
Loss of vigour

SHBG is mainly explained by the effects of obesity-induced insulin resistance, resulting in higher insulin levels (compensatory *hyperinsulinaemia*) that subsequently suppresses hepatic production of SHBG [12, 13] that would then result in reduced delivery of T to the peripheral tissues and increased availability of free T as a substrate for aromatase to convert into oestradiol. Male obesity is associated with increased aromatase activity within *adipocytes* [14], and oestradiol in turn exerts a negative feedback effect on LH secretion from the pituitary [15]. This may in turn worsen obesity and promote increased fat mass that represents a vicious circle perpetuating the hypogonadal state thus resulting in a reduction in muscle mass and an increase in the volume of visceral fat [16]. Another mechanism that mediates obesity-related effects on the male hypothalamic–pituitary–testicular axis (HPT) is influenced by increased plasma leptin levels that exert a direct negative action on LH/hCG-stimulated testicular androgen production and decrease Leydig cell responsiveness to gonadotrophin stimulation [17]. Increased levels of leptin may therefore play an important role in the pathogenesis of *male obesity secondary hypogonadism* (MOSH) [18]. Inflammatory mediators, such as C-reactive protein (CRP), have been demonstrated to contribute to the suppression of the HPT function and to the development of male SH, and the presence of inflammatory mediators may also worsen insulin resistance thus contributing to the development of benign prostate hyperplasia [19, 20] (Fig. 10.1).

10.2 Male Obesity Secondary Hypogonadism and Associated Metabolic Disturbances

Emerging data suggest that bone mass, energy metabolism and reproduction may be coordinately regulated. There has been a growing interest towards the non-classical effects of 25-hydroxycholecalciferol 25(OH)D (*vitamin D*), based on the presence of its receptors in tissues other than the bone, gut and kidneys [21]. Furthermore, several studies have suggested the involvement of vitamin D in the pathogenesis of CVD, cancer and MetS [22–24]. The association of low vitamin D levels and MetS is more pronounced in overweight and obese than in

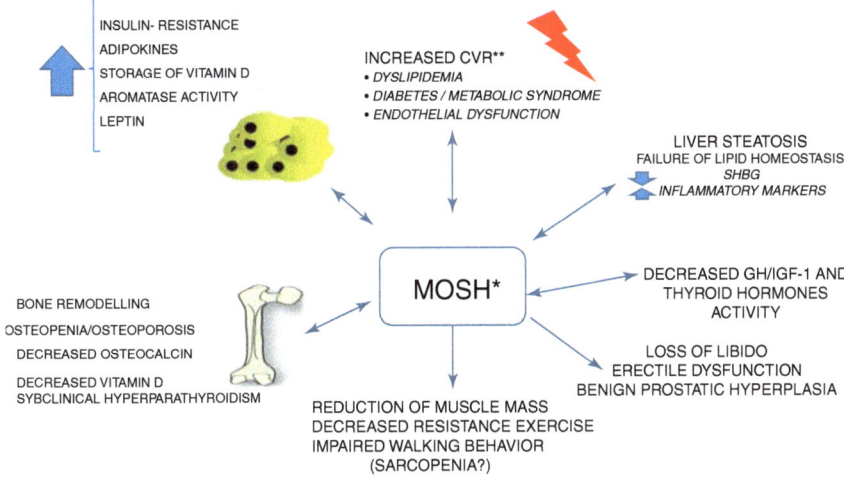

Fig. 10.1 Relationship between endocrinometabolic disturbances, obesity and testicular function

normal-weight individuals [25]. A recent study confirmed the lowest vitamin D concentrations and the highest prevalence of vitamin D deficiency in T2DM patients with hypogonadism, particularly in those with SH [26]. Several mechanisms have been proposed to explain the role of vitamin D in the pathogenesis of insulin resistance, and adiponectin has been proposed as a major player with its strong association with impaired glucose tolerance, independent from adiposity [27]. Adiponectin and glucose homeostasis are both correlated to *osteocalcin* (OSCA) levels, an osteoblast hormone linked to vitamin D metabolism [28]. Interesting animal studies suggest that bone may be a positive regulator of male fertility and that this action may be mediated through OSCA, via binding to a specific receptor present on Leydig cells that favours T biosynthesis. OSCA-deficient mice show a decrease in testicular, epididymal and seminal vesicle weights and sperm count, and Leydig cell maturation appears to be halted in absence of OSCA [29]. Androgens favour periosteal bone formation in men and maintain trabecular bone mass and integrity by inhibiting IL6 production [30]. Also, they stimulate the proliferation of osteoblast progenitors and the differentiation of mature osteoblasts by decreasing osteoclast formation and bone resorption, via increased production of osteoprotegerin by osteoblasts [31]. The net result of these functions leads to an accrual in bone formation [32]. In agreement with animal data, our group has recently demonstrated an association between visceral fat mass, insulin sensitivity, OSCA and T levels in ageing males that are significantly correlated with skeletal health. In this view, OSCA may be considered a new important marker of metabolic and gonadic function, other than the well-established function as marker of bone remodelling [33].

10.3 Obesity or Hypogonadism: Which Comes First?

The cause–effect relationship between obesity, insulin resistance, MetS, T2DM and TDS remains unclear. Data from the Massachusetts Male Aging Study showed that lower levels of total T and SHBG were predictive of the development of the MetS, particularly in men with BMI <25 kg/m^2 [34]. By contrast, other data suggests that the MetS is an independent risk factor for hypogonadism in middle-aged men, and relative T deficiency appears to be a marker, rather than the cause of MetS or T2DM in older men [35]. Recently we demonstrated that in hypogonadal men with MetS, TRT improves body composition and insulin sensitivity independently from diet and physical exercise [36]. Follow-up for 2 years in these men demonstrated also a significant reduction of *cardiovascular risks* (CVRs) without any serious adverse event [37]. However, it is not clear whether after TRT withdrawal there is a stabilisation of clinical patterns associated with CVR over the time and recovery from hypogonadism. We then investigated whether TRT combined with diet and physical exercise is better than diet plus physical exercise alone in achieving a reduction of CVR in a cohort of severely obese male subjects and whether T withdrawal was able to maintain outcomes evaluated. In this study, we demonstrated for the first time that TRT is beneficial on cardiac function in severely obese patients and that withdrawal is not a good prevention strategy for reducing CVR. The new protective effects of T on endothelial function and its inverse relationship with epicardial fat thickness clearly suggest that T reduction plays a critical role in the pathogenesis of cardiac dysfunction associated with obesity [38]. If male hypogonadism remains clinically unrecognised or underinvestigated, this can subsequently lead to significantly higher morbidity and mortality. Therefore, it is important that this condition is managed appropriately with TRT along with weight reduction and lifestyle changes [39]. However, encouragement of weight reduction alone (without TRT) cannot be endorsed and recommended as an effective treatment for SH and its associated sequelae, unless clear evidence is produced to demonstrate this. On the basis of our studies, we believe that TDS may be antecedent to visceral fat accumulation in ageing men, and in fact, once TRT is withdrawn, many of the advantages determined by TRT are lost in the short term thus suggesting that T decline comes first instead of being the consequence of central obesity. In conclusion, the available data suggest that hypoandrogenism may represent an early marker for glico-metabolic disturbances that may progress to MetS or T2DM and may in turn contribute to vicious cycle maintaining visceral obesity and its associated metabolic and andrologic disturbances.

10.4 Treatment of Male Obesity in the Presence of Hypogonadism

Generalized symptoms and signs of androgen deficiency vary depending on age of onset, duration and severity of the TDS. When severe obesity occurs, T serum level below 3.45 ng/mL (12 nmol/L) should be considered pathognomonic of

TDS as stated by International Guidelines and clinical questionnaires [40]. The Endocrine Society Guidelines recommend measurement of T levels in men with T2DM and endorse the early prescription of TRT in hypogonadal men with ED [41] especially because of the reduced success rate of phosphodiesterase type 5 (PDE5) inhibitors. Interestingly, in obese men with ED who do not respond to treatment with PDE5 inhibitors alone, the addition of T is recommended and even makes PDE5 inhibitors redundant in a number of cases. The use of a PDE5 inhibitor before T normalisation may be recommended until time-course effects on penile erection are achieved [42] keeping in mind that its efficacy is reduced because of low T levels [43].

In men with 'severe' TDS (total T less than 8 nmol/l), significant improvements in ED and sexual desire are expected. In symptomatic men with 'moderate' TDS, men falling within the 'grey area' (total T between 8 and 12 nmol/l or 180 and 250 pmol/l for free T), a trial of 3–6 months is also recommended. A target level of 15–21 nmol/l for total T during TRT is suggested [44]. Recent evidence suggests that long-term T treatment of obese diabetic men with low T levels produces important clinical benefits for up to 6 years [45]; improves glycaemic control, lipid profiles and bone mineral density [46]; and may prove useful in reducing CVR. Similar results were reported in a controlled study by our group [47], suggesting that TRT therapy ameliorates MetS components, MOSH and CVR without prostate adverse events [48]. Accurate evaluation of absolute contraindications (Table 10.2) and regular follow-up is needed in patients receiving TRT, as potentially androgen-dependent adverse events may occur suddenly (Table 10.3). The primary aim of TRT is to alleviate the clinical symptoms of TDS. Careful monitoring of changes in the clinical manifestations of T deficiency should therefore be an essential part of every follow-up visit. Effects of TRT on sexual drive may already appear after 3 weeks of treatment and reach a plateau at 6 weeks. Improvements in ED and ejaculation may require up to 6 months. Effects on quality of life and also on depressive mood may become detectable within 1 month, but the maximum effect may take longer [42]. In severely obese men, TRT appears to be a promising treatment leading to persistent results on body composition and cardiac performance than lifestyle changes alone. In addition, attrition rates without T supplementation seem to be higher and lead to poor adherence to diet and physical exercise in the long term.

Table 10.2 Absolute contraindications against testosterone treatment

Prostate cancer
PSA >4 ng/ml
Male breast cancer
Severe sleep apnoea
Male infertility
Haematocrit >50 %
Severe lower urinary tract symptoms due to benign prostatic hyperplasia

Table 10.3 Monitoring of patients receiving testosterone replacement therapy (TRT)

The response to treatment should be assessed 3, 6 and 12 months after the onset of treatment and thereafter annually
In men with an abnormal BMD, BMD measurements should be repeated 6 and 12 months after the start of TRT and thereafter annually
Haematocrit: at 3, 6 and 12 months and thereafter annually. The testosterone dosage should be decreased or therapy discontinued if the haematocrit increases above normal levels
Healthy prostate should be assessed by digital rectal examination and PSA before the start of TRT. Follow-up by PSA at 3, 6 and 12 months and thereafter annually
Routine screening of potential cardiovascular side effects is not indicated in men receiving TRT
Men with cardiovascular co-morbidity should be assessed by a cardiologist before TRT is initiated, and there should be close cardiovascular monitoring during TRT

References

1. Wu FW, Tajar A, Beynon JM, EMAS Group et al (2010) Identification of late-onset hypogonadism in middle-aged and elderly men. N Engl J Med 363:123–136
2. Dhindsa S, Prabhakar S, Sethi M et al (2004) Frequent occurrence of hypogonadotrophic hypogonadism in type 2 diabetes. J Clin Endocrinol Metab 89:5462–5468
3. Kapoor D, Aldred H, Clark S et al (2007) Clinical and biochemical assessment of hypogonadism in men with type 2 diabetes. Correlations with bioavailable testosterone and visceral adiposity. Diabetes Care 30:911–917
4. Gray A, Feldman HA, Mckinlay JB et al (1991) Age, disease, and changing sex hormone levels in middle-aged men: results of the Massachusetts male aging study. J Clin Endocrinol Metab 73:1016–1025
5. Kaufman JM, Vermeulen A (2005) The decline of androgen levels in elderly men and its clinical and therapeutic implications. Endocr Rev 26:833–876
6. Dhindsa S, Miller MG, McWhirter CL et al (2010) Testosterone concentrations in diabetic and non-diabetic obese men. Diabetes Care 33:1186–1192
7. Grossmann M, Thomas MC, Panagiotopoulos S et al (2008) Low testosterone levels are common and associated with insulin resistance in men with diabetes. J Clin Endocrinol Metab 93:1834–1840
8. Derby CA, Zilber S, Brambilla D et al (2006) Body mass index, waist circumference and waist to hip ratio and change in sex steroid hormones: the Massachusetts Male Ageing Study. Clin Endocrinol (Oxford) 65:125–131
9. Svartberg J, Von Muhlen D, Sundsfjord J et al (2004) Waist circumference and testosterone levels in community dwelling men. The Tromso study. Eur J Epidemiol 19:657–663
10. Seidell JC, Bjorntorp P, Sjostrom L (1990) Visceral fat accumulation in men is positively associated with insulin, glucose, and C-peptide levels, but negatively with testosterone levels. Metabolism 39:897–901
11. Pasquali R, Casimirri F, Cantobelli S et al (1991) Effect of obesity and body fat distribution on sex hormones and insulin in men. Metabolism 40:101–104
12. Hautanen A (2000) Synthesis and regulation of sex hormone-binding globulin in obesity. Int J Obes Relat Metab Disord 24(Suppl 2):S64–S70
13. Kalme T, Koistinen H, Loukovaara M et al (2003) Comparative studies on the regulation of insulin-like growth factor-binding protein-1 (IGFBP-1) and sex hormone-binding globulin (SHBG) production by insulin and insulin like growth factors in human hepatoma cells. J Steroid Biochem Mol Biol 86:197–200
14. Dandona P, Dhindsa S (2011) Update: hypogonadotropic hypogonadism in type 2 diabetes and obesity. J Clin Endocrinol Metab 96:2643–2651

15. Pitteloud N, Dwyer AA, DeCruz S et al (2008) The relative role of gonadal sex steroids and gonadotropin-releasing hormone pulse frequency in the regulation of follicle-stimulating hormone secretion in men. J Clin Endocrinol Metab 93:2686–2692
16. Caprio M, Fabbrini E, Isidori AM et al (2001) Leptin in reproduction. Trends Endocrinol Metab 12:65–72
17. Isidori AM, Caprio M, Strollo F et al (1999) Leptin and androgens in male obesity: evidence for leptin contribution to reduced androgen levels. J Clin Endocrinol Metab 84:3673–3680
18. Saboor Aftab SA, Kumar S, Barber TM (2013) The role of obesity and type 2 diabetes mellitus in the development of male obesity-associated secondary hypogonadism. Clin Endocrinol 78:330–337
19. Dandona P, Aljada A, Bandyopadhyay A (2004) Inflammation: the link between insulin resistance, obesity and diabetes. Trends Immunol 25:4–7
20. Corona G, Vignozzi L, Rastrelli G et al (2014) Benign prostatic hyperplasia: a new metabolic disease of the aging male and its correlation with sexual dysfunctions. Int J Endocrinol 2014(2014):Article ID 329456, 14 p
21. Bikle D (2009) Nonclassic actions of vitamin D (review). J Clin Endocrinol Metab 94:26–34
22. Wang TJ, Pencina MJ, Booth SL et al (2008) Vitamin D deficiency and risk of cardiovascular disease. Circulation 117:503–511
23. Lappe JM, Travers-Gustafson D, Davies KM et al (2007) Vitamin D and calcium supplementation reduces cancer risk: results of a randomized trial. Am J Clin Nutr 85:1586–1591
24. Martini LA, Wood RJ (2006) Vitamin D status and the metabolic syndrome. Nutr Rev 64:479–486
25. Lu L, Yu Z, Pan A et al (2009) Plasma 25-hydroxyvitamin D concentration and metabolic syndrome among middle-aged and elderly Chinese individuals. Diabetes Care 32:1278–1283
26. Bellastella G, Maiorino MI, Olita L et al (2014) Vitamin D deficiency in Type 2 diabetic patients with hypogonadism. J Sex Med 11:536–542
27. Nimitphong H, Chanprasertyothin S, Jongjaroenprasert W et al (2009) The association between vitamin D status and circulating adiponectin independent of adiposity in subjects with abnormal glucose tolerance. Endocrinology 36:205–210
28. Lee NK, Sowa H, Hinoi E et al (2007) Endocrine regulation of energy metabolism by the skeleton. Cell 130:456–469
29. Oury F, Sumara G, Sumara O et al (2011) Endocrine regulation of male fertility by the skeleton. Cell 144(5):796–809
30. Jilka RL, Hangoc G, Girasole G et al (1992) Increased osteoclast development after estrogen loss: mediation by interleukin-6. Science 257:88–91
31. Manolagas SC, Kousteni S, Jilka RL (2002) Sex steroids and bone. Recent Prog Horm Res 57:385–409
32. Michael H, Harkonen PL, Vaananen HK et al (2005) Estrogen and testosterone use different cellular pathways to inhibit osteoclastogenesis and bone resorption. J Bone Miner Res 20:2224–2232
33. Migliaccio S, Francomano D, Bruzziches R et al (2013) Trunk fat negatively influences skeletal and testicular functions in obese men: clinical implications for the aging male. Int J Endocrinol. doi:10.1155/2013/182753, Epub 2013 Nov 20
34. Kupelian V, Page ST, Araujo AB et al (2006) Low sex hormone-binding globulin, total testosterone, and symptomatic androgen deficiency are associated with development of the metabolic syndrome in nonobese men. J Clin Endocrinol Metab 91:843–850
35. Chen RY, Wittert GA, Andrews GR (2006) Relative androgen deficiency in relation to obesity and metabolic status in older men. Diabetes Obes Metab 8:429–435
36. Aversa A, Bruzziches R, Francomano D et al (2010) Efficacy and safety of two different testosterone undecanoate formulations in hypogonadal men with metabolic syndrome. J Endocrinol Invest 33:776–783
37. Aversa A, Bruzziches R, Francomano D et al (2010) Effects of testosterone undecanoate on cardiovascular risk factors and atherosclerosis in middle-aged men with late onset hypogonadism and metabolic syndrome: results from a 24-months, randomized, double-blind, placebo-controlled study. J Sex Med 7:3495–3503

38. Francomano D, Bruzziches R, Barbaro G et al (2014) Effects of testosterone undecanoate replacement and withdrawal on cardio-metabolic, hormonal and body composition outcomes in severely obese hypogonadal men: a pilot study. J Endocrinol Invest. doi:10.1007/s40618-014-0066-9
39. Donini LM, Cuzzolaro M, Gnessi L et al (2014) Obesity treatment: results after 4 years of a Nutritional and Psycho-Physical Rehabilitation Program in an outpatient setting. Eat Weight Disord 19:249–60
40. Lunenfeld B, Mskhalaya G, Kalinchenko S et al (2013) Recommendations on the diagnosis, treatment and monitoring of late-onset hypogonadism in men – a suggested update. Aging Male 16:143–150
41. Wang C, Nieschlag E, Swerdloff R, International Society of Andrology; International Society for the Study of Aging Male; European Association of Urology; European Academy of Andrology; American Society of Andrology et al (2009) Investigation, treatment, and monitoring of late-onset hypogonadism in males: ISA, ISSAM, EAU, EAA, and ASA recommendations. Eur Urol 55:121–130
42. Saad F, Aversa A, Isidori AM et al (2011) Onset of effects of testosterone treatment and time span until maximum effects are achieved. Eur J Endocrinol 65:675–685
43. Aversa A, Isidori AM, Spera G et al (2003) Androgens improve cavernous vasodilation and response to sildenafil in patients with erectile dysfunction. Clin Endocrinol (Oxford) 58: 632–638
44. Dohle GR, Arver S, Bettocchi C et al (2013) Guidelines on male hypogonadism. http://www.uroweb.org/gls/pdf/16_Male_Hypogonadism_LR%20II.pdf
45. Haider A, Yassin A, Doros G, Saad F et al (2014) Effects of long-term testosterone therapy on patients with "diabesity": results of observational studies of pooled analyses in obese hypogonadal men with type 2 diabetes. Int J Endocrinol 2014:Article ID 683515, 15 p
46. Haider A, Meergans U, Traish A et al (2014) Progressive improvement of T-scores in men with osteoporosis and subnormal serum testosterone levels upon treatment with testosterone over six years. Int J Edocrinol 2014:Article ID 496948, 9 p
47. Francomano D, Lenzi A, Aversa A et al (2014) Effects of five-year treatment with testosterone undecanoate on metabolic and hormonal parameters in ageing men with metabolic syndrome. Int J Endocrinol 2014:Article ID 527470, 9 p
48. Francomano D, Ilacqua A, Bruzziches R et al (2014) Effects of 5-year treatment with testosterone undecanoate on lower urinary tract symptoms in obese men with hypogonadism and metabolic syndrome. Urology 83:167–173

Obesity and Glucose Metabolism

11

Nicola Napoli and Paolo Pozzilli

Obesity is associated with multiple metabolic alterations that are risk factors for glucose homeostasis abnormalities, cardiovascular diseases, and nonalcoholic fatty liver disease [1–4]. It is believed that insulin resistance in the adipose tissue, liver, and skeletal muscle is crucial in the pathogenesis of these metabolic abnormalities [5, 6]. Adipocytes are key regulators of whole-body energy homeostasis, and altered adipose tissue glucose metabolism is also an important cause of insulin resistance and metabolic function [7]. Adipose tissue contributes to the development of obesity-related glucose abnormalities through excessive release of free fatty acids (FFA), adipokines, cytokines, and macrophage infiltration [8].

11.1 Epidemiological Link

Prevalence of glucose metabolic alterations has been reported to be related to grades of BMI or waist circumference. It is estimated that for every 1 kg increase in weight, the prevalence of diabetes increases by 9 % [9, 10]. According to NHANES, two-thirds of T2D patients in the United States have a BMI >27 [11] with a prevalence of diabetes that ranges from 2 % among subjects with BMI of 25–29.9 to 13 % in those with a BMI greater than 35 [12].

Epidemiological studies show that overweight subjects (BMI 25–30) present a 2.62 increased risk of developing diabetes (CI 2.18–3.16). This risk increases linearly with BMI in obese subjects, with a relative risk of 5.1 (CI 4.34–6.1) for subjects belonging to the classes I and II of obesity (BMI 30–40) that is doubled

---

N. Napoli (✉) • P. Pozzilli
Division of Endocrinology and Diabetes, University Campus Bio-Medico of Rome,
Via Alvaro del Portillo, Rome, Italy
e-mail: n.napoli@unicampus.it; p.pozzilli@unicampus.it

(RR 11; CI 8.61–14.04) for those belonging to the class III of obesity (BMI>40). At the same time, the probability of developing diabetes increases with physical inactivity at any BMI [13].

Abdominal fat mass is highly correlated to the risk of diabetes as well, and according to some studies, increase in waist circumference correlate with diabetes in a greater manner than BMI [14, 15].

When weight gain is achieved at a young age, the risk of developing diabetes is even worsened with an increased risk that is directly correlated to the amount of weight gained [9, 16, 17]. Studies show that in patients aged 35–60, the risk of diabetes is three times greater in those who gained 5–10 kg since the age of 18–20 compared to those who had a stable body weight [9, 10].

Physical exercise represents a protective factor: inactive subjects are at risk of insulin resistance and impaired glucose tolerance regardless of BMI [13]. Incidence of diabetes and cardiovascular mortality is in fact lower in those who are aerobically fit across a range of body adiposity [18, 19]. Ethnicity may play also a crucial role since the risk of developing diabetes is higher for Southeastern Asians than Caucasians for matched BMI [20].

11.1.1 Metabolically Normal Versus Abnormal Obesity

Obesity is associated with metabolic abnormalities like insulin resistance, T2D, and other cardiometabolic complications. However, not all obese develop complications, and about 25 % are considered "metabolically normal obese" (MNO). These subjects are metabolically healthy and present normal insulin sensitivity and ≤1 cardiometabolic abnormality [21–23]. "Metabolically abnormal obese" (MAO) are those subjects with similar body fat like MNO but with higher visceral and liver fat, abnormal insulin sensitivity inflammatory profile, and other cardiometabolic complications [21–25]. Importantly, MNO subjects are protected from metabolic abnormalities, and recent findings show that up to 11 years of follow-up do not present an increased risk of developing diabetes compared to lean subjects. On the contrary, MAO subjects have 4–11-fold increased relative risk to develop diabetes. As reviewed by Bonet, protective factors in MNO subjects include increased capacity for storing fat in adipose tissue, decreased de novo lipogenesis in liver, lower visceral adiposity, increased circulating adiponectin, decreased proinflammatory cytokines, and macrophage infiltration into adipose tissue [26].

However, recent data reveal also a possible role of the immune system. In an elegant study, Fabbrini et al., has shown that adipose tissue from MAO subjects had three to tenfold increase in numbers of T-helper 17 and Th22 compared with MNO and lean subjects. MAO subjects also had increased plasma concentrations of IL-22 and IL-6. Importantly, IL-17 and IL-22 inhibited uptake of glucose in skeletal muscle isolated from rats and reduced insulin sensitivity in cultured human hepatocytes. In other words, MAO individuals may have a peculiar immune asset with highly expressed Th17 and Th22 cells, which produce cytokines that cause metabolic dysfunction in the liver and muscle in vitro [27].

11.2 Pathophysiological Link

11.2.1 FFA

Obese subjects present an increased FFA release from adipose tissue that is considered an important cause of insulin resistance, impairing the ability of insulin to stimulate muscle glucose uptake and suppressing hepatic glucose production [28–31]. Experimental models show that high plasma FFA concentrations cause insulin resistance in skeletal muscle [30], while their reduction improves skeletal muscle insulin sensitivity [32, 33]. However, the pathogenesis of skeletal muscle insulin resistance in obese people is complex. Data from Klein's group have found that the overall rate of FFA release during both postabsorptive and simulated postprandial states accounted for less than half of the variability in skeletal muscle insulin sensitivity, indicating that other factors must be involved [8]. Studies from the same group have revaluated the possible role played by excessive rates of adipose tissue triglyceride lipolysis on the onset of skeletal muscle insulin resistance. Authors suggest that other mechanisms may be involved and metabolic dysfunction may be caused by a redirection of plasma FFA trafficking away from adipose tissue and toward skeletal muscle and subsequent alterations in fatty acid metabolism within the skeletal muscle itself [8].

Complex mechanisms involving mTOR, protein kinase C, and alteration of GLUT-4 translocation have been proposed and rely on increased deposition of fatty acid metabolites in myocytes. Other involved pathways include enhancement of inflammation through the activation of nuclear factor kappa B (IkB) mediated by PKC or by increased production of reactive oxygen species. IkB activation may impair insulin-induced glucose uptake via mTOR-mediated serine phosphorylation of IRS1 [29, 34, 35].

Other proteins regulating triglyceride distribution like lipin 1 have been studied, showing that knockout mice for the lipin 1 gene are lipodystrophic and insulin resistant [36, 37]. Lipin 1 expression in the liver and adipose tissue is inversely related to insulin resistance and increases after weight loss, playing an antiinflammatory effect and enhancing TG esterification [38].

11.2.2 Genetics

Obese phenotype is the result of a gene–environment interaction that in turn influences the development of glucose metabolism abnormalities. It is estimated that genetics may account only for the 40 % of the variance of body mass while environmental factors related to increased energy intake and sedentary lifestyle play a main role [39]. In obesity, genetic traits do not follow the simple Mendelian inheritance, and monogenic causes of obesity and insulin resistance are rare. Therefore, current scientific research has been mostly focused on single nucleotide polymorphisms (SNPs), but the large number of genes potentially involved has complicated the determination of genetic influence on the final phenotype. GWAS studies have allowed the discovery of new candidate genes and potential new metabolic pathways.

FTO

FTO gene (fat mass and obesity-associated gene) which represented a breakthrough for the strong correlations with obesity and T2D obtained in different ages and ethnic groups. The FTO gene has emerged 450 million years ago and is located on chromosome 16q12.2, spanning for nine exons [40]. FTO encodes for a 2-oxoglutarate-dependent nucleic demethylase that is mostly expressed in the brain, in a hypothalamic area that regulates energy balance. Recent studies have revealed FTO to be a member of the Fe (II)- and 2-oxoglutarate (2OG)-dependent oxygenase superfamily, involved in fatty acid metabolism, DNA repair [41], energy homeostasis [40, 42], nucleic acid demethylation, and regulation of body fat masses by lipolysis [43].

In particular, the A allele of rs9939609 SNP of the FTO gene is strongly associated with increased BMI, type 2 diabetes, and obesity. Other metabolic abnormalities in obesity are associated with FTO SNPs like higher fasting insulin, triglycerides, lower HDL cholesterol, waist circumference, and weight [5, 11–13]. The following studies have shown that the rs9939609 SNP of the FTO gene is also associated with morbidly obese patients (BMI>40) [1], high concentration of fat cells [2], and increased fat cell lipolysis. The association of FTO variants with T2DM and BMI has been clearly identified in white European populations [44] while results have not been consistent in Asians and in other ethnic groups [45–47].

FABPs

Intracellular fatty acid-binding proteins (FABPs) belong to a multigene family involved in obesity and glucose abnormalities. FABPs are expressed in the liver, intestine, and heart and are thought to participate in the uptake, intracellular metabolism, and/or transport of long-chain fatty acids.

Most studies associated with this gene have been focused on the Ala→Thr (G→A) substitution in exon 2 showing that subjects bearing the Thr allele had increased BMI, percent body fat, and plasma triglycerides [48]. Other studies have found that FABP2 Ala54Thr variants present increased risk of atherosclerosis and diabetes because of decreased insulin sensitivity, increased rate of lipid oxidation, increased fasting insulin concentration, and increased triglyceride-rich lipoprotein [49–52].

PPAR-γ

Adipogenesis is under the control of the master regulator PPAR-γ. PPARs are transcriptional regulators that form part of the ligand-activated nuclear hormone receptor superfamily [53]. The substitution of alanine for proline at codon 12 of PPAR-γ and the risk for obesity and T2DM have been widely studied [54]. A meta-analysis conducted by Ludovico found that the alanine polymorphism conferred significantly greater protection against T2DM among Asians than Caucasians [55].

11.2.3 GLUT4

GLUT4 is the major insulin-responsive glucose transporter and has a central role in systemic glucose metabolism [56–59]. Insulin resistance is characterized by the downregulation of GLUT4 in adipose tissue, but not in the muscle, the major site of insulin-stimulated glucose uptake. Animal models where adipose-specific GLUT4 is overexpressed show an improved glucose homeostasis [59]. On the contrary, when adipose-specific GLUT4 is knocked out, mice have insulin resistance and type 2 diabetes.

Previous work from Kahn's group has shown that adipose GLUT4 expression regulates systemic insulin sensitivity [58, 59] indicating that adipocytes are capable of sensing and coordinating responses to changes in glucose availability. From a recent study conducted by Herman, it is clear that adipose tissue ChREBP has a key role in integrating adipocyte and whole-body metabolic function and this may be mediated by transcriptional regulation of the potent ChREBP-b isoform [60].

11.2.4 Oxidative Stress

Obesity and diabetes are associated with increased oxidative stress [61, 62]. A low-grade inflammation present in obesity and the abnormal activation of resident macrophages in the adipose tissues increase the levels of reactive oxygen species (ROS). A main source of ROS is the increased exposure of target the tissue to inflammatory cytokines such as IL-1, TNF, and IL-6 which are increased in obesity. ROS may also directly regulate the activity of transcription factors, such as NF-κB, thus controlling proinflammatory gene expression [63]. Moreover, dysglycemia frequently observed in obesity is associated with increased release of ROS by enhanced NADPH oxidase activity [61].

Previous data have shown that uric acid (UA) concentration is a strong predictor for developing diabetes in obese subjects [64], and a strong correlation between serum UA and insulin resistance in subjects with a metabolic syndrome has been found [65, 66],

Based on these data, Fabbrini et al. have investigated the effect of a marked decrease in serum UA levels in obese subjects. Interestingly, subjects with high serum UA levels had 20–90 % greater nonenzymatic antioxidant capacity (NEAC) but lower insulin sensitivity (40 %) and levels of markers of oxidative stress (30 %) than subjects with normal UA. Acute UA reduction caused a 45–95 % decrease in NEAC and a 25–40 % increase in levels of systemic and muscle markers of oxidative stress [67].

However, the increase in oxidative stress did not have a significant effect on insulin sensitivity. According to authors, these findings demonstrate that circulating UA is a potent antioxidant and may play a protective mechanism to prevent systemic oxidative damage by free radicals [67].

11.2.5 Inflammation and Adipokines

Both animal models and data from human studies have clearly shown that obesity is characterized by an increased release of TNFα and in general by a chronic low-grade inflammation, which is responsible for the metabolic dysfunction [68]. Obesity is also associated with increased adipose tissue macrophage infiltration [69, 70] in conjunction with a switch in macrophage population from an anti-inflammatory to a proinflammatory state [71]. In this complex scenario, data from animal models indicate also that hepatic T lymphocytes may also have an important role in obesity-related adipose tissue inflammation and metabolic dysfunction [72].

Adiponectin

Exclusively produced by fat tissue, adiponectin circulates in much higher concentrations than other adipokines. In contrast to leptin, adiponectin is negatively correlated with visceral fat mass and BMI in humans, and low levels are described in patients affected by diabetes or myocardial infarction [73–76]. Adiponectin is structurally similar to TNF and RANKL [76].

Resistin

It is a recently discovered adipocyte-secreted factor [77]. Resistin has rarely been found to be produced by fat tissue [78]. It is expressed by the bone marrow and produced by peripheral mononuclear cells as an inflammatory cytokine [79]. Resistin is involved in the atherogenic process, and serum levels are higher in diabetic and obese patients [77, 80, 81].

IL6

One-third of the circulating levels of IL-6 is produced by adipocytes and adipose tissue matrix [82]. This is consistent with the evidence that serum IL-6 is increased in overweight and obese individuals [83, 84]. IL-6 may affect glucose homeostasis and energy expenditure either directly or indirectly by acting on adipocytes, hepatocytes, skeletal muscle, and pancreatic β-cells [85].

MCP-1

MCP-1 is a factor involved in macrophagic activation during the inflammation response and recently has been recognized as a new protagonist of the complex interaction between insulin resistance, diabetes, and inflammatory disease. Experimental studies in vivo performed on obese mice demonstrate that mice with higher levels of MCP-1 in adipose tissue were at higher risk of fat inflammation and future insulin resistance both in the adipose tissue and in the liver in comparison with mice with lower levels of MCP-1.

11.2.6 Sex Hormones

The adipose tissue can contribute significantly to the circulating pool of estrogens. Aromatase expression in adipose tissue primarily accounts for the peripheral formation of estrogen and increases as a function of body weight and advancing age [86]. Estrogen deficiency is associated with marrow adiposity in postmenopausal women [87], and estrogen administration can reverse marrow adiposity in the ovariectomized rat model [88–90].

Observational studies support an association between estrogen metabolism and BMI [91], suggesting that obesity is associated with significant decreases in hydroxylation of estrone at C-2. This results in reduced production of less active or inactive estrogenic metabolites, which can possibly sustain bone mass in obesity. Indeed, a recent study showed that in postmenopausal women, an increase in the metabolism of estrogen toward the inactive metabolites is associated with lower body fat and higher lean mass than those with predominance of the metabolism toward the active metabolites [92].

11.3 RANKL System and Insulin Resistance

RANKL is a member of the TNF superfamily and, after binding to its cognate receptor RANK, acts as a potent stimulator of NF-κB. There are evidences supporting a role of this system in diabetes and associated diseases [93]. Both liver tissues [94] and β-cells express RANKL and RANK [95]. Moreover, levels of OPG, which competes for RANK/RANKL interaction, are elevated in T2D, especially in those with poor glycemic control and relates with fat mass and atherosclerosis parameters [96–99]. Recently, Kiechl et al. showed that increased levels of soluble RANKL are associated with the development of diabetes in 844 subjects from the Brunek study (OR = 3.37; 95 % CI: 1.63–6.97). Besides the epidemiologic finding, the authors showed that RANKL interacted with glucose homeostasis by acting on hepatocyte function and insulin resistance. Indeed, mice selectively lacking RANK in the hepatocyte (*Rank*LKO) were protected by high-fat diet-induced insulin resistance and showed fasting glucose and insulin concentrations similar to those of *Rank*WT mice fed with a normal-fat diet [95]. These data suggest the RANKL involvement in the pathogenesis of hepatic insulin resistance and T2D and provide a link between inflammation and disrupted glucose homeostasis.

11.3.1 Osteocalcin

Osteocalcin (OCN), an osteoblast-synthesized hormone, has been shown to regulate glucose homeostasis by stimulating beta cell proliferation and increasing insulin secretion and action (Fig. 11.1).

Karsenty's group has indicated that OCN-knockout mice display decreased β-cell proliferation, glucose intolerance, and insulin resistance. In ex vivo studies, when pancreatic β-cells isolated from wild-type mice were cocultured with wild-type osteoblasts or in the presence of supernatants from cultured osteoblasts, insulin secretion increased, suggesting the presence of an osteoblast-derived circulating factor that regulates β-cell function. Administration of OCN significantly decreased glycemia and increased insulin secretion. Furthermore, OCN function was exerted

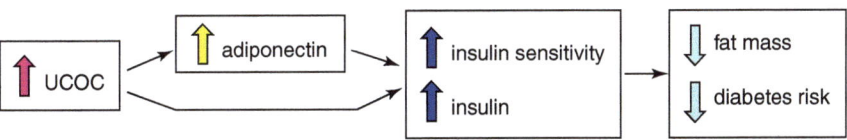

Fig. 11.1 Role of osteocalcin in glucose metabolism homeostasis. Adapted from Motyl et al. [109]

through adiponectin – coculture of wild-type osteoblasts with adipocytes increased adiponectin expression and action [100, 101]. A number of human studies have also explored the relationship between OCN and glucose homeostasis. OCN levels have been reported to be lower in T2D compared to healthy subjects [102], inversely related to body mass index, fat mass, and plasma glucose [103–106] but also to atherosclerosis and inflammatory parameters such as high sensitive C-reactive protein and IL-6 [107].

Ferron et al. have also shown that in mice fed with a high-fat diet (HFD), daily injections of osteocalcin partially restored insulin sensitivity and glucose tolerance. Intermittent osteocalcin injections displayed additional mitochondria in their skeletal muscle, with increased energy expenditure and improved insulin sensitivity.

Lifestyle Intervention

Lifestyle intervention is considered the golden standard for treating obesity and preventing cardiometabolic-related events. In a recent study, Villareal's group has randomized 107 obese elderly subjects to control group, diet group, exercise group, and diet–exercise group for 1 year. At the end of the study, the diet–exercise and diet groups had similar improvements in insulin area under the curve (AUC), glucose AUC, visceral fat, tumor necrosis factor, and adiponectin while no changes in these parameters occurred in both exercise and control groups [108]. Importantly, the combination of these two interventions reduced insulin sensitivity and the cardiometabolic syndrome prevalence by 40 % [108]. These data confirmed previous findings showing that exercise training per se may have a neutral effect on insulin sensitivity while it becomes detrimental when associated to weight loss.

References

1. Klein S, Wadden T, Sugerman HJ (2002) AGA technical review on obesity. Gastroenterology 123(3):882–932
2. Kragelund C, Hassager C, Hildebrandt P, Torp-Pedersen C, Kober L (2005) Impact of obesity on long-term prognosis following acute myocardial infarction. Int J Cardiol 98(1):123–131
3. McAuley P, Myers J, Abella J, Froelicher V (2007) Body mass, fitness and survival in veteran patients: another obesity paradox? Am J Med 120(6):518–524
4. Alberti KG, Eckel RH, Grundy SM, Zimmet PZ, Cleeman JI, Donato KA et al (2009) Harmonizing the metabolic syndrome: a joint interim statement of the International Diabetes Federation Task Force on Epidemiology and Prevention; National Heart, Lung, and Blood Institute; American Heart Association; World Heart Federation; International Atherosclerosis Society; and International Association for the Study of Obesity. Circulation 120(16):1640–1645
5. DeFronzo RA (2010) Insulin resistance, lipotoxicity, type 2 diabetes and atherosclerosis: the missing links. The Claude Bernard Lecture 2009. Diabetologia 53(7):1270–1287
6. Groop LC, Bonadonna RC, DelPrato S, Ratheiser K, Zyck K, Ferrannini E et al (1989) Glucose and free fatty acid metabolism in non-insulin-dependent diabetes mellitus. Evidence for multiple sites of insulin resistance. J Clin Invest 84(1):205–213
7. Fabbrini E, Magkos F, Mohammed BS, Pietka T, Abumrad NA, Patterson BW et al (2009) Intrahepatic fat, not visceral fat, is linked with metabolic complications of obesity. Proc Natl Acad Sci U S A 106(36):15430–15435

8. Magkos F, Fabbrini E, Conte C, Patterson BW, Klein S (2012) Relationship between adipose tissue lipolytic activity and skeletal muscle insulin resistance in nondiabetic women. J Clin Endocrinol Metab 97(7):E1219–E1223
9. Colditz GA, Willett WC, Rotnitzky A, Manson JE (1995) Weight gain as a risk factor for clinical diabetes mellitus in women. Ann Intern Med 122(7):481–486
10. Chan JM, Rimm EB, Colditz GA, Stampfer MJ, Willett WC (1994) Obesity, fat distribution, and weight gain as risk factors for clinical diabetes in men. Diabetes Care 17(9):961–969
11. Flegal KM, Troiano RP (2000) Changes in the distribution of body mass index of adults and children in the US population. Int J Obes Relat Metab Disord 24(7):807–818
12. Cowie CC, Rust KF, Ford ES, Eberhardt MS, Byrd-Holt DD, Li C et al (2009) Full accounting of diabetes and pre-diabetes in the U.S. population in 1988–1994 and 2005–2006. Diabetes Care 32(2):287–294
13. Sullivan PW, Morrato EH, Ghushchyan V, Wyatt HR, Hill JO (2005) Obesity, inactivity, and the prevalence of diabetes and diabetes-related cardiovascular comorbidities in the U.S., 2000–2002. Diabetes Care 28(7):1599–1603
14. Ohlson LO, Larsson B, Svardsudd K, Welin L, Eriksson H, Wilhelmsen L et al (1985) The influence of body fat distribution on the incidence of diabetes mellitus. 13.5 years of follow-up of the participants in the study of men born in 1913. Diabetes 34(10):1055–1058
15. Kaye SA, Folsom AR, Sprafka JM, Prineas RJ, Wallace RB (1991) Increased incidence of diabetes mellitus in relation to abdominal adiposity in older women. J Clin Epidemiol 44(3):329–334
16. Willett WC, Manson JE, Stampfer MJ, Colditz GA, Rosner B, Speizer FE et al (1995) Weight, weight change, and coronary heart disease in women. Risk within the 'normal' weight range. JAMA 273(6):461–465
17. Rimm EB, Stampfer MJ, Giovannucci E, Ascherio A, Spiegelman D, Colditz GA et al (1995) Body size and fat distribution as predictors of coronary heart disease among middle-aged and older US men. Am J Epidemiol 141(12):1117–1127
18. Wei M, Gibbons LW, Mitchell TL, Kampert JB, Lee CD, Blair SN (1999) The association between cardiorespiratory fitness and impaired fasting glucose and type 2 diabetes mellitus in men. Ann Intern Med 130(2):89–96
19. Lee CD, Blair SN, Jackson AS (1999) Cardiorespiratory fitness, body composition, and all-cause and cardiovascular disease mortality in men. Am J Clin Nutr 69(3):373–380
20. Yoon KH, Lee JH, Kim JW, Cho JH, Choi YH, Ko SH et al (2006) Epidemic obesity and type 2 diabetes in Asia. Lancet 368(9548):1681–1688
21. Karelis AD (2008) Metabolically healthy but obese individuals. Lancet 372(9646):1281–1283
22. Iacobellis G, Ribaudo MC, Zappaterreno A, Iannucci CV, Leonetti F (2005) Prevalence of uncomplicated obesity in an Italian obese population. Obes Res 13(6):1116–1122
23. Stefan N, Kantartzis K, Machann J, Schick F, Thamer C, Rittig K et al (2008) Identification and characterization of metabolically benign obesity in humans. Arch Intern Med 168(15):1609–1616
24. Karelis AD, Faraj M, Bastard JP, St-Pierre DH, Brochu M, Prud'homme D et al (2005) The metabolically healthy but obese individual presents a favorable inflammation profile. J Clin Endocrinol Metab 90(7):4145–4150
25. Aguilar-Salinas CA, Garcia EG, Robles L, Riano D, Ruiz-Gomez DG, Garcia-Ulloa AC et al (2008) High adiponectin concentrations are associated with the metabolically healthy obese phenotype. J Clin Endocrinol Metab 93(10):4075–4079
26. Samocha-Bonet D, Chisholm DJ, Tonks K, Campbell LV, Greenfield JR (2012) Insulin-sensitive obesity in humans - a 'favorable fat' phenotype? Trends Endocrinol Metab 23(3):116–124
27. Fabbrini E, Cella M, McCartney SA, Fuchs A, Abumrad NA, Pietka TA et al (2013) Association between specific adipose tissue CD4+ T-cell populations and insulin resistance in obese individuals. Gastroenterology 145(2):366–374, e1–3
28. Shulman GI (2000) Cellular mechanisms of insulin resistance. J Clin Invest 106(2):171–176

29. Boden G (2006) Fatty acid-induced inflammation and insulin resistance in skeletal muscle and liver. Curr Diab Rep 6(3):177–181
30. Kelley DE, Mokan M, Simoneau JA, Mandarino LJ (1993) Interaction between glucose and free fatty acid metabolism in human skeletal muscle. J Clin Invest 92(1):91–98
31. Ferrannini E, Barrett EJ, Bevilacqua S, DeFronzo RA (1983) Effect of fatty acids on glucose production and utilization in man. J Clin Invest 72(5):1737–1747
32. Santomauro AT, Boden G, Silva ME, Rocha DM, Santos RF, Ursich MJ et al (1999) Overnight lowering of free fatty acids with Acipimox improves insulin resistance and glucose tolerance in obese diabetic and nondiabetic subjects. Diabetes 48(9):1836–1841
33. Kleiber H, Munger R, Jallut D, Tappy L, Felley C, Golay A et al (1992) Interaction of lipid and carbohydrate metabolism after infusions of lipids or of lipid lowering agents: lack of a direct relationship between free fatty acid concentrations and glucose disposal. Diabete Metab 18(2):84–90
34. Um SH, D'Alessio D, Thomas G (2006) Nutrient overload, insulin resistance, and ribosomal protein S6 kinase 1, S6K1. Cell Metab 3(6):393–402
35. Itani SI, Ruderman NB, Schmieder F, Boden G (2002) Lipid-induced insulin resistance in human muscle is associated with changes in diacylglycerol, protein kinase C, and IkappaB-alpha. Diabetes 51(7):2005–2011
36. Reue K, Xu P, Wang XP, Slavin BG (2000) Adipose tissue deficiency, glucose intolerance, and increased atherosclerosis result from mutation in the mouse fatty liver dystrophy (fld) gene. J Lipid Res 41(7):1067–1076
37. Phan J, Reue K (2005) Lipin, a lipodystrophy and obesity gene. Cell Metab 1(1):73–83
38. Takeuchi K, Reue K (2009) Biochemistry, physiology, and genetics of GPAT, AGPAT, and lipin enzymes in triglyceride synthesis. Am J Physiol Endocrinol Metab 296(6):E1195–E1209
39. Bouchard C, Perusse L (1993) Genetics of obesity. Annu Rev Nutr 13:337–354
40. Fredriksson R, Hagglund M, Olszewski PK, Stephansson O, Jacobsson JA, Olszewska AM et al (2008) The obesity gene, FTO, is of ancient origin, up-regulated during food deprivation and expressed in neurons of feeding-related nuclei of the brain. Endocrinology 149(5): 2062–2071
41. Clifton IJ, McDonough MA, Ehrismann D, Kershaw NJ, Granatino N, Schofield CJ (2006) Structural studies on 2-oxoglutarate oxygenases and related double-stranded beta-helix fold proteins. J Inorg Biochem 100(4):644–669
42. Stratigopoulos G, Padilla SL, LeDuc CA, Watson E, Hattersley AT, McCarthy MI et al (2008) Regulation of Fto/Ftm gene expression in mice and humans. Am J Physiol Regul Integr Comp Physiol 294(4):R1185–R1196
43. Wahlen K, Sjolin E, Hoffstedt J (2008) The common rs9939609 gene variant of the fat mass- and obesity-associated gene FTO is related to fat cell lipolysis. J Lipid Res 49(3):607–611
44. Dina C, Meyre D, Gallina S, Durand E, Korner A, Jacobson P et al (2007) Variation in FTO contributes to childhood obesity and severe adult obesity. Nat Genet 39(6):724–726
45. Li H, Wu Y, Loos RJ, Hu FB, Liu Y, Wang J et al (2008) Variants in the fat mass- and obesity-associated (FTO) gene are not associated with obesity in a Chinese Han population. Diabetes 57(1):264–268
46. Hotta K, Nakata Y, Matsuo T, Kamohara S, Kotani K, Komatsu R et al (2008) Variations in the FTO gene are associated with severe obesity in the Japanese. J Hum Genet 53(6): 546–553
47. Ng MC, Park KS, Oh B, Tam CH, Cho YM, Shin HD et al (2008) Implication of genetic variants near TCF7L2, SLC30A8, HHEX, CDKAL1, CDKN2A/B, IGF2BP2, and FTO in type 2 diabetes and obesity in 6,719 Asians. Diabetes 57(8):2226–2233
48. Hegele RA, Harris SB, Hanley AJ, Sadikian S, Connelly PW, Zinman B (1996) Genetic variation of intestinal fatty acid-binding protein associated with variation in body mass in aboriginal Canadians. J Clin Endocrinol Metab 81(12):4334–4337
49. Yamada K, Yuan X, Ishiyama S, Koyama K, Ichikawa F, Koyanagi A et al (1997) Association between Ala54Thr substitution of the fatty acid-binding protein 2 gene with insulin resistance and intra-abdominal fat thickness in Japanese men. Diabetologia 40(6):706–710

50. Agren JJ, Vidgren HM, Valve RS, Laakso M, Uusitupa MI (2001) Postprandial responses of individual fatty acids in subjects homozygous for the threonine- or alanine-encoding allele in codon 54 of the intestinal fatty acid binding protein 2 gene. Am J Clin Nutr 73(1):31–35
51. Baier LJ, Bogardus C, Sacchettini JC (1996) A polymorphism in the human intestinal fatty acid binding protein alters fatty acid transport across Caco-2 cells. J Biol Chem 271(18): 10892–10896
52. Marin C, Perez-Jimenez F, Gomez P, Delgado J, Paniagua JA, Lozano A et al (2005) The Ala54Thr polymorphism of the fatty acid-binding protein 2 gene is associated with a change in insulin sensitivity after a change in the type of dietary fat. Am J Clin Nutr 82(1):196–200
53. Tontonoz P, Spiegelman BM (2008) Fat and beyond: the diverse biology of PPARgamma. Annu Rev Biochem 77:289–312
54. Yen CJ, Beamer BA, Negri C, Silver K, Brown KA, Yarnall DP et al (1997) Molecular scanning of the human peroxisome proliferator activated receptor gamma (hPPAR gamma) gene in diabetic Caucasians: identification of a Pro12Ala PPAR gamma 2 missense mutation. Biochem Biophys Res Commun 241(2):270–274
55. Ludovico O, Pellegrini F, Di Paola R, Minenna A, Mastroianno S, Cardellini M et al (2007) Heterogeneous effect of peroxisome proliferator-activated receptor gamma2 Ala12 variant on type 2 diabetes risk. Obesity (Silver Spring) 15(5):1076–1081
56. Shepherd PR, Kahn BB (1999) Glucose transporters and insulin action–implications for insulin resistance and diabetes mellitus. N Engl J Med 341(4):248–257
57. Attie AD, Scherer PE (2009) Adipocyte metabolism and obesity. J Lipid Res 50(Suppl): S395–S399
58. Abel ED, Peroni O, Kim JK, Kim YB, Boss O, Hadro E et al (2001) Adipose-selective targeting of the GLUT4 gene impairs insulin action in muscle and liver. Nature 409(6821):729–733
59. Shepherd PR, Gnudi L, Tozzo E, Yang H, Leach F, Kahn BB (1993) Adipose cell hyperplasia and enhanced glucose disposal in transgenic mice overexpressing GLUT4 selectively in adipose tissue. J Biol Chem 268(30):22243–22246
60. Herman MA, Peroni OD, Villoria J, Schon MR, Abumrad NA, Bluher M et al (2012) A novel ChREBP isoform in adipose tissue regulates systemic glucose metabolism. Nature 484(7394):333–338
61. West IC (2000) Radicals and oxidative stress in diabetes. Diabet Med 17(3):171–180
62. Stadler K (2012) Oxidative stress in diabetes. Adv Exp Med Biol 771:272–287
63. Zmijewski JW, Zhao X, Xu Z, Abraham E (2007) Exposure to hydrogen peroxide diminishes NF-kappaB activation, IkappaB-alpha degradation, and proteasome activity in neutrophils. Am J Physiol Cell Physiol 293(1):C255–C266
64. Bhole V, Choi JW, Kim SW, de Vera M, Choi H (2010) Serum uric acid levels and the risk of type 2 diabetes: a prospective study. Am J Med 123(10):957–961
65. Vuorinen-Markkola H, Yki-Jarvinen H (1994) Hyperuricemia and insulin resistance. J Clin Endocrinol Metab 78(1):25–29
66. Yoo TW, Sung KC, Shin HS, Kim BJ, Kim BS, Kang JH et al (2005) Relationship between serum uric acid concentration and insulin resistance and metabolic syndrome. Circ J 69(8): 928–933
67. Fabbrini E, Serafini M, Colic Baric I, Hazen SL, Klein S (2014) Effect of plasma uric acid on antioxidant capacity, oxidative stress, and insulin sensitivity in obese subjects. Diabetes 63(3):976–981
68. Rodriguez-Hernandez H, Simental-Mendia LE, Rodriguez-Ramirez G, Reyes-Romero MA (2013) Obesity and inflammation: epidemiology, risk factors, and markers of inflammation. Int J Endocrinol 2013:678159
69. Weisberg SP, McCann D, Desai M, Rosenbaum M, Leibel RL, Ferrante AW Jr (2003) Obesity is associated with macrophage accumulation in adipose tissue. J Clin Invest 112(12): 1796–1808
70. Curat CA, Miranville A, Sengenes C, Diehl M, Tonus C, Busse R et al (2004) From blood monocytes to adipose tissue-resident macrophages: induction of diapedesis by human mature adipocytes. Diabetes 53(5):1285–1292

71. Lumeng CN, Bodzin JL, Saltiel AR (2007) Obesity induces a phenotypic switch in adipose tissue macrophage polarization. J Clin Invest 117(1):175–184
72. Tang Y, Bian Z, Zhao L, Liu Y, Liang S, Wang Q et al (2011) Interleukin-17 exacerbates hepatic steatosis and inflammation in non-alcoholic fatty liver disease. Clin Exp Immunol 166(2):281–290
73. Weyer C, Funahashi T, Tanaka S, Hotta K, Matsuzawa Y, Pratley RE et al (2001) Hypoadiponectinemia in obesity and type 2 diabetes: close association with insulin resistance and hyperinsulinemia. J Clin Endocrinol Metab 86(5):1930–1935
74. Pischon T, Girman CJ, Hotamisligil GS, Rifai N, Hu FB, Rimm EB (2004) Plasma adiponectin levels and risk of myocardial infarction in men. JAMA 291(14):1730–1737
75. Nakashima R, Kamei N, Yamane K, Nakanishi S, Nakashima A, Kohno N (2006) Decreased total and high molecular weight adiponectin are independent risk factors for the development of type 2 diabetes in Japanese-Americans. J Clin Endocrinol Metab 91(10):3873–3877
76. Shinoda Y, Yamaguchi M, Ogata N, Akune T, Kubota N, Yamauchi T et al (2006) Regulation of bone formation by adiponectin through autocrine/paracrine and endocrine pathways. J Cell Biochem 99(1):196–208
77. Steppan CM, Bailey ST, Bhat S, Brown EJ, Banerjee RR, Wright CM et al (2001) The hormone resistin links obesity to diabetes. Nature 409(6818):307–312
78. Fain JN, Cheema PS, Bahouth SW, Lloyd Hiler M (2003) Resistin release by human adipose tissue explants in primary culture. Biochem Biophys Res Commun 300(3):674–678
79. Patel L, Buckels AC, Kinghorn IJ, Murdock PR, Holbrook JD, Plumpton C et al (2003) Resistin is expressed in human macrophages and directly regulated by PPAR gamma activators. Biochem Biophys Res Commun 300(2):472–476
80. Vendrell J, Broch M, Vilarrasa N, Molina A, Gomez JM, Gutierrez C et al (2004) Resistin, adiponectin, ghrelin, leptin, and proinflammatory cytokines: relationships in obesity. Obes Res 12(6):962–971
81. Yannakoulia M, Yiannakouris N, Bluher S, Matalas AL, Klimis-Zacas D, Mantzoros CS (2003) Body fat mass and macronutrient intake in relation to circulating soluble leptin receptor, free leptin index, adiponectin, and resistin concentrations in healthy humans. J Clin Endocrinol Metab 88(4):1730–1736
82. Fain JN, Madan AK, Hiler ML, Cheema P, Bahouth SW (2004) Comparison of the release of adipokines by adipose tissue, adipose tissue matrix, and adipocytes from visceral and subcutaneous abdominal adipose tissues of obese humans. Endocrinology 145(5):2273–2282
83. Fernandez-Real JM, Ricart W (2003) Insulin resistance and chronic cardiovascular inflammatory syndrome. Endocr Rev 24(3):278–301
84. Das UN (2001) Is obesity an inflammatory condition? Nutrition 17(11–12):953–966
85. Kristiansen OP, Mandrup-Poulsen T (2005) Interleukin-6 and diabetes: the good, the bad, or the indifferent? Diabetes 54(Suppl 2):S114–S124
86. Nelson LR, Bulun SE (2001) Estrogen production and action. J Am Acad Dermatol 45(3 Suppl):S116–S124
87. Okazaki R, Inoue D, Shibata M, Saika M, Kido S, Ooka H et al (2002) Estrogen promotes early osteoblast differentiation and inhibits adipocyte differentiation in mouse bone marrow stromal cell lines that express estrogen receptor (ER) alpha or beta. Endocrinology 143(6):2349–2356
88. Benayahu D, Shur I, Ben-Eliyahu S (2000) Hormonal changes affect the bone and bone marrow cells in a rat model. J Cell Biochem 79(3):407–415
89. Elbaz A, Rivas D, Duque G (2009) Effect of estrogens on bone marrow adipogenesis and Sirt1 in aging C57BL/6J mice. Biogerontology 10(6):747–755
90. Somjen D, Katzburg S, Kohen F, Gayer B, Posner GH, Yoles I et al (2011) The effects of native and synthetic estrogenic compounds as well as vitamin D less-calcemic analogs on adipocytes content in rat bone marrow. J Endocrinol Invest 34(2):106–110
91. Matthews CE, Fowke JH, Dai Q, Leon Bradlow H, Jin F, Shu XO et al (2004) Physical activity, body size, and estrogen metabolism in women. Cancer Causes Control 15(5):473–481

92. Napoli N, Vattikuti S, Yarramaneni J, Giri TK, Nekkalapu S, Qualls C et al (2012) Increased 2-hydroxylation of estrogen is associated with lower body fat and increased lean body mass in postmenopausal women. Maturitas 72(1):66–71
93. Anderson DM, Maraskovsky E, Billingsley WL, Dougall WC, Tometsko ME, Roux ER et al (1997) A homologue of the TNF receptor and its ligand enhance T-cell growth and dendritic-cell function. Nature 390(6656):175–179
94. Sakai N, Van Sweringen HL, Schuster R, Blanchard J, Burns JM, Tevar AD et al (2012) Receptor activator of nuclear factor-kappaB ligand (RANKL) protects against hepatic ischemia/reperfusion injury in mice. Hepatology 55(3):888–897
95. Kiechl S, Wittmann J, Giaccari A, Knoflach M, Willeit P, Bozec A et al (2013) Blockade of receptor activator of nuclear factor-kappaB (RANKL) signaling improves hepatic insulin resistance and prevents development of diabetes mellitus. Nat Med 19(3):358–363
96. Walus-Miarka M, Katra B, Fedak D, Czarnecka D, Miarka P, Wozniakiewicz E et al (2011) Osteoprotegerin is associated with markers of atherosclerosis and body fat mass in type 2 diabetes patients. Int J Cardiol 147(2):335–336
97. Secchiero P, Corallini F, Pandolfi A, Consoli A, Candido R, Fabris B et al (2006) An increased osteoprotegerin serum release characterizes the early onset of diabetes mellitus and may contribute to endothelial cell dysfunction. Am J Pathol 169(6):2236–2244
98. Grigoropoulou P, Eleftheriadou I, Zoupas C, Tentolouris N (2011) The role of the osteoprotegerin/RANKL/RANK system in diabetic vascular disease. Curr Med Chem 18(31):4813–4819
99. Venuraju SM, Yerramasu A, Corder R, Lahiri A (2010) Osteoprotegerin as a predictor of coronary artery disease and cardiovascular mortality and morbidity. J Am Coll Cardiol 55(19):2049–2061
100. Lee NK, Sowa H, Hinoi E, Ferron M, Ahn JD, Confavreux C et al (2007) Endocrine regulation of energy metabolism by the skeleton. Cell 130(3):456–469
101. Ferron M, Hinoi E, Karsenty G, Ducy P (2008) Osteocalcin differentially regulates beta cell and adipocyte gene expression and affects the development of metabolic diseases in wild-type mice. Proc Natl Acad Sci U S A 105(13):5266–5270
102. Oz SG, Guven GS, Kilicarslan A, Calik N, Beyazit Y, Sozen T (2006) Evaluation of bone metabolism and bone mass in patients with type-2 diabetes mellitus. J Natl Med Assoc 98(10):1598–1604
103. Kanazawa I, Yamaguchi T, Yamauchi M, Yamamoto M, Kurioka S, Yano S et al (2011) Serum undercarboxylated osteocalcin was inversely associated with plasma glucose level and fat mass in type 2 diabetes mellitus. Osteoporos Int 22(1):187–194
104. Kanazawa I, Yamaguchi T, Yamamoto M, Yamauchi M, Kurioka S, Yano S et al (2009) Serum osteocalcin level is associated with glucose metabolism and atherosclerosis parameters in type 2 diabetes mellitus. J Clin Endocrinol Metab 94(1):45–49
105. Kindblom JM, Ohlsson C, Ljunggren O, Karlsson MK, Tivesten A, Smith U et al (2009) Plasma osteocalcin is inversely related to fat mass and plasma glucose in elderly Swedish men. J Bone Miner Res 24(5):785–791
106. Zhou M, Ma X, Li H, Pan X, Tang J, Gao Y et al (2009) Serum osteocalcin concentrations in relation to glucose and lipid metabolism in Chinese individuals. Eur J Endocrinol 161(5):723–729
107. Pittas AG, Harris SS, Eliades M, Stark P, Dawson-Hughes B (2009) Association between serum osteocalcin and markers of metabolic phenotype. J Clin Endocrinol Metab 94(3):827–832
108. Bouchonville M, Armamento-Villareal R, Shah K, Napoli N, Sinacore DR, Qualls C et al (2014) Weight loss, exercise or both and cardiometabolic risk factors in obese older adults: results of a randomized controlled trial. Int J Obes (Lond) 38(3):423–431
109. Motyl KJ, McCabe LR, Schwartz AV. Bone and glucose metabolism: a two-way street. Arch Biochem Biophys. 2010;503(1):2–10

Dyslipidemia and Cardiovascular Risk in Obesity

12

Marcello Arca

12.1 Introduction

Obesity is a major public health problem due to its increasing prevalence in both developed and developing countries [1]. The increase in the prevalence of obesity is occurring not only in adults but also in children and adolescents, in whom relative increases in obesity prevalence are particularly striking [2]. The exploding obesity epidemic has put this emerging risk factor at the front of cardiovascular risk assessment and management. Accordingly, the American Heart Association has published several position papers to document and emphasize the health hazards of obesity [3]. Although it is clear that more obesity is associated with more type 2 diabetes mellitus and with a greater risk of developing a variety of cardiovascular health outcomes, this condition is complex and heterogeneous as a phenotype. It is well established that visceral obesity may be a driver of an increased risk of coronary heart disease (CHD). Recent reviews of the strength of the prospective relationship between adiposity in adult life (measured as body mass index [BMI]) and CHD risk have suggested that a 1 kg/m^2 higher BMI is associated with increases in CHD risk of approximately 7–5 % [4–6]. The association is largely independent of confounding by cigarette smoking [5] but is partly mediated by blood pressure and dyslipidemia. Therefore, the current review will mainly focus on the changes in lipoprotein metabolisms seen in obesity and their implication into atherogenesis. In addition, the pharmacological and non-pharmacological interventions to control dyslipidemia in obesity will be examined.

M. Arca, MD
Dipartimento di Medicina Interna e Specialità Mediche,
Sapienza Università di Roma – Centro Aterosclerosi,
Azienda Policlinico Umberto I Viale del Policlinico, 155-00161 Rome, Italy
e-mail: marcelloarca@libero.it

12.2 Dyslipidemia in Obesity: The Pathophysiological Mechanisms

Obesity significantly affects lipoprotein metabolism. The typical plasma lipid abnormality associated with visceral obesity is characterized by increased plasma concentration of triglycerides (TG), reduced concentration of high-density lipoprotein cholesterol (HDL-C), and qualitative alteration of low-density lipoprotein (LDL) fraction due to the preponderance of the small and dense LDL (sdLDL) (Fig. 12.1). There is a large agreement that these alterations have a great pro-atherogenic potential so that this form of dyslipidemia has been, more appropriately, defined as atherogenic dyslipidemia (AD) [7].

It is thought that atherogenic dyslipidemia is caused by a multiple array of metabolic abnormalities such as: (1) increased production of TG-rich lipoproteins from the liver and intestine, (2) increased cholesterol synthesis, (3) delayed clearance of TG-rich lipoproteins, and (4) increased HDL catabolism. However, an important question is which of these abnormalities is the more relevant in determining the typical lipid phenotype of AD. Several lines of evidence indicate that the pivotal role is played by the increased production of very-low-density lipoproteins (VLDL) by the liver. In vivo turnover studies have, in fact, shown that the dominant feature of AD is the increased production rate of VLDL-apo B by the liver, mainly as large VLDL particles (VLDL1) [8]. The VLDL1 production rate is the strongest determinant of TG concentration in the plasma and is significantly related to indices of insulin sensitivity [8].

The enhanced influx of VLDL particles into the bloodstream not only determines hypertriglyceridemia but is the major cause of the other lipid abnormalities of AD since it will lead to delayed clearance of the TG-rich lipoproteins and formation of sdLDL [9, 10]. In the presence of hypertriglyceridemia, the cholesterol-ester content of LDL decreases, whereas that of TG increases due to the enhanced activity of

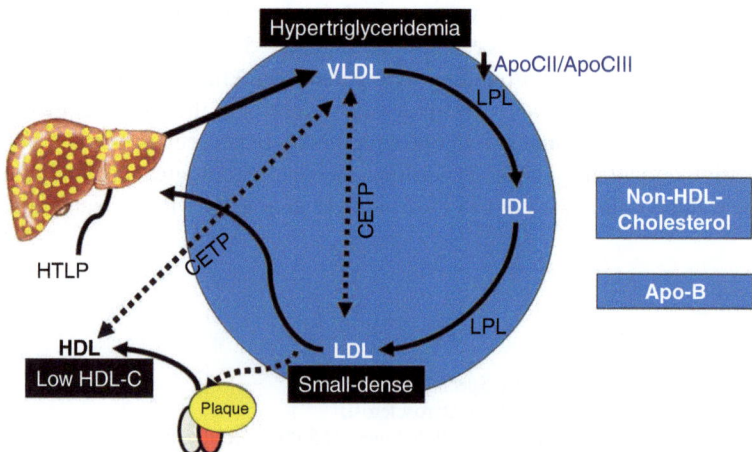

Fig. 12.1 Schematic representation of metabolic changes characterizing dyslipidemia in obesity

the cholesteryl ester transfer protein (CETP), the circulating enzyme that promotes the exchange of cholesterol esters (CE) with TGs between VLDL and LDL. However, the increased TG content within the LDL is hydrolyzed by hepatic lipase, which leads to the formation of sdLDL particles [11]. The development of sdLDL in obesity is mainly due to increased TG concentrations and does not depend on total body fat mass [12].

Lipolysis of TG-rich lipoproteins is also impaired in obesity by reduced activity of lipoprotein lipase (LPL), the enzyme that regulated the lipolysis of TGs in VLDL and intestinal-derived chylomicron [13]. Studies using stable isotopes have shown a decreased catabolism of chylomicron remnants in obese subjects with the waist/hip ratio as the best predictor for the fractional catabolic rate [14]. Additionally, prolonged postprandial lipemia leads to elevated levels of FFA, resulting in detachment of LPL from its endothelial surface [15], further reducing the postprandial catabolism of TG-rich lipoproteins. It has been well demonstrated that postprandial hyperlipidemia with accumulation of atherogenic remnants is especially linked to visceral obesity [16]. Van Oostrom et al. have shown that diurnal triglyceridemia in obese subjects correlates better to waist circumference than to body mass index [17], which is in agreement with the hypothesis that the distribution of adipose tissue modulates postprandial lipemia. There are reports suggesting that also the metabolism of LDL might be altered in obese individuals mainly due to the reduced expression of LDL receptors [18].

The increased number of remnants of chylomicrons and VLDL together with impaired lipolysis in obesity also significantly affects the HDL metabolism. As mentioned before, the increased number of TG-rich lipoproteins results in increased CETP activity, which exchanges CE from HDL for TG from VLDL and LDL [19]. Moreover, lipolysis of these TG-rich HDLs occurs by hepatic lipase resulting in small HDL with a reduced affinity for apo A-I, which leads to dissociation of apo A-I from HDL. This will ultimately lead to lower levels of HDL-C and a reduction in circulating HDL particles with impairment of reversed cholesterol transport [20].

12.3 The Atherogenic Potential of Lipoprotein Abnormalities in Obesity

The resulting effect of all abovementioned abnormalities in the lipoprotein metabolism in obesity is the accumulation of pro-atherogenic lipoproteins and the impairment of HDL function. In fact, sdLDLs are relatively slowly metabolized with a 5-day (instead of 2-day) residence time, which enhances its atherogenicity [11]. In addition, sdLDLs have an increased affinity for arterial proteoglycans resulting in enhanced subendothelial lipoprotein retention [21]. Finally, it has been described that sdLDLs are more susceptible to oxidation, in part due to less free cholesterol and anti-oxidative content [19]. Remnants of chylomicrons and VLDL are also involved in the development of atherosclerosis. Several investigations have documented an association between TG-rich lipoproteins and remnant cholesterol levels with the presence of coronary atherosclerosis [22]. This has been explained by the fact that chylomicron remnants and LDL may migrate into the vessel wall and become trapped in the subendothelial space where they can be taken up by monocytes/macrophages [23]. This mechanism may be facilitated by the fact that subendothelial remnants of chylomicrons and VLDL do not need to become modified to allow uptake by scavenger receptors of macrophages in contrast to native LDL [23]. Even though LDL particles migrate more easily than chylomicron remnants into the subendothelial space, the number of migrated particles does not necessarily translate into more cholesterol deposition since chylomicron remnants contain approximately 40 times more cholesterol per particle than LDL [23]. Other mechanisms of remnant-mediated atherogenesis, which may play a role in obesity, comprise the postprandial activation of leukocytes, generation of oxidative stress, and production of cytokines [24]. On the other side, the abnormality in HDL concentration and composition is thought to have an important impact in deteriorating the contribution of this particle to the cholesterol efflux from the cells. The capacity of cholesterol efflux, which is the first step in the reverse cholesterol transport, has been associated with increased risk of coronary artery disease and with the flow-mediated vasodilation in diabetic obese patients [25]. It has been also reported that HDL isolated from obese diabetic patients shows a reduced capacity to promote ex vivo cholesterol efflux from cells and that this may be related to a lower expression of ABCA1, which is the membrane transporter responsible for the first step of transfer of cholesterol from cell membrane to HDL particle [26].

12.4 Lipid Targets for Treatment of Dyslipidemia in Obesity

The EAS/ESC guidelines recommend testing lipids in obese subjects in order to assess their cardiovascular risk [27]. However, the necessity to initiate pharmacological treatment next to lifestyle intervention in obese subjects with dyslipidemia depends on the comorbidity, the potential underlying primary lipid disorders, and the calculated cardiovascular risk [13, 27]. Irrespective of increased body weight, LDL-C is the primary target for the treatment of dyslipidemia in obesity [27] (Table 12.1). Nevertheless, the presence of obesity can affect treatment targets since obesity may contribute to increased remnant cholesterol, higher TG levels, and lower HDL-C concentrations. Therefore, apo B or non-HDL-C levels are recommended as secondary treatment targets next to LDL-C levels in the presence of AD [13, 27]. Apo B represents the total *number* of atherogenic particles (chylomicrons, chylomicron remnants, VLDL, IDL, and LDL), whereas non-HDL-C represents the *amount of cholesterol* in both the TG-rich lipoproteins and LDL. Recently, a meta-analysis has shown that implementation of non-HDL-C or apo B as treatment target over LDL-C would prevent an additional 300,000–500,000 cardiovascular events in the US population over a 10-year period [28]. However, others did not describe any benefit of apo B or non-HDL-C over LDL-C levels to assess cardiovascular risk [29]. The treatment target for non-HDL-C should be 30 mg/dl higher than the target for LDL-C, which corresponds with non-HDL-C levels of 160 mg/dl and 130 mg/dL for subjects at moderate and high risk, respectively.

Table 12.1 Targets, therapeutic goals, and suggested strategies to control dyslipidemia in patients with obesity

Targets	Parameters	Therapeutic goals	Suggested strategies
Primary target ↓ LDL	LDL-C	High risk <100 mg/dl	Statin as first choice
		Moderate risk <130 mg/dl	Titrate according to guidelines
		Lower risk <160 mg/dl	
Secondary target ↓ non-HDL	Non-HDL-C	High risk <130 mg/dl	Intensify statin therapy
		Moderate risk <160 mg/dl	Consider adding fibrate mainly in high-risk individuals. Consider PUFA
		Lower risk <190 mg/dl	If TG <500 mg/dl initiate with fibrates before adding statins
Tertiary target ↑ HDL	HDL-C	Therapeutic goals ">40 mg/dl"	Maximize dietary intervention
			Increase physical activity
			Consider adding fibrates after LDL-lowering drugs

Treatment targets for apo B are approximately 0.80–1.00 g/L [27]. Specific treatment targets for TG levels are unavailable, especially since TGs are highly variable and increase during the day. However, pharmacological interventions to lower specifically TG should be initiated when TG levels exceed 800 mg/dl to reduce the risk for pancreatitis [13, 30].

12.5 Pharmacological and Non-pharmacological Interventions for Dyslipidemia in Obesity

Treatment of obesity-associated dyslipidemia should be focused on lifestyle changes including weight loss, physical exercise, and a healthy diet. Lifestyle changes synergistically improve insulin resistance and dyslipidemia [31]. Weight loss has been demonstrated to markedly reduce fasting and non-fasting TG concentrations, which can be attributed to an increase in LPL activity, and thereby an increased catabolism of TG-rich lipoproteins [32]. Besides reductions in fasting and non-fasting TG, a small reduction in LDL-C can be expected upon weight loss, which may be attributed to increased LDL receptor activity. A weight loss of 4–10 kg in obese subjects resulted in a 12 % reduction in LDL-C and a 27 % increase in LDL receptor mRNA levels [33]. The type of dietary fat also affects postprandial lipemia. In obese men, a moderate weight loss (approximately 10 %) induced by a diet low on carbohydrates and saturated (SFA) and high on monounsaturated fatty acids (MUFA), resulted in a 27–46 % reduction in postprandial TG levels [34]. Long-term intervention with MUFA resulted in a reduction in postprandial inflammation when compared to a diet rich in SF in patients with metabolic syndrome (MetS) [35].

Physical exercise has been shown to increase LPL and hepatic lipase activity, which stimulates TG lipolysis [36]. The mechanism of exercise-induced LPL activity remains unclear, but it was hypothesized that exercise stimulates especially muscular LPL activity. A 12-week walking program supplemented with fish oil (1,000 mg eicosapentaenoic acid and 700 mg docosahexaenoic acid daily) in subjects with the MetS resulted in lower fasting TG and decreased the postprandial response of TG and apoB48 [37]. More interestingly, physical activity has been reported to favorably influence ectopic fat accumulation (mainly in the liver) in obese individuals. Exercise training for 16 weeks in obese subjects with non-alcoholic fatty liver disease (NAFLD) resulted in a small reduction in intrahepatic TG content, although no changes in VLDL-TG or apoB100 secretion were observed [38]. Exercise-induced reductions in intrahepatic TG content have also been reported even in the absence of weight loss [39]. Moreover, intrahepatic TG content was reduced in overweight men after a low-fat diet for 3 weeks, whereas a high-fat diet increased intrahepatic TG [40]. The plasma TG-lowering effect of exercise and weight loss is the most consistent finding in studies concerning blood lipids [41], whereas increasing HDL-C levels by exercise remains controversial, especially in those subjects with high TG and low HDL-C levels [42]. Other dietary factors such as dietary fibers have been shown to improve nutrient absorption and have also been linked to insulin metabolism. Daily intake of resistant starch from bread, cereals, vegetables, and pastas is approximately 5 g/day in the Western world, which is highly insufficient for potential health benefits [43]. Recently, a randomized study in 15 insulin-resistant subjects has shown that 8 weeks of resistant starch supplementation (40 g/day) improved insulin resistance and subsequently FFA metabolism. Resistant starch ingestion resulted in lower fasting FFA concentrations and increased TG lipolysis by enhanced expression of genes like LPL coupled with increased FFA uptake by skeletal muscle [44]. However, no effect of resistant starch supplementation was observed on TG and cholesterol concentrations [44].

Unfortunately, lifestyle modifications are often insufficient to achieve weight loss and improvement of dyslipidemia, and, therefore, pharmacological treatment must be considered. The effects on dyslipidemia of antiobesity drugs are very limited, if present. A recent meta-analysis concerning antiobesity drugs reported a mean weight loss of 3.13 kg, but a very little improvement of dyslipidemia [45]. Orlistat, which reduces the lipolysis of TG within the gastrointestinal system and thus prevents absorption of intestinal fat by 30 %, showed only a modest reduction in LDL-C of 8 mg/dl. Sibutramine, which increases the sensation of satiety by modulating the central nervous system, showed a 12 mg/dl reduction in TG, whereas rimonabant did not show any lipid improvements [45]. Conversely, bariatric surgery-induced weight loss has been associated with decreased TG and increased HDL-C levels [46].

Obesity-associated dyslipidemia may well be treated with specific hypolidemic medications (Table 12.1). Statins are the first-choice agents to reduce LDL-C, non-HDL-C, and/or apo B. However, statins lower TG only marginally and do not fully correct the characteristic dyslipidemia seen in obesity, which may contribute to the residual risk after initiating statin therapy [47]. Statins inhibit the enzyme 3-hydroxy-3-methylglutaryl-coenzyme A (HMG-CoA), which is the rate-limiting step in the hepatic cholesterol synthesis. This, in turn, increases the fractional catabolic rate of VLDL and LDL together with a slight reduction in hepatic secretion of VLDL. Therefore, statins lower both remnant cholesterol and LDL-C levels [48]. Recently, strategies for combination therapies with statins to achieve even lower cholesterol levels have been reviewed [47]. Combinations can be made with ezetimibe, which inhibits the intestinal cholesterol absorption by interaction with NPC1L1, which results in an additional 20 % lowering effect on LDL-C, but without affecting TG or HDL-C concentrations [49]. On the contrary, fibrates are primarily indicated in the case of hypertriglyceridemia, and they reduce TG by approximately 30 % and LDL-C by 8 %, whereas HDL-C is increased by an average of 9 % [50]. Fibrates are peroxisome proliferator-activated receptor-α agonists, which transcriptionally regulate lipid metabolism-related genes. Fibrates as monotherapy have been shown to reduce cardiovascular mortality, especially in subjects with characteristics of the MetS with TG levels >190 mg/dl [51]. However, there is controversy about the effectiveness of fibrate therapy on top of statin therapy since the ACCORD trial was unable to confirm a beneficial effect on cardiovascular end points by fenofibrate combined with statins in diabetic patients [52]. Nevertheless, It must be mentioned that subgroup analyses suggested a beneficial effect of combination therapy of fibrates with statins in patients with AD [52]. Omega-3 fatty acids, which decrease the hepatic synthesis and accumulation of TG [53], have been shown to reduce plasma TG by 25–30 % by effectively reducing the hepatic secretion of VLDL in insulin-resistant subjects [54]. Omega-3 fatty acids have also been shown to increase the conversion of VLDL into IDL, which suggests an additional benefit for combining omega-3 fatty acids with statins by increased catabolism of VLDL, IDL, and LDL. Drugs that increase insulin sensitivity like metformin or thiazolidinedione derivatives have no or minimal effects on lipoprotein profile in obesity [55].

Conclusions

The pathophysiology of the typical dyslipidemia observed in obesity is multifactorial and includes hepatic overproduction of VLDL, decreased circulating TG lipolysis and impaired peripheral FFA trapping, increased FFA fluxes from adipocytes to the liver and other tissues, and formation of sdLDL. Treatment should be aimed at weight loss by increasing exercise and improving dietary habits with a reduction in total calorie intake and reduced SFA intake. Medical therapy can be initiated if lifestyle changes are insufficient. Statins are the primary lipid-lowering drugs with effective reductions in LDL and remnant cholesterol levels. Moreover, the addition of fibrates may be considered in case of residual dyslipidemia in subjects with diabetes mellitus, elevated TG, and reduced HDL-C levels. Apo B and/or non-HDL-C concentrations reflect the atherogenic lipid burden more accurately than LDL-C alone in obesity and should be used as treatment targets.

References

1. Knight JA (2011) Diseases and disorders associated with excess body weight. Ann Clin Lab Sci 41:107–121
2. Ebbeling CB, Pawlak DB, Ludwig DS (2002) Childhood obesity: public-health crisis, common sense cure. Lancet 360:473–482

3. Poirier P, Giles TD, Bray GA, American Heart Association; Obesity Committee of the Council on Nutrition, Physical Activity, and Metabolism et al (2006) Obesity and cardiovascular disease: pathophysiology, evaluation, and effect of weight loss: an update of the 1997 American Heart Association Scientific Statement on Obesity and Heart Disease from the Obesity Committee of the Council on Nutrition, Physical Activity, and Metabolism. Circulation 113: 898–918
4. Whitlock G, Lewington S, Mhurchu CN (2002) Coronary heart disease and body mass index: a systematic review of the evidence from larger prospective cohort studies. Semin Vasc Med 2: 369–381
5. Bogers RP, Bemelmans WJ, Hoogenveen RT et al (2007) Association of overweight with increased risk of coronary heart disease partly independent of blood pressure and cholesterol levels: a meta-analysis of 21 cohort studies including more than 300 000 persons. Arch Intern Med 167:1720–1728
6. Whitlock G, Lewington S, Sherliker P et al (2009) Body-mass index and cause-specific mortality in 900.000 adults: collaborative analyses of 57 prospective studies. Lancet 373:1083–1096
7. Grundy SM (2006) Atherogenic dyslipidemia associated with metabolic syndrome and insulin resistance. Clin Cornerstone 8(Suppl 1):S21–S27
8. Adiels M, Borén J, Caslake MJ et al (2005) Overproduction of VLDL1 driven by hyperglycemia is a dominant feature of diabetic dyslipidemia. Arterioscler Thromb Vasc Biol 25:1697–1703
9. Castro Cabezas M, de Bruin TW, Jansen H et al (1993) Impaired chylomicron remnant clearance in familial combined hyperlipidemia. Arterioscler Thromb 13:804–814
10. Hokanson JE, Krauss RM, Albers JJ et al (1995) LDL physical and chemical properties in familial combined hyperlipidemia. Arterioscler Thromb Vasc Biol 15:452–459
11. Packard CJ (2003) Triacylglycerol-rich lipoproteins and the generation of small, dense low-density lipoprotein. Biochem Soc Trans 31:1066–1069
12. Tchernof A, Lamarche B, Prud'Homme D et al (1996) The dense LDL phenotype. Association with plasma lipoprotein levels, visceral obesity, and hyperinsulinemia in men. Diabetes Care 19:629–637
13. Klop B, Jukema JW, Rabelink TJ, Castro Cabezas M (2012) A physician's guide for the management of hypertriglyceridemia: the etiology of hypertriglyceridemia determines treatment strategy. Panminerva Med 54:91–103
14. Taskinen MR, Adiels M, Westerbacka J et al (2011) Dual metabolic defects are required to produce hypertriglyceridemia in obese subjects. Arterioscler Thromb Vasc Biol 31: 2144–2150
15. Karpe F, Olivecrona T, Walldius G, Hamsten A (1992) Lipoprotein lipase in plasma after an oral fat load: relation to free fatty acids. J Lipid Res 33:975–984
16. Couillard C, Bergeron N, Prud'homme D, Bergeron J et al (1998) Postprandial triglyceride response in visceral obesity in men. Diabetes 47:953–960
17. Van Oostrom AJ, Castro Cabezas M, Ribalta J et al (2000) Diurnal triglyceride profiles in healthy normolipidemic male subjects are associated to insulin sensitivity, body composition and diet. Eur J Clin Invest 30:964–971
18. Mamo JC, Watts GF, Barrett PH et al (2001) Postprandial dyslipidemia in men with visceral obesity: an effect of reduced LDL receptor expression? Am J Physiol Endocrinol Metab 281:E626–E632
19. Subramanian S, Chait A (2012) Hypertriglyceridemia secondary to obesity and diabetes. Biochim Biophys Acta 1821:819–825
20. Deeb SS, Zambon A, Carr MC et al (2003) Hepatic lipase and dyslipidemia: interactions among genetic variants, obesity, gender, and diet. J Lipid Res 44:1279–1286
21. Tabas I, Williams KJ, Boren J (2007) Subendothelial lipoprotein retention as the initiating process in atherosclerosis: update and therapeutic implications. Circulation 116:1832–1844
22. Jorgensen AB, Frikke-Schmidt R, West AS et al (2012) Genetically elevated non-fasting triglycerides and calculated remnant cholesterol as causal risk factors for myocardial infarction. Eur Heart J doi:10.1093/eurheartj/ehs431

23. Proctor SD, Vine DF, Mamo JC (2002) Arterial retention of apolipoprotein B(48)- and B(100)-containing lipoproteins in atherogenesis. Curr Opin Lipidol 13:461–470
24. Van Oostrom AJ, van Wijk J, Castro Cabezas M (2004) Lipaemia, inflammation and atherosclerosis: novel opportunities in the understanding and treatment of atherosclerosis. Drugs 64:19–41
25. Zhou H, Shiu SW, Wong Y, Tan KC (2009) Impaired serum capacity to induce cholesterol efflux is associated with endothelial dysfunction in type 2 diabetes mellitus. Diabetes Vasc Dis Res 6:238–243
26. Patel DC, Albrecht C, Pavitt D et al (2011) Type 2 diabetes is associated with reduced ATP-binding cassette transporter A1 gene expression, protein and function. PLoS One 6:e22142
27. Catapano AL, Reiner Z, de Backer G et al (2011) ESC/EAS guidelines for the management of dyslipidaemias: the task force for the management of dyslipidaemias of the European Society of Cardiology (ESC) and the European Atherosclerosis Society (EAS). Atherosclerosis 217:1–44
28. Sniderman, AD, Williams, K, Contois, JH, et al (2011) A meta-analysis of low-density lipoprotein cholesterol, non-high-density lipoprotein cholesterol, and apolipoprotein B as markers of cardiovascular risk. Circ. Cardiovasc. Qual. Outcomes 4:337–345
29. Boekholdt, SM, Arsenault, BJ, Mora, S, et al (2012) Association of LDL cholesterol, non-HDL cholesterol, and apolipoprotein B levels with risk of cardiovascular events among patients treated with statins: A meta-analysis. JAMA 307:1302–1309
30. Brunzell JD (2007) Clinical practice. Hypertriglyceridemia. N Engl J Med 357:1009–1017
31. Klop B, Castro Cabezas M (2012) Chylomicrons: a key biomarker and risk factor for cardiovascular disease and for the understanding of obesity. Curr Cardiovasc Risk Rep 6:27–34
32. Patalay M, Lofgren IE, Freake HC et al (2005) The lowering of plasma lipids following a weight reduction program is related to increased expression of the LDL receptor and lipoprotein lipase. J Nutr 135:735–739
33. James AP, Watts GF, Barrett PH et al (2003) Effect of weight loss on postprandial lipemia and low-density lipoprotein receptor binding in overweight men. Metabolism 52:136–141
34. Maraki MI, Aggelopoulou N, Christodoulou N et al (2011) Lifestyle intervention leading to moderate weight loss normalizes postprandial triacylglycerolemia despite persisting obesity. Obesity (Silver Spring) 19:968–976
35. Cruz-Teno C, Perez-Martinez P, Delgado-Lista J (2012) Dietary fat modifies the postprandial inflammatory state in subjects with metabolic syndrome: the LIPGENE study. Mol Nutr Food Res 56:854–865
36. Ferguson MA, Alderson NL, Trost SG et al (1998) Effects of four different single exercise sessions on lipids, lipoproteins, and lipoprotein lipase. J Appl Physiol 85:1169–1174
37. Slivkoff-Clark KM, James AP, Mamo JC (2012) The chronic effects of fish oil with exercise on postprandial lipaemia and chylomicron homeostasis in insulin resistant viscerally obese men. Nutr Metab (Lond) 9:9. doi:10.1186/1743-7075-9-9
38. Sullivan S, Kirk EP, Mittendorfer B, Patterson BW, Klein S (2012) Randomized trial of exercise effect on intrahepatic triglyceride content and lipid kinetics in nonalcoholic fatty liver disease. Hepatology 55:1738–1745
39. Magkos F (2010) Exercise and fat accumulation in the human liver. Curr Opin Lipidol 21:507–517
40. van Herpen NA, Schrauwen-Hinderling VB, Schaart G et al (2012) Three weeks on a high-fat diet increases intrahepatic lipid accumulation and decreases metabolic flexibility in healthy overweight men. J Clin Endocrinol Metab 96:E691–E695
41. Mestek ML (2009) Physical activity, blood lipids, and lipoproteins. Am J Lifestyle Med 3:279–283
42. Thompson PD, Rader DJ (2001) Does exercise increase HDL cholesterol in those who need it the most? Arterioscler Thromb Vasc Biol 21:1097–1098
43. Maki KC, Pelkman CL, Finocchiaro ET et al (2012) Resistant starch from high-amylose maize increases insulin sensitivity in overweight and obese men. J Nutr 142:717–723
44. Robertson MD, Wright JW, Loizon E et al (2012) Insulin-sensitizing effects on muscle and adipose tissue after dietary fiber intake in men and women with metabolic syndrome. J Clin Endocrinol Metab 97:3326–3332

45. Zhou YH, Ma XQ, Wu C et al (2012) Effect of anti-obesity drug on cardiovascular risk factors: a systematic review and meta-analysis of randomized controlled trials. PLoS One 7:e39062. doi:10.1371/journal.pone.0039062
46. Aron-Wisnewsky J, Julia Z, Poitou C et al (2011) Effect of bariatric surgery-induced weight loss on SR-BI-, ABCG1-, and ABCA1-mediated cellular cholesterol efflux in obese women. J Clin Endocrinol Metab 96:1151–1159
47. Watts GF, Karpe F (2011) Triglycerides and atherogenic dyslipidaemia: extending treatment beyond statins in the high-risk cardiovascular patient. Heart 97:350–356
48. Chan DC, Watts GF (2011) Dyslipidaemia in the metabolic syndrome and type 2 diabetes: pathogenesis, priorities, pharmacotherapies. Expert Opin Pharmacother 12:13–30
49. Dujovn CA, Williams CD, Ito MK (2011) What combination therapy with a statin, if any, would you recommend? Curr Atheroscler Rep 13:12–22
50. Rubenfire M, Brook RD, Rosenson RS (2010) Treating mixed hyperlipidemia and the atherogenic lipid phenotype for prevention of cardiovascular events. Am J Med 123:892–898
51. Tenenbaum A, Fisman EZ (2012) Fibrates are an essential part of modern anti-dyslipidemic arsenal: spotlight on atherogenic dyslipidemia and residual risk reduction. Cardiovasc Diabetol. 11:125 doi:10.1186/1475-2840-11-125
52. Ginsberg HN, Elam MB, Lovato LC et al (2010) Effects of combination lipid therapy in type 2 diabetes mellitus. N Engl J Med 362:1563–1574
53. Watts GF, Chan DC, Ooi EM et al (2006) Fish oils, phytosterols and weight loss in the regulation of lipoprotein transport in the metabolic syndrome: lessons from stable isotope tracer studies. Clin Exp Pharmacol Physiol 33:877–882
54. Chan, DC, Watts, GF, Barrett, PH, et al (2002) Regulatory effects of HMG CoA reductase inhibitor and fish oils on apolipoprotein B-100 kinetics in insulin-resistant obese male subjects with dyslipidemia. Diabetes 51:2377–2386
55. Van Wijk JP, de Koning EJ, Martens EP, Rabelink TJ (2003) Thiazolidinediones and blood lipids in type 2 diabetes. Arterioscler Thromb Vasc Biol 23:1744–1749

Pulmonary Complications of Obesity

Dinkar Bhasin, Animesh Sharma, and Surendra K. Sharma

13.1 Introduction

Obesity is one of the greatest public health problems and a pandemic that continues to grow despite increasing awareness. The World Health Organization projects that by 2015, there will be more than 700 million obese people [1]. Obesity has several health consequences including a particularly well-established role in the pathogenesis of pulmonary diseases like obstructive sleep apnea and obesity hypoventilation syndrome. These in turn increase the risk of cardiovascular and metabolic complications severalfold. There is also emerging evidence of association between obesity and asthma where studies have shown that obesity may predate asthma, and severity of symptoms increases with increasing body mass index (BMI) [2].

Obesity impacts airway and respiratory muscle function in multiple ways. There is evidence indicating that inspiratory and expiratory muscle function is potentially compromised in obesity even in the absence of underlying lung disease [3]. In obese subjects, airway dysfunction is attributed to reduction in lung volume with airway compression. Inflammation due to circulating cytokines, vascular congestion, and intrinsic airway disease may also play a role [4].

D. Bhasin
Department of Medicine, All India Institute of Medical Sciences,
Ansari Nagar, New Delhi, Delhi 110029, India
e-mail: dinkarbhasin@gmail.com

A. Sharma
Medical School, Smt. Kashibai Navale Medical College and General Hospital,
Pune, Maharastra 411 041, India
e-mail: sharmanimesh666@gmail.com

S.K. Sharma, MD, PhD (✉)
Division of Pulmonary, Critical Care and Sleep Medicine, Department of Medicine,
All India Institute of Medical Sciences, Ansari Nagar, New Delhi, Delhi 110029, India
e-mail: sksharma.aiims@gmail.com; sksharma@aiims.ac.in

Table 13.1 Pulmonary complications of obesity

Obesity-related dyspnea
Sleep-disordered breathing
Snoring
Upper airway resistance syndrome
Obstructive sleep apnea (OSA)
Obesity hypoventilation syndrome
Obesity-related respiratory failure
Severe OSA with associated hypercapnia
Lone obesity hypoventilation syndrome (OHS)
Combined OHS and OSA
Asthma
Increased severity of symptoms
Possible role in etiology
Chronic obstructive pulmonary disease (COPD)
Decreased mortality
Overlap syndrome (COPD and OSA)
Anesthesia-related complication
Difficult bag and mask ventilation
Difficult endotracheal intubation
Perioperative atelectasis and hypoxemia

In this chapter, we will discuss in detail the mechanisms underlying pulmonary dysfunction in obesity and the clinical manifestations and management of obesity-related lung disorders. The pulmonary complications of obesity are summarized in Table 13.1.

13.2 Role of Fat Distribution

Studies have shown that the effects of obesity on the respiratory system are influenced more by the distribution of fat rather than the absolute value of weight or BMI. *Central obesity* (upper body fat distribution) is more common in males and is caused by deposition of adipose tissue in the abdomen, anterior abdominal wall, and anterior chest wall while *peripheral obesity* (lower body fat distribution) is associated with excess subcutaneous fat. The two can be distinguished by *waist circumference to hip ratio* (WHR) with ratios greater than 0.95 being indicative of central obesity. *Subscapular* and *biceps skinfold thickness* can also be used as indirect measures of upper body fat distribution [5]. Higher values of WHR and abdominal height correlate well with decline in lung function [6–8]. Central obesity increases the resistive load on the respiratory muscles and decreases diaphragmatic excursion, thereby, limiting expansion of basal lung units and premature closure of peripheral lung airways. In contrast, peripheral obesity is associated with minimal compromise of lung function and, thereby, less obesity-related complications.

13.3 Effect of Obesity on Pulmonary Mechanics

Obesity affects virtually all parameters of lung function testing. Obese patients have lower *lung compliance*, chest wall compliance, and total respiratory compliance [9, 10]. Among the static lung volumes, a consistent relationship has been established with increase in BMI and reduction in expiratory reserve volume (ERV) and hence the functional residual capacity (FRC) [11] (Fig. 13.1). Weight loading of the thoracic chest wall causes normal tidal respiration to occur at lower levels of FRC. Intra-abdominal fat deposition decreases diaphragmatic movements resulting in micro-atelectasis and early closure of small airways in the basal juxta-diaphragmatic lung units and, therefore, volume loss and reduction in FRC and ERV. Figure 13.1 illustrates the effect of obesity on static lung volumes. Among the dynamic lung volumes, forced expiratory volume in first second (FEV_1) and forced vital capacity (FVC) are generally well preserved until extreme elevations in BMI [12]. Excessively obese patients tend to have low FEV_1 and FVC with FEV_1/FVC ratio being normal (>70 %) suggestive of a restrictive pattern [13].

Airway resistance is higher in obese individuals compared to normal controls. This can be explained in part by the low lung volumes at which normal tidal respiration occurs in these patients leading to closure of small airways [14]. Studies have shown that corrected for lung volume, the airway conductance (inverse of airway resistance) is normal in obese subjects [15]. A positive correlation between airway conductance and FRC has been established; however, there is no conclusive evidence to support a

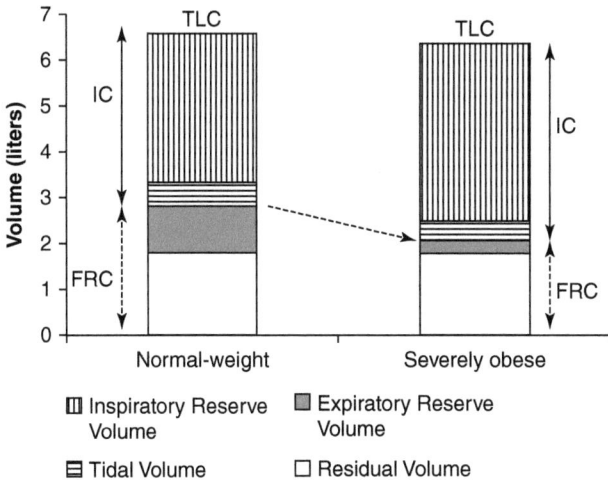

Fig. 13.1 Effect of obesity on lung volumes: Expiratory reserve volume (*ERV*) decreases in obesity. The functional residual capacity (*FRC*), sum of ERV and residual volume, is reduced, often approaching residual volume (see *arrow*). The decline in FRC in obese subjects is primarily the result of reduced ERV. Compensatory increase in inspiratory reserve volume may occur so that the total lung capacity (*TLC*, the sum of FRC and inspiratory capacity or *IC*) is often normal (Reproduced with permission from Sood [11])

relation between absolute BMI and airway conductance [16]. Inflammatory cytokines (*adipokines*) released by adipose tissue have also been hypothesized to contribute to airway inflammation and increased airway resistance [17].

Obese individuals generally have normal arterial oxygen pressure (PaO_2), but *alveolar-arterial oxygen gradient* [$P(A-a)O_2$] is often widened, especially in morbidly obese subjects who may also have hypoxemia. This is explained by *ventilation-perfusion (V/Q) mismatch* secondary to premature closure of airways in dependent portions of the lungs which have good perfusion but are underventilated [18]. These changes are more marked in the supine position while $P(A-a)O_2$ gradient and PaO_2 improve during exercise which is explained by recruitment of the collapsed basal units [19]. Recent studies have shown a correlation between WHR and changes in PaO_2, $PaCO_2$, and $P(A-a)O_2$ gradient [20]. Gas exchange is generally normal in obese subjects with some studies showing that DLco when corrected for lung volume in extremely obese (height/weight ratio > 1.10) may actually be elevated [21].

Obese individuals have higher basal oxygen consumption which can be attributed to the increased *work of breathing* caused by higher resistive loads of the anterior chest wall, overstretching of the diaphragm resulting in lower efficiency, and increased basal body requirement when compared with lean subjects [22]. Therefore, resting *minute ventilation* is higher in obese subjects, at the expense of higher respiratory rates as obese patients cannot significantly increase tidal volume [22, 23]. Minute ventilation increases during exercise, and the increase is more marked as compared to normal subjects which can be explained by the recruitment of basal atelectatic lung units during exercise [19].

The effects of obesity on *pulmonary physiology* are summarized in Table 13.2.

Table 13.2 Altered resting respiratory physiology in obesity

Physiologic parameter	Effect of obesity
Respiratory compliance	Decreased
Respiratory muscle strength	Decreased
Work of breathing at rest	Increased
Vital capacity (VC)	Normal or decreased
Forced expiratory volume in one second (FEV_1)	Normal or decreased
Ratio (FEV_1/VC)	Normal, increased, or decreased
Maximal expiratory flow rates at low lung volumes	Decreased
Expiratory reserve volume (ERV)	Decreased
Residual volume (RV)	Normal
Inspiratory capacity (IC)	Normal or increased
Total lung capacity	Normal or slightly decreased
Airway resistance	Decreased
Specific airway conductance	Normal
Diffusion capacity	Variable
Alveolar-arterial oxygen tension gradient [$P(A-a)O2$]	Decreased

Adapted with permission from Sood [11]

13.4 Obesity and Dyspnea

Overweight and obese subjects are more likely to have self-reported dyspnea at rest and exertion compared with lean individuals even in the absence of an underlying pulmonary disease [24, 25]. Prior studies have suggested that the increased perception of dyspnea in obese patient may be related to increased work of breathing and lower efficiency of respiratory muscles [24, 26]. Weight loss can reverse these symptoms; however, it still remains to be explained why only some obese subjects complain of exertional dyspnea [25].

13.5 Obesity and Sleep-Disordered Breathing

Sleep-disordered breathing (SDB) refers to a set of conditions associated with narrowing of the upper airways. As the upper airway resistance increases, the severity of SDB increases. The least severe presentation is in the form of simple *snoring* during sleep without sleep fragmentation and daytime somnolence. At the other end of the spectrum is *obstructive sleep apnea* (OSA) wherein patients have episodes of apnea and/or hypopnea followed by arousal from sleep and, therefore, sleep fragmentation leading to excessive daytime somnolence. The presentation of patients with *upper airway resistance syndrome* (UARS) is intermediate of normal subjects and those with OSA as characterized by sleep fragmentation and daytime somnolence but without the typical apneic and hypopneic episodes of OSA. Epidemiological studies have shown obesity to be a major risk factor for OSA, and nearly 50 % of patients with this syndrome have a BMI > 30 kg/m^2. Further, in obese subjects, the risk of developing OSA increases with rising BMI, and morbidly obese individuals have 55–90 % risk of developing OSA [27]. In newer studies, *neck circumference* has been demonstrated to correlate better with risk of OSA than absolute BMI while *abdominal circumference* may be a superior predictor than both neck circumference and BMI [28, 29].

Obesity predisposes to development of SDB by increasing collapsibility of the upper airway (UA). The airway passes through a partly closed maxillomandibular bony enclosure, and increased deposition of adipose tissue in this region causes narrowing of the pharyngeal airway, resulting in an increase in *critical pressure* (P_{crit}) which is defined as the pressure inside the airway at which airway collapse occurs. As P_{crit} increases, severity of OSA increases and effective therapy of OSA requires application of continuous positive airway pressure (CPAP) higher than P_{crit}. Obese persons also have higher basal oxygen consumption and consequently greater fall in oxygen saturation during apneas/hypopneas as compared to nonobese patients with OSA of same severity [30]. Further, as OSA causes fatigue and increased daytime somnolence, the level of physical activity is likely to be lower making weight loss difficult. Studies have also shown that decreased sleep at night increases daytime intake of carbohydrates thereby promoting obesity [31]. Hence, the relationship between OSA and obesity is bidirectional, setting up a vicious cycle. Consequences of SDB can result either from sleep fragmentation and excessive daytime sleepiness

Table 13.3 Consequences of obstructive sleep apnea

Cardiovascular
Hypertension
Coronary artery disease
Nocturnal angina
Myocardial infarction
Heart failure
Arrhythmias especially bradyarrhythmias
Pulmonary hypertension
Chronic cor pulmonale
Sudden cardiac death
Neurological and neuropsychiatric
Morning headache
Refractory epilepsy
Stroke
Anxiety
Depression
Acute delirium
Endocrine
Insulin resistance
Diabetes mellitus
Impotence and erectile dysfunction
Metabolic syndrome
Automobile accidents
Miscellaneous
Hoarse voice
Nocturia
Gastroesophageal reflux disease
Polycythemia

or from nocturnal hypoxemia/hypercapnia during apneic and hypopneic episodes. Table 13.3 summarizes the consequences of SDB.

The clinical features of SDB depend on the severity of upper airway obstruction. Patients with OSA commonly present with complaints of snoring, apneas witnessed by partners, fatigue, chronic sleep deprivation, excessive daytime sleepiness, and morning headaches. Diagnosis of obstructive sleep apnea can only be confirmed by overnight multichannel *polysomnography (PSG)* which includes electrocardiogram, electroencephalogram for staging sleep, electrooculogram for detecting rapid eye movements, chin electromyogram to measure muscle tone, respiratory inductance plethysmography to measure respiratory muscle effort, nasal airflow sensors, and pulse oximetry for recording arterial oxygen saturation. *Apnea* is defined as reduction in airflow by 90 % or more for at least 10 s and *hypopnea* is defined as 30–90 % reduction in airflow for a minimum of 10 s with either a reduction in baseline oxygen saturation by 3 % or an event-associated arousal from sleep [32]. *Apnea-hypopnea index (AHI)* measures the average number of obstructive sleep events (apnea and hypopnea) per hour of sleep time and AHI $\geq$ 5 events/h in the presence of symptoms, or AHI ≥ 15 events/h in the absence of symptoms is diagnostic of OSA. Severity of OSA is also graded based on AHI: ≥ 5 to 15 events/h - mild OSA, ≥ 15-30 events/h - moderate OSA and > 30 events/h - severe OSA. Obstructive sleep apnea syndrome (OSAS) is classically defined as OSA (diagnosed by polysomnography) with *excessive daytime sleepiness* (*EDS*). *Epworth Sleepiness Scale* (*ESS*) is a subjective test, and a score greater than 10 out of 24 denotes EDS. Objective tests include multiple sleep latency test or maintenance of wakefulness test but are seldom needed. EDS is not synonymous with OSA and also associated with several other conditions. However, all patients with unexplained EDS should be tested for OSA.

PSG has critical limitations in being expensive, requiring specially trained personnel, and a well-equipped sleep laboratory. In patients without major medical complications such as heart failure, coronary artery disease, and respiratory failure, home testing using portable monitors that measure oxygen saturation and airflow has been validated and is equally reliable for diagnosis and monitoring response to treatment [33].

Sleep apnea, even when asymptomatic, confers an increased risk of associated medical complications, most importantly cardiovascular diseases [34]. Although the literature has reported conflicting results, snoring alone has been associated with hypertension, angina, and insulin resistance [35, 36]. *Continuous positive airway pressure* (*CPAP*) at night acts as a pneumatic splint, preventing airway collapse, and is the most beneficial treatment modality reducing both the AHI and risk of complications. The pressure requirement is calculated by CPAP titration during polysomnography, and modern machines have facility of *auto-CPAP* which detects changing obstruction and makes automatic adjustments to CPAP. *Bi-level positive airway pressure* (*BPAP*) machines use higher pressures during inspiration compared with expiration, and this therapy is indicated in patients with high PAP titration pressures (>13–14 cm H_2O), type II respiratory failure, and coexistent obesity hypoventilation syndrome. PAP therapy for OSA is provided with room air except for complications such as pulmonary hypertension and respiratory failure when supplemental oxygen therapy or formal *noninvasive positive pressure ventilation* (*NIPPV*) is needed. The choice of delivery system depends upon patient comfort and includes full face masks, oral masks, nasal masks, and nasal pillows. Nasal masks have greater tolerance and are generally preferred as the first choice. However, the drawback of PAP is discomfort to the patient from the delivery system and difficulty in daily adherence. Surgical procedures like *uvulopalatopharyngoplasty* may benefit patients with mild disease, but cure rate is reported to be less than 20 % [37]. Oral appliances including *tongue repositioning devices* and *mandibular advancing devices* can be used as primary therapy in patients with mild to moderate OSA or as adjunct to PAP in severe OSA [38]. Weight loss through lifestyle changes or *bariatric surgery* results in both subjective and objective (AHI) improvement in patients with OSA [39, 40].

13.6 Obesity Hypoventilation Syndrome

Obesity is central to the pathogenesis of *obesity hypoventilation syndrome* (*OHS*) which is defined by BMI ≥ 30 kg/m², chronic daytime *hypoxemia* and *hypercapnia* ($PaO_2 < 70$ mmHg and $PaCO_2 \geq 45$ mmHg), and sleep-disordered breathing (SDB) [41, 42]. Other causes of hypoventilation such as underlying pulmonary, neuromuscular, skeletal, and metabolic diseases need to ruled out [43]. The most common form of SDB in OHS is OSA, occurring in nearly 90 % of the patients [44]. The remaining 10 % of the patients have "lone" OHS with an AHI < 5 events/h. SDB in this subgroup is termed as *sleep hypoventilation* and is defined by an increase in $PaCO_2$ by 10 mmHg during sleep or significant decline in oxygen saturation not explained by apnea or hypopnea [41, 43]. While majority of OHS patients have OSA, a causal relationship between the two has not been established [44]. Among patients with OSA only 10 % have features of OHS [45, 46].

As discussed previously in this chapter, obesity causes restrictive lung functions and increased basal demands. Normal obese subjects can meet these demands by increasing their respiratory drive. However, patients with OHS have greater respiratory restriction and have poor central responsiveness to hypoxemia and hypercapnia resulting in chronic hypoventilation [47]. Leptin has been shown to increase central responsiveness in obese individuals, and patients with OHS have high *leptin* levels indicative of *leptin resistance* [48]. In addition to hypoventilation, V/Q mismatch secondary to physiologic effects of obesity, as already mentioned, also contributes to the daytime hypoxemia and increased $P(A-a)O_2$. Nonetheless, why some obese patients develop OHS and others do not is still not clearly understood.

As most patients with OHS have OSA, they are predisposed to all its ensuing consequences (Table 13.3). However, the risk for cardiovascular disease and mortality is significantly higher in patients with OHS when compared with pure OSA, with a particularly increased incidence of *pulmonary hypertension, chronic cor pulmonale,* and *right heart failure* [47]. The term *Pickwickian syndrome,* first used in 1956, represents patients with severe manifestation of OHS who have morbid obesity, dyspnea at rest, excessive daytime sleepiness, cyanosis (hypoxemia) and facial plethora (secondary to polycythemia), hypoxemia and hypercapnia on arterial gases, pulmonary hypertension, and right heart failure [49].

Treatment for OHS is multimodal requiring *noninvasive ventilation (NIV)*, weight loss, and rehabilitation. NIV is the first-line of treatment, and as most patients have coexistent OSA, *CPAP* is the preferred initial mode. Patients not able to tolerate CPAP (because of high pressures) or where no therapeutic response is seen with CPAP are likely to benefit from *BPAP*, which may be the preferred modality of treatment in patient with "pure" OHS. Weight reduction can be achieved using lifestyle modifications; however, *bariatric surgery* has a significant impact on improvement in both diurnal hypoventilation and spirometric variables postsurgery [50].

Pharmacotherapeutic agents studied for the treatment of OHS include *medroxyprogesterone* and *acetazolamide*. Medroxyprogesterone is a respiratory stimulant that increases respiratory drive while acetazolamide depletes bicarbonate and increases sensitivity of respiratory centers to hypercapnia [51, 52]. These drugs increase alveolar ventilation; however, they do not reverse the underlying pathophysiology of OHS, and their long-term safety has not been studied. The doses of medroxyprogesterone used in OHS may increase the risk of *DVT* [53].

13.7 Obesity and Asthma

Obese subjects have greater frequency of self-reported symptoms of dyspnea and wheezing and are often erroneously diagnosed with asthma. The dyspnea in obese individuals is attributable to low lung volumes during tidal ventilation which decreases the caliber of airways and produces obstructive symptoms. However, epidemiological studies suggest the prevalence of asthma to be higher in overweight and obese subjects when compared to normal population even though a causal relationship between the two has been difficult to establish [54]. This could possibly be explained by common respiratory symptomatology of dyspnea and wheezing between the two disease states. Further studies have shown that obesity is not associated with increased *airway hyperresponsiveness*, elevated IgE levels, and raised eosinophil counts [55, 56]. Nonetheless, obese patients are more likely to have severe manifestation of asthma with more acute exacerbations, increased requirement of bronchodilators, more frequent emergency admissions, and longer durations of hospital stay [57]. In the obese asthmatic patient, weight loss has been associated with improvement in morbidity, mortality, and overall health status [58]. The systemic inflammatory effects of obesity mediated by IL-6, IL-8 and TNF-alpha, and *adipokines* such as *leptin* have been suggested to increase airway inflammation resulting in increased symptoms and glucocorticoid insensitivity seen in some patients with asthma [59, 60].

13.8 Obesity and COPD

Obesity has paradoxical effects on both symptoms and mortality in patients with COPD. Obese and overweight patients with COPD have a lower mortality when compared with normal-weight patients while underweight patients have the highest mortality [61]. The possible explanation for this lies in that weight loss in COPD patients is because of loss of skeletal muscle mass, in the setting of chronic systemic inflammation, which results in respiratory muscle weakness and deterioration of lung function. Hence, *fat-free muscle (FFM)* index may provide added information in COPD patients than measuring the BMI alone. Further, nutritional supplementation in COPD has been shown to increase body weight, decrease airflow limitation, and improve overall quality of life [62].

Studies have also shown that for the same airflow limitation, obese patients with COPD are likely to have less dyspnea and greater exercise tolerance. The restrictive effects of obesity on the lungs decrease compliance and reduce FRC, thereby, mitigating the dynamic hyperinflation associated with small airway obstruction in COPD resulting in improved exercise tolerance [63]. It is still not clearly understood if the beneficial effects of obesity, as defined by BMI, are related to the greater fat-free muscle mass or weight loading effects of obesity on respiratory mechanics, but the effect on mortality is consistent across studies especially for patients with severe COPD. Further, among COPD patients undergoing pulmonary rehabilitation, outcomes are similar in obese and nonobese patients, even though obese patients are often referred at an earlier stage of the disease [64].

While obesity confers survival advantage in patients with COPD, the scenario is different for patients who have COPD with coexistent OSA, described as *overlap syndrome*. The overlap syndrome is reported to occur in around 1 % of adult males; however, subclinical forms are likely to be more prevalent [65]. These patients not only have greater morbidity but increased overall mortality and cardiovascular mortality when compared to patients with either OSA or COPD alone [66]. Nocturnal hypoxemia and daytime hypercapnia is more severe and the risk for *pulmonary hypertension* and *chronic cor pulmonale* is higher [67]. Obese patients with COPD should be screened for OSA, and those at high risk should undergo PSG to establish diagnosis, as timely initiation of CPAP therapy improves outcomes including mortality [66, 68]. Hypoxemic patients may need supplemental oxygen therapy in addition to CPAP.

13.9 Obesity and Anesthesia

Obese patients pose a challenge to the anesthetist right from the point of induction to postoperative recovery. *Airway management* is often difficult in view of increased neck circumference, narrower upper airway, larger tongue size, and diminished neck flexibility. The increased collapsibility of the upper airway in obese patients, especially those with OSA, can prevent proper *bag and mask ventilation*. BMI greater than 30 kg/m^2, snoring, sleep apnea, and thick neck are known predictors of difficult intubation [69]. Also, as obese patients have lower respiratory reserves and greater oxygen requirement, oxygen saturation is likely to fall more rapidly following preoxygenation. Elevating the head end up by 25° during preoxygenation or delivering oxygen to the nasopharynx at 5 L/min via a 10 F catheter during direct laryngoscopy may delay the rapid desaturation during airway *intubation* [70, 71].

Mechanical ventilation disrupts the normal physiology of the lungs resulting in basal atelectasis. This is more marked in obese individuals because of lower resting lung volumes, smaller airway caliber, and cephalad displacement of the diaphragm in the supine position. Atelectasis leads to *V/Q mismatch* causing intraoperative hypoxemia for which *recruitment maneuvers* such as increasing the inspiratory pressures to 40–50 cm of H$_2$O immediately after induction in addition to application of PEEP of 8–10 cm of H$_2$O can improve oxygenation [72]. There is no difference in outcomes with volume-controlled ventilation (VCV) or pressure-controlled ventilation (PCV) mode of ventilation [72]. Preoxygenation with CPAP of 10 cm of H$_2$O also decreases intraoperative atelectasis [72].

Morbidly obese patients are especially prone to upper airway obstruction following extubation, increasing the risk of re-intubation and necessitating close monitoring. Postoperative lung atelectasis is often prolonged in obese patients compared to lean subjects resulting in frequent desaturation. Simple measures such as incentive spirometry and supplemental oxygen at 3 L/min should be provided to all obese patients following extubation. Noninvasive positive pressure ventilation or CPAP can significantly improve post-extubation spirometric parameters and oxygenation and should be considered in morbidly obese patients [73, 74].

References

1. Ryan S, Crinion SJ, McNicholas WT (2014) Obesity and sleep-disordered breathing – when two "bad guys" meet. QJM [Internet]. Available from: http://www.qjmed.oxfordjournals.org/cgi/doi/10.1093/qjmed/hcu029
2. Arteaga-Solis E, Kattan M (2014) Obesity in asthma: location or hormonal consequences? J Allergy Clin Immunol 133:1315–1316, [Internet]. Available from: http://linkinghub.elsevier.com/retrieve/pii/S0091674914002024
3. Arena R, Cahalin LP (2014) Evaluation of cardiorespiratory fitness and respiratory muscle function in the obese population. Prog Cardiovasc Dis 56:457–464
4. Oppenheimer BW, Berger KI, Segal LN, Stabile A, Coles KD, Parikh M et al (2014) Airway dysfunction in obesity: response to voluntary restoration of end expiratory lung volume. PLoS One 9:e88015
5. Collins LC, Hoberty PD, Walker JF, Fletcher EC, Peiris AN (1995) The effect of body fat distribution on pulmonary function tests. Chest 107:1298–1302
6. Ochs-Balcom HM, Grant BJB, Muti P, Sempos CT, Freudenheim JL, Trevisan M et al (2006) Pulmonary function and abdominal adiposity in the general population. Chest 129:853–862
7. Wannamethee SG, Shaper AG, Whincup PH (2005) Body fat distribution, body composition, and respiratory function in elderly men. Am J Clin Nutr 82:996–1003
8. Leone N, Courbon D, Thomas F, Bean K, Jégo B, Leynaert B et al (2009) Lung function impairment and metabolic syndrome: the critical role of abdominal obesity. Am J Respir Crit Care Med 179:509–516
9. Pelosi P, Croci M, Ravagnan I, Vicardi P, Gattinoni L (1996) Total respiratory system, lung, and chest wall mechanics in sedated-paralyzed postoperative morbidly obese patients. Chest 109:144–151
10. Sharp JT, Henry JP, Sweany SK, Meadows WR, Pietras RJ (1964) The total work of breathing in normal and obese men. J Clin Invest 43:728–739
11. Sood A (2009) Altered resting and exercise respiratory physiology in obesity. Clin Chest Med 30:445, vii
12. Littleton SW (2012) Impact of obesity on respiratory function. Respirology 17:43–49
13. Abbas Q, Kooragayalu S, Vasudevan V, Vasudevan V, Shahzad S, Arjomand F et al (2011) Pft pattern of restrictive ventilatory defect in obesity and its diagnostic value. Chest J 140:684A
14. Zerah F, Harf A, Perlemuter L, Lorino H, Lorino AM, Atlan G (1993) Effects of obesity on respiratory resistance. Chest 103:1470–1476
15. Rubinstein I, Zamel N, DuBarry L, Hoffstein V (1990) Airflow limitation in morbidly obese, nonsmoking men. Ann Intern Med 112:828–832
16. King GG, Brown NJ, Diba C, Thorpe CW, Muñoz P, Marks GB et al (2005) The effects of body weight on airway calibre. Eur Respir J 25:896–901
17. Salome CM, King GG, Berend N (2010) Physiology of obesity and effects on lung function. J Appl Physiol 108:206–211
18. Douglas FG, Chong PY (1972) Influence of obesity on peripheral airways patency. J Appl Physiol 33:559–563
19. Whipp BJ, Davis JA (1984) The ventilatory stress of exercise in obesity. Am Rev Respir Dis 129:S90–S92
20. Zavorsky GS, Murias JM, Kim DJ, Gow J, Sylvestre J-L, Christou NV (2007) Waist-to-hip ratio is associated with pulmonary gas exchange in the morbidly obese. Chest 131:362–367
21. Biring MS, Lewis MI, Liu JT, Mohsenifar Z (1999) Pulmonary physiologic changes of morbid obesity. Am J Med Sci 318:293–297
22. Babb TG, Korzick D, Meador M, Hodgson JL, Buskirk ER (1991) Ventilatory response of moderately obese women to submaximal exercise. Int J Obes 15:59–65
23. Li J, Li S, Feuers RJ, Buffington CK, Cowan GS (2001) Influence of body fat distribution on oxygen uptake and pulmonary performance in morbidly obese females during exercise. Respirol Carlton Vic 6:9–13
24. Gibson GJ (2000) Obesity, respiratory function and breathlessness. Thorax 55:S41–S44

25. El-Gamal H, Khayat A, Shikora S, Unterborn JN (2005) Relationship of dyspnea to respiratory drive and pulmonary function tests in obese patients before and after weight loss. Chest 128:3870–3874
26. Laghi F, Tobin MJ (2003) Disorders of the respiratory muscles. Am J Respir Crit Care Med 168:10–48
27. Lettieri CJ, Eliasson AH, Greenburg DL (2008) Persistence of obstructive sleep apnea after surgical weight loss. J Clin Sleep Med 4:333–338
28. Isono S (2009) Obstructive sleep apnea of obese adults: pathophysiology and perioperative airway management. Anesthesiology 110:908–921
29. Schäfer H, Pauleit D, Sudhop T, Gouni-Berthold I, Ewig S, Berthold HK (2002) Body fat distribution, serum leptin, and cardiovascular risk factors in men with obstructive sleep apnea. Chest 122:829–839
30. Sato M, Suzuki M, Suzuki J, Endo Y, Chiba Y, Matsuura M et al (2008) Overweight patients with severe sleep apnea experience deeper oxygen desaturation at apneic events. J Med Dent Sci 55:43–47
31. Crummy F, Piper AJ, Naughton MT (2008) Obesity and the lung: 2 obesity and sleep-disordered breathing. Thorax 63:738–746
32. Berry RB, Budhiraja R, Gottlieb DJ, Gozal D, Iber C, Kapur VK et al (2012) Rules for scoring respiratory events in sleep: update of the 2007 AASM Manual for the Scoring of Sleep and Associated Events. J Clin Sleep Med 8:597–619
33. Off Publ Am Acad Sleep Med (2009) Clinical guideline for the evaluation, management and long-term care of obstructive sleep apnea in adults. J Clin Sleep Med 15:263–276
34. Kohler M, Craig S, Nicoll D, Leeson P, Davies RJO, Stradling JR (2008) Endothelial function and arterial stiffness in minimally symptomatic obstructive sleep apnea. Am J Respir Crit Care Med 178:984–988
35. Koskenvuo M, Partinen M, Sarna S, Kaprio J, Langinvainio H, Heikkilä K (1985) Snoring as a risk factor for hypertension and angina pectoris. Lancet 325:893–896
36. Shin C, Kim J, Kim J, Lee S, Shim J, In K et al (2005) Association of habitual snoring with glucose and insulin metabolism in nonobese Korean adult men. Am J Respir Crit Care Med 171:287–291
37. Holty J-EC, Guilleminault C (2010) Surgical options for the treatment of obstructive sleep apnea. Med Clin North Am 94:479–515
38. Cistulli PA, Gotsopoulos H, Marklund M, Lowe AA (2004) Treatment of snoring and obstructive sleep apnea with mandibular repositioning appliances. Sleep Med Rev 8:443–457
39. Anandam A, Akinnusi M, Kufel T, Porhomayon J, El-Solh AA (2013) Effects of dietary weight loss on obstructive sleep apnea: a meta-analysis. Sleep Breath 17:227–234
40. Greenburg DL, Lettieri CJ, Eliasson AH (2009) Effects of surgical weight loss on measures of obstructive sleep apnea: a meta-analysis. Am J Med 122:535–542
41. The Report of an American Academy of Sleep Medicine Task Force (1999) Sleep-related breathing disorders in adults: recommendations for syndrome definition and measurement techniques in clinical research. Sleep 22:667–689
42. Olson AL, Zwillich C (2005) The obesity hypoventilation syndrome. Am J Med 118: 948–956
43. Mokhlesi B (2010) Obesity hypoventilation syndrome: a state-of-the-art review. Respir Care 55:1347–1362
44. Kessler R, Chaouat A, Schinkewitch P, Faller M, Casel S, Krieger J et al (2001) The obesity-hypoventilation syndrome revisited: a prospective study of 34 consecutive cases. Chest 120: 369–376
45. Resta O, Foschino-Barbaro MP, Bonfitto P, Talamo S, Legari G, De Pergola G et al (2000) Prevalence and mechanisms of diurnal hypercapnia in a sample of morbidly obese subjects with obstructive sleep apnoea. Respir Med 94(3):240–246
46. Laaban J-P, Chailleux E (2005) Daytime hypercapnia in adult patients with obstructive sleep apnea syndrome in France, before initiating nocturnal nasal continuous positive airway pressure therapy. Chest 127:710–715

47. Teichtahl H (2001) The obesity-hypoventilation syndrome revisited. Chest J 120:336–339
48. Makinodan K, Yoshikawa M, Fukuoka A, Tamaki S, Koyama N, Yamauchi M et al (2007) Effect of serum leptin levels on hypercapnic ventilatory response in obstructive sleep apnea. Respiration 75:257–264
49. Bickelmann AG, Burwell CS, Robin ED, Whaley RD (1956) Extreme obesity associated with alveolar hypoventilation; a Pickwickian syndrome. Am J Med 21:811–818
50. Lumachi F, Marzano B, Fanti G, Basso SMM, Mazza F, Chiara GB (2010) Hypoxemia and hypoventilation syndrome improvement after laparoscopic bariatric surgery in patients with morbid obesity. In Vivo 24:329–331
51. Lyons HA, Huang CT (1968) Therapeutic use of progesterone in alveolar hypoventilation associated with obesity. Am J Med 44:881–888
52. Raurich J-M, Rialp G, Ibáñez J, Llompart-Pou JA, Ayestarán I (2010) Hypercapnic respiratory failure in obesity-hypoventilation syndrome: CO2 response and acetazolamide treatment effects. Respir Care 55:1442–1448
53. Vasilakis C, Jick H, del Mar Melero-Montes M (1999) Risk of idiopathic venous thromboembolism in users of progestogens alone. Lancet 354:1610–1611
54. Beuther DA, Sutherland ER (2007) Overweight, obesity, and incident asthma: a meta-analysis of prospective epidemiologic studies. Am J Respir Crit Care Med 175:661–666
55. Tantisira KG, Litonjua AA, Weiss ST, Fuhlbrigge AL, Childhood Asthma Management Program Research Group (2003) Association of body mass with pulmonary function in the Childhood Asthma Management Program (CAMP). Thorax 58:1036–1041
56. Aaron SD, Vandemheen KL, Boulet L-P, McIvor RA, Fitzgerald JM, Hernandez P et al (2008) Overdiagnosis of asthma in obese and nonobese adults. Can Med Assoc J 179:1121–1131
57. Rodrigo GJ, Plaza V (2007) Body mass index and response to emergency department treatment in adults with severe asthma exacerbations: a prospective cohort study. Chest 132:1513–1519
58. Juel CT-B, Ali Z, Nilas L, Ulrik CS (2012) Asthma and obesity: does weight loss improve asthma control? a systematic review. J Asthma Allergy 5:21–26
59. Sin DD, Sutherland ER (2008) Obesity and the lung: 4. Obesity and asthma. Thorax 63:1018–1023
60. Shore SA, Schwartzman IN, Mellema MS, Flynt L, Imrich A, Johnston RA (2005) Effect of leptin on allergic airway responses in mice. J Allergy Clin Immunol 115:103–109
61. Cao C, Wang R, Wang J, Bunjhoo H, Xu Y, Xiong W (2012) Body mass index and mortality in chronic obstructive pulmonary disease: a meta-analysis. PLoS One 24:e43892
62. Ferreira IM, Brooks D, White J, Goldstein R (2012) Nutritional supplementation for stable chronic obstructive pulmonary disease. Cochrane Database Syst Rev (12):CD000998.
63. Ora J, Laveneziana P, Ofir D, Deesomchok A, Webb KA, O'Donnell DE (2009) Combined effects of obesity and chronic obstructive pulmonary disease on dyspnea and exercise tolerance. Am J Respir Crit Care Med 180:964–971
64. Dreher M, Kabitz H-J (2012) Impact of obesity on exercise performance and pulmonary rehabilitation: exercise and rehabilitation in obesity. Respirology 17:899–907
65. McNicholas WT (2009) Chronic obstructive pulmonary disease and obstructive sleep apnea: overlaps in pathophysiology, systemic inflammation, and cardiovascular disease. Am J Respir Crit Care Med 180:692–700
66. Marin JM, Soriano JB, Carrizo SJ, Boldova A, Celli BR (2010) Outcomes in patients with chronic obstructive pulmonary disease and obstructive sleep apnea: the overlap syndrome. Am J Respir Crit Care Med 182:325–331
67. Chaouat A, Weitzenblum E, Krieger J, Ifoundza T, Oswald M, Kessler R (1995) Association of chronic obstructive pulmonary disease and sleep apnea syndrome. Am J Respir Crit Care Med 151:82–86
68. Machado M-CL, Vollmer WM, Togeiro SM, Bilderback AL, Oliveira M-VC, Leitão FS et al (2010) CPAP and survival in moderate-to-severe obstructive sleep apnoea syndrome and hypoxaemic COPD. Eur Respir J 35:132–137
69. Kheterpal S, Han R, Tremper KK, Shanks A, Tait AR, O'Reilly M et al (2006) Incidence and predictors of difficult and impossible mask ventilation. Anesthesiology 105:885–891

70. Dixon BJ, Dixon JB, Carden JR, Burn AJ, Schachter LM, Playfair JM et al (2005) Preoxygenation is more effective in the 25 degrees head-up position than in the supine position in severely obese patients: a randomized controlled study. Anesthesiology 102:1110–1115
71. Baraka AS, Taha SK, Siddik-Sayyid SM, Kanazi GE, El-Khatib MF, Dagher CM et al (2007) Supplementation of pre-oxygenation in morbidly obese patients using nasopharyngeal oxygen insufflation. Anaesthesia 62:769–773
72. Aldenkortt M, Lysakowski C, Elia N, Brochard L, Tramèr MR (2012) Ventilation strategies in obese patients undergoing surgery: a quantitative systematic review and meta-analysis. Br J Anaesth 109:493–502
73. Gaszynski T, Tokarz A, Piotrowski D, Machala W (2007) Boussignac CPAP in the postoperative period in morbidly obese patients. Obes Surg 17:452–456
74. El-Solh AA, Aquilina A, Pineda L, Dhanvantri V, Grant B, Bouquin P (2006) Noninvasive ventilation for prevention of post-extubation respiratory failure in obese patients. Eur Respir J 28:588–595

Sexual Distress in Obesity

14

Erika Limoncin, Giacomo Ciocca, Daniele Mollaioli, and Emmanuele A. Jannini

14.1 Sexuality and Alimentation: Libido and Hunger

Sexual and eating behaviors have a double common matrix from a psychological and neurophysiological perspective. Psychoanalysis has linked the concept of libido to the concept of hunger, highlighting the same function of these primary instincts, i.e., satisfaction [1]. Moreover, the same neuroanatomic areas, localized in the hypothalamic regions, are involved in the regulation of sexuality and alimentation [2, 3]. Therefore, the pathological declinations of these basilar behaviors inevitably regard alimentation and sexual function, as in anorexia, bulimia, binge eating disorder (BED), and also obesity. In fact, many studies have investigated the relationship between alimentation disorders and sexual problems, with particular attention given to differential analysis between obese people with or without binge eating disorder, pointing to emotional and psychopathological aspects characterizing these patients [4].

The psychoanalytic perspective of desire states that a lack of sexual activity is the main motive for an increase in libido, on the basis of the biological parallel of hunger [1]. In other words, lacking food or lacking sex activates the behavioral response that induces one to search for food or a sexual partner.

More recently, evidences on the role of sexual activity on testosterone production changed this unilateral paradigm of desire induced by the absence of the stimulus [5].

E. Limoncin • G. Ciocca • D. Mollaioli
Department of Biotechnological and Applied Clinical Sciences,
University of L'Aquila, L'Aquila, Italy

E.A. Jannini (✉)
Department of Biotechnological and Applied Clinical Sciences,
University of L'Aquila, L'Aquila, Italy

Department of Systems Medicine, University of Rome Tor Vergata, Rome, Italy
e-mail: Emmanuele.jannini@uniroma2.it

© Springer International Publishing Switzerland 2015
A. Lenzi et al. (eds.), *Multidisciplinary Approach to Obesity:
From Assessment to Treatment*, DOI 10.1007/978-3-319-09045-0_14

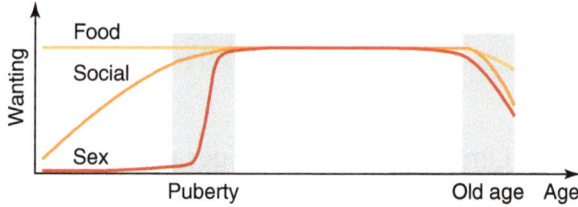

Fig. 14.1 Sex, social, and food pleasures in the cycle of life [2]

Physiologically, androgens decrease with little sexual activity, but they increase with the presence of sexual stimuli and the resumption of regular sexual activity [6–9]. Hypothalamus and the cross talk with the pituitary gonadotroph seem the site of action of the ability of sexual activity in inducing the activation of the hypothalamic-pituitary-gonadal axis [5].

This suggests for sex (but the same could be for food) that the Freudian idea about the inverse associations between a lack of sexual activity and sexual desire has to be rediscussed.

Moreover the parallelism between alimentation and sexuality was carefully examined, highlighting the similarities and the differences in these primary behaviors [2]. In particular, the authors compared three fundamental pleasures, food, sex, and social search, with interesting attention to the life cycle (Fig. 14.1). In this regard, while it is considered that sexual behavior only starts at puberty, alimentation is present from birth. From another point of view, psychodynamic theories state that a child can display specific forms of sexual behavior and hedonistic pleasure, which can be individuated in the attachment to the mother, in the sucking, in the three pregenital phases (oral, anal, and phallic), and above all during the Oedipal period [1].

Nevertheless, the phases of sexual behavior remain very similar to eating behavior. For example, the refractory period after ejaculation is very similar to the satiety after a meal, likewise the rhythmicity of vaginal thrusting and chewing food [2].

On the whole, alimentation and sexuality are composed of a motivational part, hunger and libido, and a consummatory part, i.e., the eating and the coitus.

Additionally, both the sex and the food phases are modulated by internal state, such as the blood levels of sex steroids or nutrients, prior experiences, or associations. The cerebral area involved in the reward and reinforcement processes concerning the motivation to partake in food and sex is the orbitofrontal cortex, which elaborates the associations of sex and food representations with a positive or negative judgment [2].

The other neuroanatomic areas involved in the phases of anticipation, consummation, and satiety in both sexuality and alimentation are the insula, the anterior cingulate cortex, and the amygdala ventral striatum. Moreover, it is known that the olfactory system is also central to the choice and consumption of food, and sexual behavior is also influenced by odors and perfumes. In particular, pheromones play a central role in the mating strategies of animals, and also of humans through the vomeronasal organ, which sends signals to the hypothalamic areas [2]. On the other hand, the quality of the stimuli is fundamental for choice and motivation, both in terms of sexuality and eating behavior.

14.2 Prevalence Data of Sexual Dysfunction in Obese Men and Women

In addition to medical, physical, psychosocial, and emotional consequences [10, 11], obesity is linked to both sexual dissatisfaction and/or sexual difficulties [12]. From 1966 and onwards, research studies have examined the relationship between obesity and sexual quality of life.

A US study on sexual dysfunction in obese population has reported prevalence rates of 7–22 % for women (sexual pain, arousal problems, and low desire) and 5–21 % for men [erectile dysfunction (ED) hypoactive sexual desire disorder and premature ejaculation] [13].

One of the most common sexual dysfunctions in obese men is represented by ED. Many studies have found a positive association between high levels of BMI and ED [14–16].

For example, in a cross-country study on the prevalence of ED in several countries (including the USA and five European countries), a clear relationship emerged between weight and male sexual function [15]. In fact, the prevalence in normal-weight men was inversely related to ED, whereas among overweight men there was no relation to ED while obesity is directly related, indicating that there is a correlation only among obese men.

A higher prevalence of ED in obese men has also been indicated in data from other surveys. For instance, it was reported by some follow-up studies [17, 18] that body weight was an independent risk factor for ED, with a risk exceeding 90 % of controls (odds ratio between 1.93 and 1.96, respectively).

Another study [18] shows that among younger Danish men, the odds of having ED and/or retarded ejaculation were greater for those with high BMI than for those with low BMI. Results were significant for ED in relation to BMI >30 kg/m^2, whereas premature ejaculation and sexual desire were unrelated to BMI. The association between ED and a BMI >30 kg/m^2 remained significant for younger, but not older men (See Table 14.1).

Although overweight and obesity are clearly implicated in sexual dysfunction in men, the relationship between female sexual function and obesity is not well known yet. Evidence linking female sexual disorders (FSD) to obesity is insufficient. In a study with postmenopausal women [19], it was reported that the degree of reduced sexual interest is significantly related to body weight.

On the other hand, Esposito et al. [20] discovered a negative relationship between body weight and sexual function in 52 women with abnormal values of FSFI (score <23), showing that obesity affects several areas of sexual function unlike healthy women with FSD: arousal, lubrication, satisfaction, and orgasm, but not desire and pain (Fig. 14.2).

Data from a study based on a sample of obese women preparing for bariatric surgery [21] confirm the results of Esposito's study, except for the area of desire, which is significantly lower in the sample of obese women than in the control group.

Finally, a study concerning gender differences regarding sexual quality of life in obesity [22] compared Sexual Life item responses by BMI category (Class I, II, and

Table 14.1 BMI and sexual functioning among 1,181 Danish men aged 20–45 and 50–75 years [18]

Odds ratios (95 % confidence intervals)			
BMI (kg/m²)	<25	25–29.9	>30
Erectile dysfunction			
20–45 years	1 (reference)	1.22 (0.5–2.5)	2.74 (1.1–6.8)
50–75 years	1 (reference)	1.00 (0.6–1.8)	1.40 (0.6–3.1)
Premature ejaculation			
20–45 years	1 (reference)	0.86 (0.6–1.2)	1.19 (0.7–2.0)
50–75 years	1 (reference)	1.23 (0.7–2.1)	1.58 (0.7–3.4)
No sexual desire			
20–45 years	1 (reference)	1.05 (0.4–2.4)	0.39 (0.1–3.1)
50–75 years	1 (reference)	1.43 (0.6–3.6)	1.08 (0.3–4.5)
Retarded ejaculation			
20–45 years	1 (reference)	0.33 (0.1–1.2)	1.30 (0.3–4.8)
50–75 years	1 (reference)	0.97 (0.4–2.2)	0.90 (0.3–3.1)

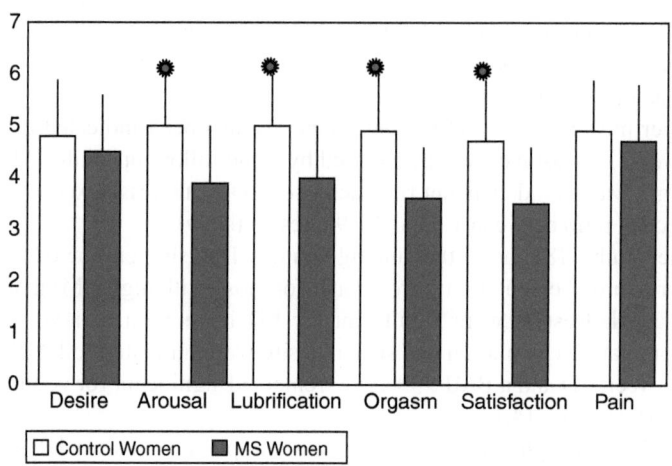

Fig. 14.2 Individual domains of female sexual function in women with metabolic syndrome (*SM*) and in control women (From Esposito et al. [20], modified)

III obesity) and sex (Table 14.2). In line with previous studies, significant differences are reported by the BMI group for all Sexual Life items, except for sexual desire. Subjects with BMI >40 kg/m², compared with the other two groups of obese subjects, had less sexual enjoyment, more difficulty with sexual performance, and greater avoidance of sexual encounters.

Women reported greater impairments than men in sexual enjoyment, desire, and avoidance of sexual encounters, but did not differ in terms of difficulties with sexual performance.

Table 14.2 IWQOL-Lite sexual life responses by BMI category [22]

	BMI category				
	Class I (30–34.9 kg/m^2) ($n=159$)	Class II (35–39.9 kg/m^2) ($n=277$)	Class III (>40 kg/m^2) ($n=722$)	p	Post hoc
Do not enjoy sexual activity					
Women	2.34±1.36	2.59±1.33	3.00±1.46	<0.001	III>II>I
Men	1.68±1.02	1.93±1.14	2.11±1.36	<0.001	F>M
Have little sexual desire					
Women	2.89±1.32	2.72±1.31	3.09±1.41	0.109	
Men	2.29±1.22	2.41±1.23	2.43±1.27	<0.001	F>M
Difficulty with sexual performance					
Women	2.31±1.37	2.55±1.36	3.08±1.41	<0.001	III>II>I
Men	2.17±1.05	2.58±1.25	2.78±1.40	0.173	
Avoid sexual encounters					
Women	2.67±1.46	2.72±1.43	3.02±1.52	0.002	III>II,I
Men	1.88±0.98	2.15±1.12	2.35±1.38	<0.00	F>M

14.3 Sexual Distress in Obese Men and Women

Obesity is a medical condition implying a series of numerous comorbidities, such as type 2 diabetes [23], hypertension [24], cardiovascular disease [25], osteoarthritis [26], certain malignancies, and premature mortality [27]. In addition, obesity is often associated with an impairment in general health-related quality of life (HRQoL) [28–30]. An important aspect of quality of life is sexual well-being. However, this aspect is often underestimated as a potential cause of distress in people affected by extreme obesity. The relationship of obesity with sexual functioning is a multifactorial phenomenon; in fact, sexuality in obese people may be jeopardized not only by weight-related comorbidities but also by reproductive hormones and many psychosocial factors.

14.3.1 Sexual Distress Due to Weight-Related Comorbidities

Literature evidence clearly shows the impact of weight-related comorbidities on sexual functioning [30, 31]. Due to a high BMI, obese people have a great probability of developing in their life type 2 diabetes, which is often preceded by insulin resistance and hyperinsulinemia. These conditions determine changes in sex hormones [31], these being a decrease in testosterone levels in men and increased levels of free testosterone, C19 steroids, and estrogen levels in women [31]. These hormone changes cause ED in men and decreased desire and decreased vaginal lubrication in women, conditions that may also have a bearing on the frequency of sexual intercourse.

Apart from type 2 diabetes, sexual functioning may also be worsened by hypertension and peripheral vascular disease. In fact, the diminished blood flow can determine the incapacity of obese persons to become sexually aroused. In addition, hypertension and cardiovascular disease are also often associated with ED. For obese women, on the other hand, hypertension may provoke hypo-lubrication, difficulties in achieving orgasm, and increased sexual pain [32].

In addition, some studies have evidenced the strict relationship between obesity and sexual functioning, independently of weight-related comorbidities [9, 33–35]. In particular, it was identified that obesity matched with physical inactivity increases the probability of developing sexual dysfunctions [5, 35].

14.3.2 Sexual Distress Due to Reproductive Hormones

A large literature exists regarding the effect that severe obesity has on reproduction [36–38]. Many studies have evidenced impairment of the reproductive system due to obesity [37, 38]. In fact, obese women frequently report amenorrhea, irregular menstrual cycles, polycystic ovary syndrome (PCOS), decreased rates of pregnancy, and increased risk of miscarriage. These conditions worsen women's sexual well-being, inducing sexual distress.

14.3.3 Sexual Distress Due to Psychosocial Factors

Among psychosocial factors, the aspect that mainly bears on sexual functioning in obese people is depression [39]. It was evidenced that among extremely obese people, the diagnosis of a mood disorder or lifetime history of mood disorders is very frequent [39, 40]. In addition, a study has evidenced how severely obese women have four times more risk of being depressed than women with a normal BMI [39]. Quite apart from full-blown psychopathologies, sexual dysfunctions with sexual distress are often present in obese persons because of body image, especially among obese women. Dissatisfaction with body image bearing on sexual functioning may also be present in subjects requesting bariatric surgery without monsplasty after massive weight loss [41–43].

14.3.4 Treatment of Sexual Distress in Obese People

The most obvious treatment of sexual distress related to sexual dysfunctions in obese persons is a massive weight loss, which may reactivate sexual functioning, removing weight-related comorbidities [44]. However, even after this intervention, whether made by bariatric surgery or by lifestyle changes, excess skin and fat remain in the pubic and genital area. Dissatisfaction with body image may contribute to sexual distress because of the restriction of body movements, unpleasant appearance, and difficulty in sexual performance. Therefore, some

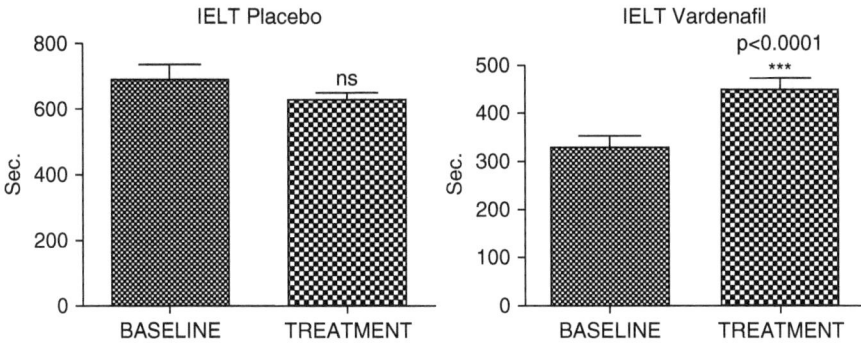

Fig. 14.3 Comparison between groups of IELT before and after treatment (vardenafil versus placebo) (Modified from Aversa et al. [45])

authors have suggested monsplasty after massive weight loss, in order to decrease distress levels.

In addition, some researchers have suggested vardenafil as a possible pharmacotherapy to improve male sexual well-being and to decrease related sexual distress levels [45]. In this study, a group of 20 healthy men with high BMI claiming not to suffer from ED, premature ejaculation, or hypogonadism were evaluated for sexual distress levels, intravaginal ejaculatory latency time (IELT), and self-esteem. Sexual distress was measured with the Sexual Distress Evaluation Questionnaire-Male (SDEQ). Half of the participants were randomly selected to take vardenafil for a specific period, while the remaining group had to take a placebo [46].

Interestingly, results have evidenced the efficacy of vardenafil for improving IELT, Fig. 14.3, self-esteem levels, and, most importantly, for decreasing sexual distress. Hence, based on this pilot study, it is possible to hypothesize that the employment of PDE-5 inhibitors, such as vardenafil, in general clinical practice, will improve global sexual well-being and prevent sexual distress.

Conclusions

Basing on literature evidences, it is possible to affirm that sexual well-being is considerably worsened in people affected by severe obesity. The reasons for this deterioration lie in weight-related comorbidities, in impairment of the reproductive system, and in many psychosocial factors related to obesity. Hence, the general clinical practice should also include the evaluation of sexuality and related sexual distress in obese people, in order to improve, through a specific psychosexological and pharmacological treatment, the obese people's quality of life.

References

1. Freud S (1905) Tre saggi sulla teoria sessuale. In: Opere, vol. IV. Boringhieri, Torino
2. Georgiadis JR, Kringelbach ML (2012) The human sexual response cycle: brain imaging evidence linking sex to other pleasures. Prog Neurobiol 98(1):49–81

3. Kringelbach ML, Stein A, van Hartevelt TJ (2012) The functional human neuroanatomy of food pleasure cycles. Physiol Behav 106(3):307–316
4. Castellini G, Mannucci E, Mazzei C, Lo Sauro C, Faravelli C, Rotella CM, Mario M, Ricca V (2010) Sexual function in obese women with and without binge eating disorder. J Sex Med 7:3969–3978
5. Carosa E, Benvenga S, Trimarchi F, Lenzi A, Pepe M, Simonelli C, Jannini EA (2002) Sexual inactivity results in reversible reduction of LH bioavailability. Int J Impot Res 14:1–7
6. Carosa E, Martini P, Brandetti F, Di Stasi SM, Lombardo F, Lenzi A, Jannini EA (2004) Type V phosphodiesterase inhibitor treatments for erectile dysfunction increase testosterone levels. Clin Endocrinol (Oxford) 61:382–386
7. Jannini EA, Fisher WA, Bitzer J, McMahon CG (2009) Is sex just fun? How sexual activity improves health. J Sex Med 6(10):2640–2648
8. Jannini EA, Screponi E, Carosa E, Pepe M, Lo Giudice F, Trimarchi F, Benvenga S (1999) Lack of sexual activity from erectile dysfunction is associated with a reversible reduction in serum testosterone. Int J Androl 22:385–392
9. Balercia G, Boscaro M, Lombardo F, Carosa E, Lenzi A, Jannini EA (2007) Sexual symptoms in endocrine diseases: psychosomatic perspectives. Psychother Psychosom 76:134–140
10. Field AE, Coakley EH, Must A et al (2001) Impact of overweight on the risk of developing common chronic diseases during a 10-year period. Arch Intern Med 161:1581–1586
11. Fontaine KR, Barofsky I (2001) Obesity and health-related quality of life. Obes Rev 2:173–182
12. Laumann EO, Paik A, Rosen RC (1999) Sexual dysfunction in the United States: prevalence and predictors. JAMA 281:537–544
13. Giugliano F, Esposito K, Di Palo C, Ciotola M, Giugliano G, Marfella R et al (2004) Erectile dysfunction associates with endothelial dysfunction and raised proinflammatory cytokine levels in obese men. J Endocrinol Invest 27:665–669
14. Larsen SH, Wagner G, Heitmann BL (2007) Sexual function and obesity. Int J Impot Res 31:1189–1198
15. Gunduz MI, Gumus BH, Sekuri C (2004) Relationship between metabolic syndrome and erectile dysfunction. Asian Soc Androl 6:355–358
16. Feldman HA, Johannes CB, Derby CA, Kleinman KP, Mohr BA, Araujo AB (2000) Erectile dysfunction and coronary risk factors: prospective results from the Massachusetts male aging study. Prev Med 30:328–338
17. Fung MM, Bettencourt R, Barrett-Connor H (2004) Heart disease risk factors predict erectile dysfunction 25 years later. J Am Coll Cardiol 43:1405–1411
18. Andersen I, Heitmann BL, Wagner G (2008) Obesity and sexual dysfunction in younger Danish men. J Sex Med 5(9):2053–2060
19. Kirchengast S, Hartmann B, Gruber D, Huber J (1996) Decreased sexual interest and its relationship to body build in post menopausal women. Maturitas 23:63–71
20. Esposito K, Ciotola M, Marfella R, Di Tommaso D, Cobellis L, Giugliano D (2005) The metabolic syndrome: a cause of sexual dysfunction in women. Int J Impot Res 17:224–226
21. Assimakopoulos K, Panayiotopoulos S, Iconomou G, Karaivazoglou K, Matzaroglou C, Vagenas K, Kalfarentzos F (2006) Assessing sexual function in obese women preparing for bariatric surgery. Obes Surg 16:1087–1091
22. Kolotkin RL, Binks M, Crosby RD, Østbye T, Gress RE, Adams TD (2006) Obesity and sexual quality of life. Obesity 14:472–479
23. Via MA, Mechanick JI (2013) The role of bariatric surgery in the treatment of type 2 diabetes: current evidence and clinical guidelines. Curr Atheroscler Rep 15(11):366
24. Kang YS (2013) Obesity associated hypertension: new insights into mechanism. Electrolyte Blood Press 11(2):46–52
25. Yao L, Herlea-Pana O, Heuser-Baker J, Chen Y, Barlic-Dicen J (2014) Roles of the chemokine system in development of obesity, insulin resistance, and cardiovascular disease. J Immunol Res 2014(2014):181450
26. Green JA, Hirst-Jones KL, Davidson RK, Jupp O, Bao Y, Macgregor AJ, Donell ST, Cassidy A, Clark IM (2014) The potential for dietary factors to prevent or treat osteoarthritis. Proc Nutr Soc 73(2):278–288

27. Borrell LN, Samuel L (2014) Body mass index categories and mortality risk in US adults: the effect of overweight and obesity on advancing death. Am J Public Health 104(3):512–519
28. Kolotkin RL, Crosby RD, Pendleton R, Strong M, Gress RE, Adams T (2003) Health-related quality of life in patients seeking gastric bypass surgery vs nontreatment-seeking controls. Obes Surg 13(3):371–377
29. Kolotkin RL, Crosby RD, Gress RE, Hunt SC, Engel SG, Adams TD (2008) Health and health related quality of life: differences between men and women who seek gastric bypass surgery. Surg Obes Relat Dis 4:651–658
30. Heo M, Allison DB, Faith MS, Zhu S, Fontaine KR (2003) Obesity and quality of life: mediating effects of pain and comorbidities. Obes Res 11:209–216
31. Sarwer DB, Spitzer JC, Wadden TA, Rosen RC, Mitchell JE, Lancaster K, Courcoulas A, Gourash W, Christian NJ (2013) Sexual functioning and sex hormones in persons with extreme obesity and seeking surgical and nonsurgical weight loss. Surg Obes Relat Dis 9(6):997–1007
32. Niskanen L, Laaksonen DE, Punnonen K, Mustajoki P, Kaukua J, Rissanen A (2004) Changes in sex hormone-binding globulin and testosterone during weight loss and weight maintenance in abdominally obese men with the metabolic syndrome. Diabetes Obes Metab 6(3):208–215
33. Kolotkin RL, Zunker C, Østbye T (2012) Sexual functioning and obesity: a review. Obesity (Silver Spring) 20(12):2325–2333
34. Esposito K, Giugliano D (2011) Obesity, the metabolic syndrome, and sexual dysfunction in men. Clin Pharmacol Ther 90(1):169–173
35. Corona G, Rastrelli G, Monami M, Melani C, Balzi D, Sforza A, Forti G, Mannucci E, Maggi M (2011) Body mass index regulates hypogonadism-associated CV risk: results from a cohort of subjects with erectile dysfunction. J Sex Med 8(7):2098–2105
36. Pasquali R, Patton L, Gambineri A (2007) Obesity and fertility. Curr Opin Endocrinol Diabetes Obes 14(6):482–487
37. Gosman GG, Katcher HI, Legro RS (2006) Obesity and the role of gut and adipose hormones in female reproduction. Hum Reprod Update 2(5):585–601
38. MacDonald AA, Herbison GP, Showell M, Farquhar CM (2010) The impact of body mass index on semen parameters and reproductive hormones in human males: a systematic review with meta-analysis. Hum Reprod Update 16(3):293–311
39. Kasen S, Cohen P, Chen H, Must A (2008) Obesity and psychopathology in women: a three decade prospective study. Int J Obes 32(3):558–566
40. Onyike CU, Crum RM, Lee HB, Lyketsos CG, Eaton WW (2003) Is obesity associated with major depression? Results from the Third National Health and Nutrition Examination Survey. Am J Epidemiol 158(12):1139–1147
41. Dixon JB, Dixon ME, O'Brien PE (2003) Depression in association with severe obesity: changes with weight loss. Arch Intern Med 163:2058–2065
42. Gilmartin J (2013) Body image concerns amongst massive weight loss patients. J Clin Nurs 22(9-10):1299–1309
43. Wadden TA, Sarwer DB, Fabricatore AN, Jones L, Stack R, Williams NS (2007) Psychosocial and behavioral status of patients undergoing bariatric surgery: what to expect before and after surgery. Med Clin N Am 91:451–469
44. Bocchieri LE, Meana M, Fisher BL (2002) A review of psychosocial outcomes of surgery for morbid obesity. J Psychosom Res 52:155–165
45. Aversa A, Bruzziches R, Francomano D, Greco EA, Violi F, Lenzi A, Donini LM (2013) Weight loss by multidisciplinary intervention improves endothelial and sexual function in obese fertile women. J Sex Med 10(4):1024–1033
46. Aversa A, Francomano D, Bruzziches R, Natali M, Guerra A, Latini M, Donini LM, Lenzi A (2012) A pilot study to evaluate the effects of vardenafil on sexual distress in men with obesity. Int J Impot Res 24(3):122–125

Part III
Evaluation of Obese Subjects

Clinical Evaluation

15

Luca Busetto and Fabio De Stefano

15.1 Introduction

Obesity is a complex chronic disease with extended and highly variable effects on individual health and function. As for any chronic disorder, a cure of the condition is the ultimate goal, but difficult to achieve. We can manage obesity but to date have no cure, and we need to use a range of partially effective long-term therapies. Combining interventions and scaling up therapy for serious or resistant disease are usual parts of the continuum of care for chronic diseases. All interventions have a range of benefits and risks, and this need to be balanced for each individual health burden and risk. This clinical balance requires a precise and complete evaluation of any individual obese patient, covering both the severity of obesity itself and the effects that obesity has on critical body systems and functions. This large body of information needs to be integrated in a general scheme guiding the therapeutic choices at the individual level.

15.2 Body Composition and Fat Distribution

A crude measure of overweight and obesity is the *body mass index* (BMI), a person's weight (in kilogrammes) divided by the square of his height (in metres). Height and weight should be measured by appropriate and calibrated scales with the subject wearing only light clothes without shoes. BMI (kg/m^2) is used in epidemiology and in clinical practice to define underweight, normal weight, overweight (pre-obesity) and severity of obesity [1]. At a population level, different and progressively increasing risks of comorbidity are observed for increasing BMI values (Table 15.1). BMI

L. Busetto (✉) • F. De Stefano
Department of Medicine, University of Padova, Via Giustiniani 2,
Padova 35128, Italy
e-mail: luca.busetto@unipd.it

© Springer International Publishing Switzerland 2015
A. Lenzi et al. (eds.), *Multidisciplinary Approach to Obesity:
From Assessment to Treatment*, DOI 10.1007/978-3-319-09045-0_15

Table 15.1 The classification of weight category by BMI in adults

Classification	BMI (kg/m^2) cut-off points	Comorbidity risk
Underweight	<18.5	–
Normal range	18.5–24.9	Normal
Pre-obese	25.0–29.9	Increased
Obese class I	30.0–34.9	Moderate
Obese class II	35.0–39.9	High
Obese class III	≥40.0	Very high

Source: Adapted from WHO [1]

cut-offs in adults are independent from age and similar in both genders. However, different cut-off points have been introduced for some particular ethnic groups, notably Asian populations, in which the relationship between BMI and risk of morbidity seems to be steeper than in Caucasian, with an increase of metabolic derangements appearing at lower BMI levels [2].

The use of BMI as a proxy for adiposity, the true determinant of the obese state, has been criticised, given that body weight is the sum of individual organs and tissues and therefore it includes adipose tissue, skeletal muscle mass and organs mass. On a population level, a strong positive correlation between BMI and overall body fat content has been reported [3]. However, at an individual level, a substantial variation in percentage body fat may be observed for any given BMI value [4]. Therefore, a high BMI may correspond to a low *fat-free mass* and a substantial fat accumulation in an obese patient, or to a large skeletal muscle mass and normal *fat mass* in a healthy athlete, in which high BMI simply reflects increased muscle mass, which has nothing to do with obesity and associated diseases. Visual inspection is usually sufficient to discriminate these extremes in body composition, but in some subjects the distinction may be more subtle, and a more precise determination of body composition may be requested. Fat mass and fat-free mass may be reliably distinguished and measured by direct densitometric methods (underwater weighing; total body densitometry). *Dual-energy X-ray absorptiometry (DEXA)* has a good reproducibility for total body fat mass (coefficient of variation: 2–3 %) and total body fat-free mass or lean soft tissue (1–2 %), and it is sensitive in assessing minimal changes in body composition [5]. Unfortunately, DEXA is not applicable in routine office practice; it is costly and exposes patients to a low dose of radiations. *Bioelectrical impedance analysis (BIA)* is an indirect method that derives body composition values from electrical data (reactance, resistance, impedance) measured during the passage of a small electrical current through the patient's body [6]. The method is applicable also in the outpatient setting and does not have virtually potential side effects, and it is relatively not expensive. However, the reliability of BIA in the accurate determination of fat mass and fat-free mass may be questioned. BIA measurements must be standardised in order to obtain reproducible results (reported mean coefficients of variation for within-day measurements: 1–2 %), and overall reproducibility/precision is estimated around 2.7–4.0 %, with prediction errors for FFM ranging from 3 % to 8 % [7]. These large errors may be even larger in obese patients and limit the utility of BMI in clinical evaluation.

A further important limitation for BMI is that this index does not convey any information on *fat distribution* (e.g. visceral fat accumulation and fatty infiltrations in individual organs) that is considered now an important determinant of metabolic and cardiovascular risk [8]. A clear evidence in favour of the inclusion of fat distribution in the clinical evaluation comes from the observation of normal-weight or slightly overweight subjects with low subcutaneous but increased visceral fat mass. This TOFI (thin-on-the-outside fat-on-the-inside) sub-phenotype has been observed in both male and female subjects and increases an individual's risk of metabolic disease [4]. The elevated *visceral fat* found in individuals classified as TOFI is accompanied by increased levels of ectopic fat deposition both in the liver and in the skeletal muscle. Lipid accumulation in non-adipose cells (ectopic fat) may impair the normal function of some tissues through a process known as "lipotoxicity". Ectopic storage of excess lipids in organs such as the liver, skeletal muscle, and pancreatic beta cells may be the causative link between fat distribution and the metabolic syndrome or cardiovascular diseases [9]. Similar findings have been already reported in obese individuals, where obese subjects with a disproportionate accumulation of visceral fat had increased incidence of metabolic disorders and cardiovascular events [10].

Visceral fat accumulation may be measured precisely with CT and MRI, but it may be difficult to quantify at a clinical level, and surrogate anthropometric indexes have been proposed. In particular, the *waist circumference* has been selected as a reliable clinical indicator of visceral fat accumulation, and having a large waist is associated to a higher prevalence of metabolic disorders and cardiovascular diseases [11]. Therefore, the measurement of the waist circumference is suggested for the determination of cardiovascular risk of overweight and obese patients, and the integration of BMI and waist values may be used to better stratify their health risk [11] (Table 15.2). Waist circumference should be measured with a plastic stretch-resistant tape on the subject in the standing position, at the end of a gentle expiration, without constricting the abdomen. Different anatomic landmarks have been suggested for waist measurement [12]. According to WHO guidelines, waist circumference should be measured at the approximate midpoint between the lower margin of the

Table 15.2 Classification of overweight and obesity by BMI, waist circumference and associated disease risk

		Disease risk relative to normal	
		Men waist <102 cm	Men waist >102 cm
BMI	Obesity class	Women waist <88 cm	Women waist >88 cm
<18.5	Underweight	–	–
18.5–24.9	Normal range	–	–
25.0–29.9	Overweight	Increased	High
30.0–34.9	Obese class I	High	Very high
35.0–39.9	Obese class II	Very high	Extremely high
≥40.0	Obese class III	Extremely high	Extremely high

Source: Adapted from NIH [11]

last palpable rib and the top of the iliac crest [13]. The US National Institutes of Health (NIH), by applying the same method used for the US National Health and Nutrition Examination Survey (NHANES) III, indicates that waist circumference measurement should be made at the top of the iliac crest [11]. The two methods did not produce the same results, with the WHO method underestimating waist values in respect to the NIH method, particularly in women [12]. It should be emphasised that the cut-off values proposed for "at-risk" waist values (Table 15.2) and utilised for the original ATP-III definition of the *metabolic syndrome* are those proposed by the NIH. The simple measurement of waist circumference has replaced the use of the *waist-to-hip circumference ratio (WHR)*, originally proposed as a powerful marker of fat distribution. More recently, on the basis of several epidemiological studies showing that having a large hip circumference may confer some BMI-independent protection from metabolic and cardiovascular diseases, particularly in women, a return to the measurement of hip circumference has been proposed [14]. The reliability of waist circumference in assessing visceral fat accumulation may be reduced in obese women, particularly at higher BMI levels [15]. Other anthropometric indexes have been therefore suggested as more effective than waist circumference for the prediction of visceral fat depots, with the *sagittal abdominal diameter (SAD)* being the more promising one [16]. SAD is determined at the highest point of the abdominal surface with the subject in the supine position and during normal breathing by means of a specifically made instrument. Abdominal ultrasonography is another reliable, repeatable and less expensive method which has been proposed to detect visceral fat deposition without radiation exposure [17]. *Peritoneal fat thickness* is considered the gold standard echographic index for visceral fat prediction in abdominal ultrasonography, and it corresponds to the distance from the internal face of the recto-abdominal muscle and the anterior wall of the aorta, measured with the echographic probe transversely placed perpendicular to the skin in the midline of the abdomen [17]. The increasing availability of portable low-cost ultrasonographic instruments will probably stimulate the applicability of ultrasonographic measurements of visceral fat accumulation in clinical practice.

The presence of *ectopic fat deposition* in the relevant organs may be even more difficult to quantify than visceral fat accumulation in clinical practice. However, liver fat infiltration (hepatic steatosis) may be roughly, albeit imprecisely, estimated by ultrasound [18]. An alternative approach to the quantification of ectopic fat accumulation may be represented by the ultrasonographic measurement of epicardial fat, which has been suggested as a further marker of metabolic and cardiovascular risk [19].

15.3 Metabolic Status and Cardiovascular Risk

Several epidemiologic studies confirmed the strict relationships between BMI and type 2 diabetes, and 65–75 % of the cases of type 2 diabetes may be attributed to the presence of overweight and obesity [1]. According to American Diabetes Association's (ADA) Standards of Medical Care, adults of any age who

Table 15.3 Criteria for the diagnosis of diabetes and prediabetes in adults

Method	Diabetes	Prediabetes
FPG	FPG > 126 mg/dL (7.0 mmol/L)	FPG 100–125 mg/dL (5.6–6.9 mmol/L) (impaired fasting glucose or IFG)
2-h PG during OGTT	2-h PG > 200 mg/dL (11.1 mmol/L)	2-h PG 140–199 mg/dL (7.8–11.0 mmol/L) (impaired glucose tolerance or IGT)
A1C	A1C > 6.5 %	A1C 5.7–6.4 %
Random PG	Random PG > 200 mg/dL (11.1 mmol/L) in a patient with classic symptoms of hyperglycaemia or hyperglycaemic crisis	–

Source: Adapted from ADA [20]
FPG fasting plasma glucose defined as no caloric intake for at least 8 h. *OGTT* oral glucose tolerance test performed using a glucose load containing the equivalent of 75 g anhydrous glucose dissolved in water. A1C, glycosylated haemoglobin performed in a laboratory using certified and standardised assay

are overweight or obese and who have one or more additional risk factors for diabetes should be tested to detect type 2 diabetes and prediabetes [20]. Additional risk factors for diabetes include physical inactivity, first-degree relative with diabetes, high-risk ethnicity, previous delivery of a macrosomic baby or previous gestational diabetes, hypertension, low HDL cholesterol level, hypertriglyceridaemia, polycystic ovarian syndrome in women, other clinical conditions associated with insulin resistance (e.g. severe obesity, acanthosis nigricans), and history of cardiovascular disease [20]. The glycosylated haemoglobin (A1C), the fasting plasma glucose (FPG) or a 2-h 75-g oral glucose tolerance test (OGTT) are all considered appropriate for testing [20]. However, the three tests do not necessarily detect diabetes in the same individuals. In particular, many obese patients may have normal FPG, but abnormal post-load glucose levels. More frequent retesting should be considered in patients testing positive for prediabetes in previous occasions. The diagnostic criteria for diabetes and prediabetes are summarised in Table 15.3. In case of diabetes, a complete screening for macro- and microvascular complications should be scheduled [20].

The association between *arterial hypertension* and obesity is very well documented. The prevalence of hypertension in adults with obesity is three to five times higher than in normal-weight subjects [1]. Arterial hypertension in obese patients is frequently unrecognised or suboptimally treated. The office measurement of systolic and diastolic blood pressure with a sphygmomanometer with a normal cuff size can grossly overestimate blood pressure levels in obese patients. The use of an appropriate cuff size is therefore of paramount importance in obese patients. In practice, a large adult size 16×36 cm should be used for arm circumferences ≥35 cm and an adult thigh size 16×42 cm for arm circumferences ≥45 cm [21]. Diagnostic criteria for arterial hypertension in overweight and obese patients did not differ from those used in the general population, and hypertension may be therefore defined as a systolic blood pressure ≥140 mmHg, or a diastolic blood pressure ≥90 mmHg or the use of any anti-hypertensive drug [22].

Obese patients, in particular in the presence of abdominal obesity or visceral fat accumulation, are frequently characterised by a particular *dyslipidaemia* with high *triglycerides* and low *HDL cholesterol* levels. LDL cholesterol levels are usually not particularly affected, but there is an increase in the proportion of a particular class of *small dense LDL particles* [1] that are considered highly atherogenic. Small dense LDL are not measured in normal clinical practice, but their presence may be indirectly estimated trough the measurement of *apo-B lipoprotein* and the ratio between apo-B lipoprotein and LDL cholesterol [1]. An alternative and more simple way to assess atherogenic dyslipidaemia in patients with abdominal obesity is the calculation of the *non-HDL-cholesterol* levels (total cholesterol minus HDL cholesterol). Non-HDL cholesterol may be used as an estimation of the total number of atherogenic particles in plasma [VLDL + intermediate-density lipoprotein (IDL) + LDL] and relates well to apo-B levels [23]. *Treatment targets for dyslipidaemia* in overweight and obese patients, as well as in the general population, are primarily based on results from clinical trials and are modulated according to the level of *total cardiovascular risk* (see below). Primary target for cardiovascular disease prevention should be a reduction in LDL cholesterol. Treatment targets for LDL cholesterol are set to less than 70 mg/dl in patients with very high cardiovascular risk, to less than 100 mg/dl in patients with high cardiovascular risk and to less than 115 mg/dl in patients with moderate cardiovascular risk [23]. Once the primary LDL target is achieved, the level of non-HDL cholesterol should be checked and targeted. Treatment targets for non-HDL cholesterol are set 30 mg/dl higher than the corresponding target for LDL cholesterol [23].

Prediabetes/diabetes, hypertension, hypertriglyceridaemia and low HDL cholesterol levels are frequently clustered in patients with abdominal obesity. This cluster of metabolic abnormalities has been labelled as the *metabolic syndrome,* and specific diagnostic criteria have been proposed [24] (Table 15.4).

Table 15.4 Clinical identification of the metabolic syndrome

Risk factor	Defining level
Abdominal obesity (waist circumference)	
Men	>102 cm (>40 in)
Women	>88 cm (>35 in)
Triglycerides	≥150 mg/dL
HDL cholesterol	
Men	<40 mg/dL
Women	<50 mg/dL
Blood pressure	≥130/85 mmHg
Fasting glucose	≥110 mg/dL

The metabolic syndrome is identified by the presence of three or more of the components listed in the table
Source: Adapted from ATP III panel [24]

The superiority of the metabolic syndrome over the combined evaluation of the single risk factors as an indicator of cardiovascular risk has been criticised, but the diagnosis of metabolic syndrome still remains useful in clinical practice for the rapid identification of overweight and obese patients with a worse cardiovascular and metabolic fate. Patients with the metabolic syndrome frequently have other accompanying metabolic abnormalities, like insulin resistance, low-grade chronic inflammation and a prothrombotic state. However, the routine measurement of insulin resistance (e.g. plasma insulin), proinflammatory state (e.g. high-sensitivity C-reactive protein) or prothrombotic state (e.g. fibrinogen or PAI-1) is not yet supported by adequate evidence, and it is not recommended [24].

All current guidelines for the prevention of cardiovascular disease in clinical practice recommend the assessment of *total cardiovascular risk*, because in most patients atherosclerotic disease is usually the product of multiple cardiovascular risk factors. Total cardiovascular risk is usually defined as the probability of having a fatal or nonfatal cardiovascular event in a given time frame (usually 10 years), and it may be estimated by using a wide array of risk assessment systems based on the occurrence of cardiovascular events in large population longitudinal studies. No specific instruments for the calculation of total cardiovascular risk has been produced for overweight and obesity, and therefore general instruments should be applied also for the clinical evaluation of these patients. In Europe, the use of the *systemic coronary risk estimation (SCORE)* system should be recommended, because it is based on a very large and representative European data set [23]. The SCORE system estimates the 10-year risk of a first fatal atherosclerotic event, and it is based on specific charts for low (Belgium, France, Greece, Italy, Luxembourg, Spain, Switzerland and Portugal) and high-risk regions in Europe. The SCORE charts are based on gender, age, smoking status, systolic blood pressure, total cholesterol and HDL cholesterol. Patients may be considered to have a very high risk when having a calculated 10-year risk SCORE $\geq$10 %, a high risk when having a 5–10 % SCORE, a moderate risk when having a 1–5 % SCORE and a low risk when having a risk SCORE <1 %. Patients with established cardiovascular disease, diabetes type 2 or type 1 with microalbuminuria or chronic renal disease should be considered high-risk patients independently from the SCORE. Patients with very high levels of individual risk factors (familial dyslipidaemia, severe hypertension) should be considered as high-risk patients independently from the SCORE. Risk will also be higher than indicated in the charts in socially deprived individuals, sedentary subjects and patients with abdominal obesity, individual with diabetes, patients with pre-clinical evidences of atherosclerosis, patients with impaired renal function or patients with positive family history of premature cardiovascular disease [23]. Considering that SCORE system estimates the 10-year risk of fatal events, the risk for total (fatal and nonfatal) events may be calculated multiplying the SCORE risk by 3.0 in men and by 4.0 in women. Alternative systems for total cardiovascular risk calculation are the Framingham Risk Score or the PROCAM Risk Score [23].

15.4 Hepatic Function

Patients with abdominal overweight or obesity and with related metabolic syndrome frequently have liver fat infiltration. *Nonalcoholic fatty liver disease (NAFLD)* corresponds to a spectrum of liver histologic findings. In most patients NAFLD is represented by a simple and uneventful steatosis, but in a proportion of cases, NAFLD may progress to *nonalcoholic steatohepatitis (NASH)*, cirrhosis and hepatocellular carcinoma [25]. Liver fat infiltration (*hepatic steatosis*) may be easily detected and, albeit imprecisely, estimated by standard abdominal ultrasonography [18]. Accompanying biochemical abnormalities are usually represented by a mild elevation of liver enzymes, with *alanine transaminase (ALT)* usually higher than *aspartate transaminase (AST)*.

The most important clinical question in the evaluation of the liver of obese patients is the distinction between the simple relatively benign hepatic steatosis and the progressive and more harmful NASH. This question remains to date substantially unresolved. The only reliable means of proving a diagnosis of NASH and separating it from simple fatty liver is a *liver biopsy*. NASH is diagnosed when histologic examination shows fat along with ballooning of hepatocytes, lobular inflammation and fibrosis. Given the rising obesity epidemic and the very large number of subjects potentially affected by NAFLD, the need for non-invasive alternative testing is rising. In the last few years, *liver stiffness measurement* (LSM) by transient elastography, with *FibroScan®* (Echosens, Paris, France), has emerged as a non-invasive test for liver fibrosis [26]. However, the reliability of LSM and its levels of correlations with histologic findings remain still debated.

15.5 Respiratory Function

The impairment of respiratory function produced by obesity is known since many years. Obese patients are affected by a restrictive respiratory impairment, with the most characteristic pulmonary function abnormality being a reduction of the *expiratory reserve volume* (ERV) [27]. The decrease of ERV and *functional vital capacity* (FVC) associated with obesity has been attributed to a mechanical effect played by visceral fat accumulation, and it is indeed more relevant in patients with abdominal fat deposition [28]. Obesity-related impairments of lungs volumes may be easily detected by standard spirometry. However, the clinical utility of spirometric testing in overweight or obese patients without respiratory symptoms may be questioned, given that the results usually do not change significantly the management of these patients.

Obstructive sleep apnoea (OSA) is a common sleep disorder characterised by repetitive episodes of apnoea and hypopnoea during sleep, accompanied by hypoventilation, oxygen desaturation, sympathetic arousal and wakening. The diagnosis of OSA is confirmed if the number of obstructive events is greater than

Table 15.5 The STOP-BANG questionnaire for the screening of obstructive sleep apnoea (*OSA*)

S = Snoring	Do you snore louder than talking or loud enough to be heard through closed doors?
T = Tiredness	Do you often feel tired, fatigued, or sleepy during daytime?
O = Observed apnoea	Has anyone observed you stop breathing during your sleep?
P = Pressure	Do you have or are you being treated for high blood pressure?
B = BMI >40 kg/m^2	
A = Age >50 years	
N = Neck circumference >40 cm	
G = Male gender	

Modified by Ref. [24]
High risk of OSA is considered if answering yes to three or more questions of the questionnaire

15 events/h of sleep or greater than 5 events/h in a patient reporting at least one of the following symptoms: unintentional sleep episodes during wakefulness; daytime sleepiness; unrefreshing sleep; fatigue; insomnia; waking up breath-holding, gasping or choking; or the bed partner describing loud snoring, breathing interruptions or both during the patient's sleep [29]. OSA severity is defined as mild for events/h ≥5 and <15, moderate for events/h ≥15 and ≤30, and severe for events/h >30 [29]. OSA is highly prevalent in the obese population and may be present in at least 40 % of patients with severe visceral obesity [28]. The screening for OSA in overweight and obese patients is therefore mandatory, given that OSA is associated with important health consequences, such as increased cardiovascular disease risk and mortality, and that these consequences can be prevented by adequate OSA management [29].

Full night *polysomnography* (PSG) is considered the gold standard for the diagnosis of OSA and sleep-disordered breathing [29]. However, PSG is a lengthy and expensive procedure and requires inhospital staying. Portable sleep monitoring devices designed for use at home have been implemented, but availability limitation frequently causes long waiting times for testing. Several screening questionnaires have been therefore proposed in order to predict which patients have the higher probability of OSA and will need PSG. The most popular of these questionnaires (Berlin Questionnaire, American Society of Anesthesiologists Checklist and STOP Questionnaire) have been recently compared and found to have a moderately high level of sensitivity and a negative predictive value [30]. The *STOP-Bang questionnaire* (Table 15.5), an extended version of the STOP Questionnaire with eight instead of four items, has a high specificity to detect moderate and severe OSA, thereby identifying the patients in which PSG is needed [31]. No screening test is perfect, and the sensitivity and specificity of these predictive tools have been criticised. However, the application of a standardised screening tool for OSA, with confirmatory PSG if screening tests are positive, should be recommended [32].

15.6 Staging

Obesity is a complex disease with extended clinical implications. Evaluation and management of any individual obese patient should be therefore based on a comprehensive characterisation of the patient's global health and on a reliable prediction of its future disease risk. On the basis of the above considerations, a more precise phenotypization of obese patients should include a determination of body composition with a reliable technique (DEXA), particularly in cases where the BMI value may be misleading, and an estimation of fat distribution and ectopic fat deposition (waist circumference, hip circumference, hepatic steatosis, epicardial fat, etc.). Phenotyping should obviously be completed by the determination of cardiovascular and metabolic risk factors and by the assessment of obesity-related comorbidities. A list of all the clinical data that should potentially be integrated in the comprehensive evaluation of the obese patients beyond BMI values is reported in Table 15.6.

Table 15.6 A list of clinical factors that should be included in a comprehensive clinical evaluation of the obese patient

Body composition	BMI (% body fat, as determined by DEXA)
Fat distribution	Waist circumference
	Hip circumference
	Visceral fat accumulation (ultrasonography)
Ectopic fat deposition	Liver fat infiltration (hepatic steatosis)
	Epicardial fat
Cardiovascular risk factors	LDL cholesterol, HDL cholesterol, triglycerides
	Fibrinogen
	hs-PCR
Obesity-related comorbidities	Type 2 diabetes
	Hypertension
	Obesity-related cardiomyopathy
	Sleep apnoea syndrome
	Obesity/hypoventilation syndrome
	Disabling weight-bearing joint disease
	Obesity-related infertility
	Urinary stress incontinence
	Severe gastro-oesophageal reflux disease
High risk for type 2 diabetes	Family history of type 2 diabetes
	Previous gestational diabetes
	Polycystic ovary syndrome
	Impaired glucose tolerance/impaired fasting glucose
	Hyperinsulinaemia/insulin resistance
Early markers of atherosclerosis	Plaques or increased intima-media thickness at carotid ultrasonography
	Low ankle-brachial index
	High coronary artery calcium score
Initial signs of organ damage	Left-sided cardiac hypertrophy
	Micro-albuminuria/proteinuria

The integration of this large set of clinical information in a comprehensive picture would be highly facilitated by the adoption of an obesity scoring system. The use of a score that could quantitatively represent the actual and future health burden that obesity induces in every single patient would be an important tool for clinicians for the phenotypization of the patients and for guiding therapeutic choices. A scoring system should also be helpful for prioritisation and resource allocation in a health system with limited resources. An integrated rating scale for the determination of the initial level of care (outpatient, partial hospitalisation, residential rehabilitation centre, inpatient hospitalisation) needed by the obese patients has been proposed by a multidisciplinary group of Italian obesity experts [33]. However, this scale has never been validated in other countries or other clinical settings. An alternative option would be the use of a more simple but integrated staging system. The *Edmonton Obesity Staging System* (EOSS) has been proposed as a clinical staging system for obesity [34]. EOSS classified obesity in five stages (0–4) accordingly to worsening clinical and functional status (Table 15.7) [34]. EOSS stage has been shown to be a more stringent predictor of total mortality than BMI levels in large epidemiological databases [35, 36]. The validation and application of EOSS or other alternative staging systems for the phenotypization of obese patients should be a focus of future clinical research in the field of overweight and obesity.

Table 15.7 Edmonton obesity scoring system: a proposed clinical and functional staging of obesity

Stage	Description
0	No apparent obesity-related risk factors (e.g. blood pressure, serum lipids, fasting glucose, etc., within normal range), no physical symptoms, no psychopathology, no functional limitations and/or impairment of well-being
1	Presence of obesity-related subclinical risk factors (e.g. borderline hypertension, impaired fasting glucose, elevated liver enzymes, etc.), mild physical symptoms (e.g. dyspnoea on moderate exertion, occasional aches and pains, fatigue, etc.), mild psychopathology, mild functional limitations and/or mild impairment of well-being
2	Presence of established obesity-related chronic disease (e.g. hypertension, type 2 diabetes, sleep apnoea, osteoarthritis, reflux disease, polycystic ovary syndrome, anxiety disorder, etc.), moderate limitations in activities of daily living and/or well-being
3	Established end-organ damage such as myocardial infarction, heart failure, diabetic complications, incapacitating osteoarthritis, significant psychopathology, significant functional limitations and/or impairment of well-being
4	Severe (potentially end-stage) disabilities from obesity-related chronic diseases, severe disabling psychopathology, severe functional limitations and/or severe impairment of well-being

Modified by Ref. [34]

References

1. WHO (2000) Obesity: preventing and managing the global epidemic. Report of a WHO consultation. World Health Organ Tech Rep Ser 894:1–253
2. WHO (2004) Appropriate body-mass index for Asian populations and its implications for policy and intervention strategies. Lancet 363:157–163
3. Okorodudu DO, Jumean MF, Montori VM et al (2010) Diagnostic performance of body mass index to identify obesity as defined by body adiposity: a systematic review and meta-analysis. Int J Obes 34:791–799
4. Thomas EL, Frost G, Taylor-Robinson SD, Bell JD (2012) Excess body fat in obese and normal-weight subjects. Nutr Res Rev 25:150–161
5. Houtkooper LB, Going SB, Sproul J, Blew RM, Lohman TG (2000) Comparison of methods for assessing body-composition changes over 1 y in postmenopausal women. Am J Clin Nutr 72:401–406
6. Foster KR, Lukaski HC (1996) Whole-body impedance. What does it measure? Am J Clin Nutr 64:388S–396S
7. Kyle UG, Bosaeus I, De Lorenzo AD et al (2004) For the ESPEN working group. Bioelectrical impedance analysis–part I: review of principles and methods. Clin Nutr 23:1226–1243
8. Müller MJ, Lagerpusch M, Enderle J, Schautz B, Heller M, Bosy-Westphal A (2012) Beyond the body mass index: tracking body composition in the pathogenesis of obesity and the metabolic syndrome. Obes Rev 13:6–13
9. Unger RH (2003) Minireview: weapons of lean body mass destruction: the role of ectopic lipids in the metabolic syndrome. Endocrinology 144:5159–5165
10. Després JP, Lemieux I (2006) Abdominal obesity and metabolic syndrome. Nature 444:881–887
11. National Institutes of Health (1998) National Heart, Lung and Blood Institute: clinical guidelines on the identification, evaluation and treatment of overweight and obesity in adults. The evidence report
12. Wang J, Thornton JC, Bari S et al (2003) Comparisons of waist circumferences measured at 4 sites. Am J Clin Nutr 77:379–384
13. WHO (2008) WHO STEPwise approach to surveillance (STEPS). World Health Organization (WHO), Geneva
14. Heitmann BL, Lissner L (2011) Hip hip hurrah! Hip size inversely related to heart disease and total mortality. Obes Rev 12:478–481
15. Busetto L, Baggio MB, Zurlo F, Carraro R, Digito M, Enzi G (1992) Assessment of abdominal fat distribution in obese patients: anthropometry versus computerized tomography. Int J Obes 16:731–736. 10
16. Armellini F, Zamboni M, Harris T, Micciolo R, Bosello O (1997) Sagittal diameter minus subcutaneous thickness. An easy to obtain parameter that improves visceral fat prediction. Obes Res 5:315–320
17. Armellini F, Zamboni M, Rigo L et al (1990) The contribution of sonography to the measurement of intra-abdominal fat. J Clin Ultrasound 18:563–567
18. Dasarathy S, Dasarathy J, Khiyami A et al (2009) Validity of real time ultrasound in the diagnosis of hepatic steatosis: a prospective study. J Hepatol 51:1061–1067
19. Iacobellis G, Malavazos AE, Corsi MM (2011) Epicardial fat: from the biomolecular aspects to the clinical practice. Int J Biochem Cell Biol 43:1651–1654
20. American Diabetes Association (2014) Standards of medical care in diabetes – 2014. Diabetes Care 37:S14–S80
21. Pickering TG, Hall JE, Appel LJ et al (2005) Subcommittee of Professional and Public Education of the American Heart Association Council on High Blood Pressure Research. Recommendations for blood pressure measurement in humans and experimental animals: Part 1: blood pressure measurement in humans: a statement for professionals from the Subcommittee of Professional and Public Education of the American Heart Association Council on High Blood Pressure Research. Hypertension 45:142–161

22. The Joint National Committee on detection, evaluation and treatment of high blood pressure: the 1984 report of the Joint National Committee on detection, evaluation and treatment of high blood pressure (1984). Arch Int Med 144:1045–1057
23. The task force for the management of dyslipidaemias of the European Society of Cardiology (ESC) and the European Atherosclerosis Society (EAS). ESC/EAS guidelines for the management of dyslipidaemias (2011). Eur Heart J 32:1769–1818
24. Third report of the National Cholesterol Education Program (NCEP) expert panel on detection, evaluation, and treatment of high blood cholesterol in adults (adult treatment panel III). Final report (2002). Circulation 106:3143–3421
25. Chalasani N, Younossi Z, Lavine J et al (2012) The diagnosis and management of nonalcoholic fatty liver disease: practice guideline by the American Association for the Study of Liver Diseases, American College of Gastroenterology, the American Gastroenterological Association. Hepatology 55:2005–2023
26. Wong VW, Vergniol J, Wong GL et al (2010) Diagnosis of fibrosis and cirrhosis using liver stiffness measurement in nonalcoholic fatty liver disease. Hepatology 51:454–462
27. Ray CS, Sue DY, Vray G, Hansen JE, Wasserman K (1983) Effects of obesity on respiratory function. Am Rev Respir Dis 128:201–206
28. Busetto L (2001) Visceral obesity and the metabolic syndrome: effects of weight loss. Nutr Metab Cardiovasc Dis 11:195–204
29. Epstein LJ, Kristo D, Strollo PJ et al (2009) Clinical guideline for the evaluation, management and long-term care of obstructive sleep apnea in adults. J Clin Sleep Med 5:263–276
30. Chung F, Yegneswaran B, Liao P et al (2008) Validation of the Berlin questionnaire and American Society of Anesthesiologists checklist as screening tools for obstructive sleep apnea in surgical patients. Anesthesiology 108:822–830
31. Chung F, Subramanyan R, Liao P et al (2012) High STOP-Bang score indicates a high probability of obstructive sleep apnoea. Br J Anaesth 108:768–775
32. Mechanick JI, Youdim A, Jones DB et al (2013) Clinical practice guidelines for the perioperative nutritional, metabolic, and nonsurgical support of the bariatric surgery patient – 2013 update: cosponsored by American Association of Clinical Endocrinologists, the Obesity Society, and American Society for Metabolic & Bariatric Surgery. Obesity 21:S1–S27
33. Donini LM, Cuzzolaro M, Spera G et al (2010) Obesity and eating disorders. Indications for the different levels of care. An Italian expert consensus document. Eat Weight Disord 15(suppl1):1–31
34. Sharma AM, Kushner RF (2009) A proposed clinical staging system for obesity. Int J Obes 33:289–295
35. Padwal RS, Pajewski NM, Allison DB et al (2011) Using the Edmonton obesity staging system to predict mortality in a population-representative cohort of people with overweight and obesity. CMAJ 183:E1059–E1066
36. Kuk JL, Ardern CI, Church TS et al (2011) Edmonton obesity staging system: association with weight history and mortality risk. Appl Physiol Nutr Metab 36:570–576

Nutritional Status Evaluation: Body Composition and Energy Balance

Massimo Pellegrini and Nino C. Battistini

Nutritional status is the anatomical, metabolic, and functional status of the body in relation to the availability of energy, nutrients, and other substances of nutritional interest; it strictly influences growth, body composition, health status, and the quality of life of the individual. In the elderly, body composition and skeletal muscle mass deficiency influence the risk of falls and the ability to lead an autonomous life. Moreover, diseases that modify the energy balance or nutrient intake can change body composition and nutritional status, and in so doing may worsen one's health status.

In obese people, a nutritional intervention will likely aim at reducing the percentage of body fat with maintenance of non-fat mass. In cases of *sarcopenic obesity*, understanding the body composition is of central importance as a lowering of the body's non-fat mass may mask increases in body fat (especially visceral fat) that are not brought into evidence with indicators such as body weight and body mass index, which may fall in the normal or overweight range. In such patients, the decrease in non-fat mass tends to affect the skeletal muscle and may result in functional deficits and a decrease in muscle strength. This condition is most commonly observed in the elderly or in patients with chronic inflammatory diseases such as chronic HIV infections. In these cases, an increased visceral fat may be associated with a lipoatrophy of the limbs [1, 2]. Recently, an abnormal distribution of adipose tissue has been also documented in anorexic patients after refeeding [3]. In all these cases, therapeutic intervention may be particularly complex and should aim at a modification of body composition through nutritional intervention, physical activity prescription, and also pharmacological therapy in selected cases.

M. Pellegrini (✉) • N.C. Battistini
Department of Diagnostic, Clinical and Public Health Medicine,
University of Modena and Reggio Emilia, Via Campi 287, 41125 Modena, Italy
e-mail: massimo.pellegrini@unimore.it

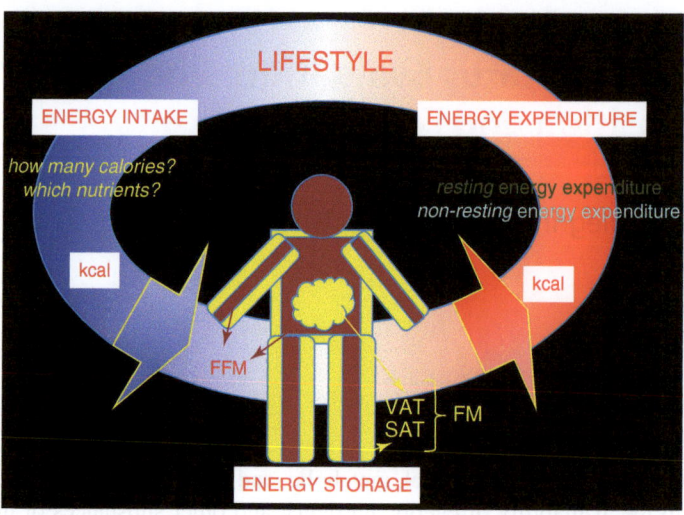

Fig. 16.1 Energy balance and body composition. *FFM* fat-free mass, *FM* fat mass, *VAT* visceral adipose tissue, *SAT* subcutaneous adipose tissue

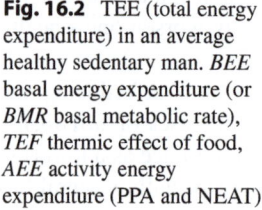

Fig. 16.2 TEE (total energy expenditure) in an average healthy sedentary man. *BEE* basal energy expenditure (or *BMR* basal metabolic rate), *TEF* thermic effect of food, *AEE* activity energy expenditure (PPA and NEAT)

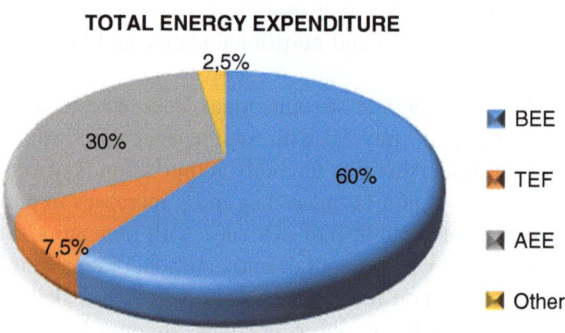

Our nutritional status, in fact, is a manifestation of the effect of our lifestyle on our body. Our lifestyle, which includes eating habits, physical activity, and sleep, is in turn, strongly influenced by psychological, social, and economic factors. In particular, nutritional status is related to the quality and quantity of the components of our diet or *energy intake* (macronutrients, micronutrients, substances of nutritional interest) and to the quantity and quality of our *energy expenditure* (Fig. 16.1). If energy balance is positive, some of the excess can be stored as fat, whereas if energy balance is negative, not just the body's fat mass (FM) but also the body's fat-free mass (FFM) that forms visceral organs and skeletal muscle can be reduced. With time, the excess or deficit of energy can modify body composition and come to be seen in biochemical testing.

Total energy expenditure (TEE) is divided into *resting* and *non-resting* energy expenditure. Resting energy expenditure includes the *basal metabolic rate* (BMR), also termed basal energy expenditure (BEE), and the *thermic effect of food* (TEF) (Figs. 16.1 and 16.2). Non-resting energy expenditure, or *activity energy*

Fig. 16.3 Nutritional status, lifestyle, and health status relationship. *Body composition*, *energy balance*, and *biochemical laboratory data* represent the main biological variables through which it is possible to investigate nutritional status

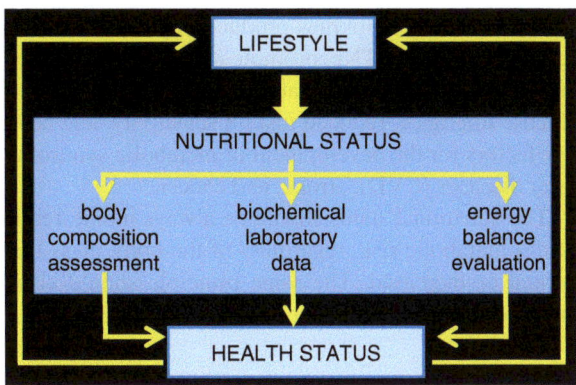

expenditure (AEE), embraces *programmed physical activity* (PPA) and *non-exercise activity thermogenesis* or NEAT (i.e., the sum of *spontaneous physical activity* plus *occupational/leisure* activities) [4, 5]. BMR is the rate of energy expenditure by human body at rest while in the postabsorptive state and is a measure of energy spent for the ongoing function of the vital organs. As such, it is operative continuously and through temporal integration plays an important part in determining one's overall energy expenditure. Equally, the BMR determines the minimum energy requirement for maintaining ongoing vital organ function. It is therefore important to know one's BMR value before planning a diet therapy.

Since energy requirements depend on the absolute and relative size of the body components (mainly skeletal muscles, organs, and skin and to a much lesser extent adipose tissue), body composition has been recognized as a more suitable basis than body weight for estimating the basal metabolic rate.

Body composition, *energy balance,* and *biochemical laboratory data* represent the main biological variables through which it is possible to investigate the nutritional status (Fig. 16.3). In undernourished people, a nutritional status evaluation helps to quantify caloric and nutrient deficits that must be addressed in an appropriate diet therapy plan. The assessment of nutritional status similarly allows us to make the diagnosis and define the severity and clinical risks of associated overweight and obesity conditions, as well as to detect the existence of a reduced muscle mass (a condition named sarcopenia), investigate the causes of weight gain, prescribe the most appropriate treatment, and assess the results of a dietetic, medical, or surgical intervention over time. Nutritional status assessment in this context goes beyond appreciating the extent of energy imbalance to quantify the excess adipose tissue or fatness (*body fat percentage*) and to specify its regional distribution. The amount of excess white adipose tissue and its central or peripheral location (respectively, *visceral adipose tissue* or *subcutaneous adipose tissue*) are important issues related to cardio-metabolic risk in obese-overweight people. While generalized and abdominal obesities are both associated with greater risk of morbidity and mortality, abdominal obesity in particular has been associated with an increased risk of myocardial infarction, stroke, and premature death. Increased visceral adipose tissue is associated with a range of metabolic abnormalities related to the secretion of proinflammatory cytokines produced by adipose tissue. These adipokines, and in particular IL-6 and TNF, promote a chronic low-grade inflammatory state linked to the obesity-associated metabolic diseases [6]. These alterations cause decreased glucose tolerance, reduced insulin sensitivity, and adverse lipid profiles, which are risk factors for the development of metabolic syndrome, type 2 diabetes, cardiovascular diseases (CVD), stroke, and cancer.

The nutritional status should be always monitored in a patient with an increased cardio-metabolic risk, regardless of the body mass index (BMI) value that may be normal or increased. The same principle should also be applied in subjects with increased BMI although apparently healthy.

16.1 Body Composition

16.1.1 Body Composition Components: FFM and FM

FFM and FM are the two generic components used in models of body composition. FFM can be divided into a more metabolically active part, mainly formed by visceral organs, skeletal muscle, and skin and a part formed by the supporting tissues, bone, and body fluids whose metabolic demands are very low. Further stratification can be made as the visceral organs consume much more energy per unit of weight than skeletal muscle. The skeletal muscle component of FFM is considered to have a much lower resting metabolic rate than the visceral organs; nevertheless, it is more abundant and its mass can be modified by our lifestyle, mainly by physical activity. The FM is not metabolically inert but it certainly represents a minor component of the BMR. These considerations have led to the development of a number of models of body composition that differ in their complexity depending on how finely the subcomponents are divided and how they account for the influence of the varying proportions of the different components of FFM and/or tissue-specific metabolic rates. Validation and use of these models in the diagnosis and prognosis of obesity and its associated comorbidities require knowledge of the percentage of FM, the relative proportion of FFM and FM, and the body composition of specific segments of the body like the trunk and limbs. Various in vivo field and laboratory methodologies have been developed to estimate or measure the compartments that represent the different constituents of the human body [7, 8]. Both these aspects of nutritional status evaluation are discussed below.

16.1.2 Body Composition Models

The information obtained from complete dissections and analyses of the composition of human cadavers has led to the establishment of reference values; the development of the concept of the *Reference Man* [9] provides the bases for developing various models of human body composition.

In the *basic two-compartment model*, the body is divided into the *fat mass* that comprises body fat and the *fat-free mass*, including all the remaining tissues. Dividing the FFM into a *lean tissue mass* (LTM) and *bone mineral content* (BMC), in combination with the FM, yields a *three-compartment model* that is particularly interesting as it can be assessed by dual X-ray absorptiometry (DXA).

The elemental, the molecular, the cellular, the functional (or tissue model), and the whole-body models of body composition represent different *multi-compartment models* of progressively higher complexity. In the *molecular model*, the FFM is subdivided in its molecular constituents, water, proteins, minerals, and glycogen, while fat is the molecular component of the FM. The body cell mass in the *cellular model* is considered the metabolically active district responsible for energy consumption at rest, in the postabsorptive state, or BMR; the other components of the cellular model are extracellular fluids, extracellular solids, and fat.

The clinician is generally interested in measuring body composition in terms of FM and FFM as the bi-compartmental model of body composition is particularly well established for the diagnosis, treatment, and prognosis of diseases related to alterations of nutritional status.

16.1.3 Field Methods and Laboratory Measurements of FFM and FM

A variety of reference *laboratory methods* have entered use for body composition analysis, including densitometry, hydrometry, in vivo neutron activation analysis (IVNAA) [10], and DXA. Estimation equations have been compiled using values obtained by different *field methods* as anthropometry (weight, height, skinfold thickness, and circumference measurement) or conductance-based techniques like body impedance assessment (BIA); these estimate equations have been validated by comparison with data obtained by *gold standard* laboratory methods.

The different densities of the FM and FFM can be used to reexpress their mass fractions in the bi-compartmental model in terms of their relative volumes. The proportions of FM and FFM obtained from cadaver analyses have led to the creation of algorithms that indirectly estimates the percentage of body FM from body density (see *Siri equation* in Table 16.1). Body density in turn can be obtained by dividing body mass by body volume. While body mass is related to body weight, body volume cannot be so easily assessed. Water displacement is one possibility, but in practice, densitometry tends to rely on either underwater weighing or air-displacement plethysmography to evaluate body volume. *Underwater weighing* is a laboratory method that compares the weight of the subject in air to that obtained while they are entirely submerged in water. In *air-displacement plethysmography* on the other hand, the subject is placed in a closed air-filled chamber that is then subjected to a pressure change in order to calculate the volume of the body. Densitometry is probably the best laboratory approach to obtaining data for the two-component model for adults.

Table 16.1 Skinfold body density (BD) predictive equations

Skinfold equations		
Durnin and Womersley [11]	$n=481$ (209 M, 272 F), 16–72 years	M: BD = $1.1765 - 0.0744 \times$ (Log SKN)
		SKN = biceps + triceps + subscapular + suprailiac
		F: BD = $1.1567 - 0.0717 \times$ (Log SKN)
		SKN = biceps + triceps + subscapular + suprailiac
Jackson and Pollock 7 skinfolds [12, 13]	$n=308$ M, 18–61 years, $n=249$ F, 18–55 years	M: BD = $1.112 - (0.00043499 \times$ SKN$) + (0.00000055 \times \sqrt{\text{SKN}}) - (0.00028826 \times \text{age})$
		SKN = chest + axilla + triceps + subscapular + abdominal + suprailiac + thigh
		F: BD = $1.097 - (0.00046971 \times$ SKN$) + (0.00000056 \times \sqrt{\text{SKN}}) - (0.00012828 \times \text{age})$
		SKN = chest + axilla + triceps + subscapular + abdominal + suprailiac + thigh
Jackson and Pollock 3 skinfolds [12, 13]	$n=308$ M, 18–61 years, $n=249$ F, 18–55 years	M: BD = $1.10938 - (0.0008267 \times$ SKN$) + (0.0000016 \times \sqrt{\text{SKN}}) - (0.0002574 \times \text{age})$
		SKN = chest + abdominal + thigh
		F: BD = $1.0994921 - (0.0009929 \times$ SKN$) + (0.0000023 \times \sqrt{\text{SKN}} - (0.0001392 \times \text{age})$
		SKN = triceps + suprailiac + thigh
Forsyth and Sinning [14]	M, 19–22 years, male athletes	M: BD = $1.103 - 0.00168 \times$ SKN$^S - 0.00127 \times$ SKN^A
		SKN^S = subscapular
		SKN^A = abdominal

SKN is the sum of the site-specific skinfold thickness measured in *mm*. The sites are specified for each equation. Age is expressed in years. BD represents the body density from which fat mass percentage (FM%) can be calculated applying the *Siri equation* [15]: FM% = $(4.95)/\text{BD} - 4.50) \times 100$
M male, *F* female

Body density can be also estimated from the measurement of skinfold thickness with the use of population-specific equations (Table 16.1).

Dilution methods are based on the principle that the volume of a body compartment can be calculated as the ratio of a tracer dose dispensed orally or intravenously to its final concentration in that compartment after a certain period of time. Since on average in healthy adults the total body water (TBW) constitutes 73 % of the FFM, the latter can be easily calculated if TBW is measured. The measurement of TBW, or *hydrometry*, is a dilution method based on deuterium [16], a stable nonradioactive isotopic tracer of hydrogen. The value of FM can then be obtained by the difference of body mass and FFM. Similarly, extracellular water can be calculated with basic dilution techniques and a nonradioactive Br tracer administered orally.

Anthropometry-based methods are good field methods. Weight, BMI, skinfold thickness, and body circumference measurements are simple, quick, inexpensive, and portable techniques.

Body weight is more a dimension of body size than a measure of body composition. Nevertheless, weight as a function of height has an essential role in the evaluation of nutritional status in children and adults. Weight is the sum in kg of the FM and FFM. In the diagnosis of overweight and obesity, it is important to know the percentage of body FM rather than the absolute amount of fat in kg, and specialists encourage a definition of obesity based on percentage of body fat or fatness. Changes in body weight over time are more often due to changes in the amount of FM, as FFM is the most stable of the two components. Daily weight fluctuations are usually caused by variations in water content, such as in edema.

Body mass index or *BMI* is calculated by dividing weight (in kilograms) by height (in meters) squared. BMI is widely used as an index of the degree of obesity or undernutrition. It is better seen as a measure of fat content (FM in kg) than of fatness (% fat) however. BMI is a compositional index that has relevant clinical and prognostic value [17]. BMI values correlate with mortality rate [18] and have developed into an indicator of risk of diseases related to adiposity like premature death, cardiovascular diseases, high blood pressure, osteoarthritis, some cancers, and diabetes. It should be remembered however that although BMI has traditionally been used as a measure of body size and composition, abdominal fat mass can vary significantly within a narrow range of total body fat and BMI.

The most widely accepted classifications for overweight and obese people are those from the World Health Organization (WHO), based on BMI (Table 16.2).

Skinfold thickness and body circumferences. Skinfold thickness is a measure of subcutaneous adipose tissue. Skinfolds themselves may be compared with reference data or used in estimation equations to derive whole-body fatness (Table 16.1).

Skinfold measurements are taken at specific sites of the body. The subscapular, triceps, biceps, and suprailiac skinfold measurements are among the most commonly used sites. After pinching the skin and subcutaneous fat tissue away from the underlying muscle, the tester uses special skinfold calipers to measure the skinfold thickness in millimeters.

Skinfold thickness has the characteristics of a good field method. It is simple and quick, and the calipers are inexpensive and portable. Since estimation equations are

Table 16.2 Classification of overweight and obesity by BMI [19, 20]

Classification of overweight and obesity and associated disease risk

Class	BMI	WC	Disease risk
Underweight	<18.5	M: <102 cm	–
		F: <88 cm	
		M: >102 cm	–
		F: >88 cm	
Normal[a]	18.5–24.9	M: <102 cm	–
		F: <88 cm	
		M: >102 cm	–
		F: >88 cm	
Overweight	25–29.9	M: <102 cm	Increased
		F: <88 cm	
		M: >102 cm	High
		F: >88 cm	
Obesity class I	30–34.9	M: <102 cm	High
		F: <88 cm	
		M: >102 cm	Very high
		F: >88 cm	
Obesity class II	35–39.9	M: <102 cm	Very high
		F: <88 cm	
		M: >102 cm	Very high
		F: >88 cm	
Obesity class III	>40	M: <102 cm	Extremely high
		F: <88 cm	
		M: >102 cm	Extremely high
		F: >88 cm	

The table shows the disease risk for type 2 diabetes, hypertension, and cardiovascular diseases associated with BMI and WC in Europid populations. Disease risk is relative to normal-weight and normal-waist circumference

In Caucasian population, a WC between 94.0 and 101.9 cm in men and 80.0–87.9 cm in women is associated with an *increased risk* of *metabolic complications* related to obesity; the risk is *substantially increased* if WC ≥ 102 cm in men and ≥ 80 cm in women or if WHR ≥ 0.90 in men and WHR ≥ 0.85 in women [19, 21]

[a]An increased *waist circumference* may denote an increased risk even in persons of *normal weight*

always specific to the population on which they have been validated (specificity concerns age, sex, ethnicity, technical origins), one must consider which of the available equations most closely fits the individual being measured. The seven- and three-skinfold equations of Jackson and Pollock [12, 13], the equations of Durnin and Womersley [11], and the equation of Forsyth and Sinning [14] are among the most used (Table 16.1).

Circumference measurement. Circumference measurement is another simple and useful anthropometric measure. The waist, hip, and mid-arm are the most frequent sites where circumferences are measured.

Waist circumference (WC) is measured at the approximate midpoint between the lower margin of the last palpable rib and the top of the iliac crest [19]. In other protocols, waist circumference has been measured at the top of the iliac crest [22], or at the level of the umbilicus or at the point of the minimal waist [23].

Hip circumference is taken around the widest portion of the buttocks.

Waist–hip ratio (WHR) is the waist circumference divided by the hip circumference.

Since waist circumference and waist–hip ratio reflect abdominal adiposity, high values for WC or WHR indicate abdominal fat accumulation [21]. They represent an additional measure of body fat distribution [24] and are a good predictor of cardio-metabolic risk [20] (Table 16.2). Unfortunately, universal cutoff points for WC, as for BMI, are not applicable as disease risk may differ between ethnic groups [19].

Mid-upper arm circumference (MUAC) is an index of nutritional status that, in conjunction with BMI, is particularly useful as a measure of chronic energy deficiency in children and hospital patients. It is highly correlated with BMI, but it does not need weight and height measuring apparatus. Used together with a triceps skinfold measurement, it is possible to obtain cross-sectional areas of adipose tissue and muscle at mid-upper arm level.

Body impedance assessment (BIA). The principle of body impedance assessment is that the resistance or impedance of the body to the flow of a weak alternating electric current (800 mA 50 kHz) is inversely proportional to the total body water (TBW). TBW composes 60 % of an adult body weight and about 73 % of the FFM of nonobese subjects [7, 25]. At low frequencies, current flows mainly through extracellular water, while at higher frequencies, it also penetrates cell membranes into intracellular water. Thus, *multifrequency instruments* can evaluate the extracellular and intracellular component of TBW.

The procedure of BIA involves the careful placement of the electrodes (signal and detecting electrodes) on the wrist and ankle. Simplified devices require merely that the subject stands barefooted on metal plates connected to the electrodes.

From appropriate well-validated estimation equations that include empirical impedance values and anthropometric variables such as height and weight, it is possible to calculate TBW and FFM, and hence FM. More involved BIA procedures give the possibility to estimate the composition of body segments, like upper and lower limbs.

BIA is a field body composition technique, it is quick and simple to use, and it has a good reproducibility. It is important to standardize the measurement conditions [26] and use appropriate well-validated estimation equations.

Dual X-ray absorptiometry (DXA). DXA is a method for *whole-body* and *regional body* composition analysis. DXA produces a bidimensional image of the entire human body. The principle behind DXA is in the differential degree of attenuation of X-ray beams of different energies by the soft tissues and bone. Subsequently, the procedure has been developed for non-osseous fat and lean tissue. This makes DXA well suited to describing the body in terms of *bone mineral content, lean tissue mass, and fat mass*, which can be used in the two-compartment model with the FFM divided into BMC and LTM. DXA technique may be used to describe the composition of the entire body or of its segments like the trunk and the limbs. Thus, DXA may be used to assess peripheral or central adipose tissue accumulation [3] or the amount of LTM in the limbs where it is mostly represented by skeletal muscle. An index obtained from the DXA has been used to diagnose sarcopenia [27].

DXA scan is relatively quick and is minimally invasive because the radiation doses are low.

The technique is quite precise, and it is increasingly used in medical practice to assess body composition even if debate continues about the status of DXA as a gold standard criterion for body composition [28].

While the DXA technique gives a bidimensional projection of body composition, whole-body techniques such as *computed tomography* (CT) and *magnetic resonance imaging* (MRI) can provide three-dimensional reconstruction. Both techniques can generate *cross-sectional volumes* and *images* of the body. CT and MRI identify FM and precisely describe its localization in terms of subcutaneous or visceral adipose tissue. CT exposes the subject to an X-ray dose greater than the DXA, and for this reason, it is more invasive and less frequently used for body composition studies than DXA. However, visceral fat distribution may be studied by a few scans at the lumbar level, limiting the dose of radiation to which the subject is exposed.

MRI does not require ionizing radiation and so is attractive for repeated measurements. It exploits the fact that elements such as hydrogen and carbon resonate in the presence of a magnetic field. After being excited by an oscillating magnetic field, the energy they dissipate is used to produce images that reflect the density of the source elements and properties of their physicochemical environment – for example, the presence of hydrogen in water or fat molecules. The disadvantages of MRI are the cost of the examination and the long scan time.

CT, MRI, and DXA are particularly helpful in regional measures of body composition allowing quantification of muscle mass and abdominal adipose tissue deposits [29–31]. Epicardial fat, a further risk factor for CVD, can be visualized by MRI and CT techniques [32].

16.2 Energy Balance

By energy balance, we mean the arithmetic difference between Ei (*energy intake*) and Eo (*energy output*).

$$\Delta E = \text{Ei} - \text{Eo}$$

In nutrition, energy is synonymous with food. Ei represents the algebraic sum of all the energy assimilated by a subject in 24 h, while Eo indicates the energy expended in the course of their physiological processes during his daily activities. We also have to consider ES (*energy storage*), which is the energy conserved by the organism during this process, especially when $\Delta E > 0$.

Under the first law of thermodynamics, energy cannot be created or destroyed, but it can be transformed from a form into another. This manifests in nutrition through biochemical processes as glycolysis, Krebs cycle, and mitochondrial respiratory chain. These reactions allow the transformation and the consequent availability of the energy conserved in food macronutrients. Each food item is composed of macromolecules that are metabolized by human cells in order to gain the energy necessary for cell metabolism and homeostasis.

In order to establish an accurate method to predict the single-person energy balance, it is fundamental to quantify the energy contained in different foods and their impact on human metabolism. Each food has a specific energy content, which is measured in *joules*. 1 J is the energy spent to move an object of a mass of 1 kg for 1 m. Although joule is the official unit of measure for energy in the SI (International System of Units), in nutrition, the kcal is the preferred unit of measure. *1 kcal*, approximately 4.2 kJ, is the energy needed to raise the temperature of 1 kg of water by 1 °C.

16.2.1 Energy Intake Evaluation

Accurate measurement of the daily Ei absorbed by an individual is essential to determining their energetic balance. There are two main approaches to this problem: retrospective methods and longitudinal ones.

Retrospective Methods
Retrospective methods consist principally of quantifying, in the most accurate manner, all the different foods eaten by patients in 24 h. *Food Frequency Questionnaires* (FFQs) are commonly used to absolve this task. Through a series of questions, FFQs gather an account of the typical daily diet of a patient. Modern FFQs may be integrated with pictures of different portions of various foods in order to increment the data accuracy.

A similar approach is the *24-h recall*, which consists of a series of questions aimed to obtain a reconstruction of the dietary intake of the day before the visit.

After data collection, the reported food intake has to be translated into a kcal intake in order to find the Ei. In this final step, the operator can take advantage of specific software packages that, together with accurate and validated food databases, give the total kcal content and the percentage content of the macronutrients and in some cases, even of the micronutrients of each food, to allow the cumulative quantities to be determined. It is fundamental for the reliability of the measurements made in these ways that validated databases be used (e.g., the INRAN food database in Italy), in which each food has been analyzed through standard chemical techniques. The retrospective methods are low cost and immediate, but do not lack disadvantages. The main problem is that the final data is only a reconstruction; the patient may have forgotten some information, could even voluntary fail to mention some food, and is unlikely to be accurate regarding portion size. For these and other reasons, the Ei obtained with retrospective methods is not very reliable. However, retrospective methods are useful for epidemiological studies.

Longitudinal Methods

Longitudinal methods give a more reliable value of an individual's Ei, so they are commonly used in clinics. A *food diary* is the most famous longitudinal method. This technique consists of making the individual write a diary in which he reports every meal with a detailed description of the quantity and the types of foods he consumes in a day. For more accurate data, the food diary should cover from 5 days to a whole week, including the weekend. In fact, it is not uncommon to find a radical diet modification during the weekend in some patients (especially in occidental culture). A food diary is also a good instrument to evaluate the psychological status associated with nutrition. In some diaries, the patient is asked to describe and report their emotional status during or after each meal. As in retrospective methods, the food data have to be transformed into micro and macronutrients and finally into kcals to find the Ei.

Although longitudinal techniques are more accurate than retrospective ones, they too have some disadvantages. First of all, patient compliance: by using a food diary, the physician or the nutritionist deeply enters into a person's life; this can be really problematic in patients affected by eating disorders with an important emotional component (e.g., anorexia, bulimia, binge eating syndrome). A food diary can be a very powerful technique for evaluating patient Ei, but it is important to recognize that a food diary's reliability is entirely based on patient compliance. A much-debated longitudinal technique is the *assisted* or *artificial nutrition*. It is the most invasive technique for Ei analysis. It is used for hospitalized patients as well as for the treatment of the severe form of anorexia. Subjects submitted to assisted nutrition are followed 24 h a day by high-qualified operators that control and report each food proposed to the patient. Considering that bromatological analysis of each food is performed a priori and each meal is accurately controlled, assisted nutrition is the most reliable technique to investigate Ei.

16.2.2 Energy Storage

An Ei major than Eo leads to an increment of ES. Overweight and obesity are strictly related to an altered mechanism of energy storage, which is mainly caused by an unhealthy and overabundant caloric intake, especially in the westernized world.

Extra energy is metabolized by human organism through biochemical processes and mainly transformed and stored into fat, glycogen, and proteins. While the energy conserved in glycogen and proteins has a physiological threshold, the quantity of exceeding energy that we can convert into fat is theoretically unlimited. This behavior seems to be a heritage from our past; throughout most of human evolution, the tendency to store calories as fat would likely have conferred an advantage by allowing energy storage during periods of abundance that enable survival during periods of prolonged caloric restriction, as well as providing greater energy stores to nourish the mother and fetus during and following pregnancy. According to

Lewis et al., the average US adult gains only 500–1,000 g of weight (approximately 2,000–2,500 kcal of stored energy) per year (more pronounced in older individuals, African Americans, Native Americans, and Hispanic Americans) despite ingestion of approximately 900,000–1,000,000 kcal/year [33]. Lewis' research points into focus an important data: energy storage is not only due to the simple difference between Ei and Eo, but this biochemical process is mastered and finely regulated by individual metabolic, neuroendocrine, and autonomic systems.

Rosenbaum and Leibel [34] investigated the mechanisms behind ES. In their study, they underline the importance of considering the bioenergetics physiologies and the hormonal impact on body weight. Several metabolic hormonal effects have been detected with leptin, involved in the hunger and satiety mechanism, playing a central role in energy storage. One must also consider the central roles of insulin, cortisol, thyroid hormones, and other important molecules implied in energy storage whose regulation is strictly correlated with the subject's nutritional behavior.

The many molecular mechanisms implicated in energy storage processes and their mutual interaction are one of the main causes of the potent *opposition* to the maintenance of reduced body weight. In addition to an increase of energy intake (increased appetite and less sense of satiety), this potent mechanism brings to a reduction of energy expenditure by an improvement of muscle efficiency especially at low levels of work, as during activities of daily life [4, 34].

16.2.3 Energy Expenditure Evaluation

Once we have investigated individual Ei, the estimation or even the measurement of the energy expenditure (Eo) is essential for the development of an efficient diet therapy.

Eo, also known as total energy expenditure (TEE), represents all the energy used by a single subject within 24 h, and it is measured in kcal/day.

In adult subjects, TEE can be represented by the following equation:

$$TEE = BEE + TEF + AEE + other$$

where BEE is the energy necessary for the conservation of vital functions (normally 60–70 % of TEE). Thermic effect of food (TEF) is the energy necessary for nutrient assimilation (5–10 % of TEE); this parameter becomes greater for a high protein intake. Finally, AEE represents the energy used during physical activity (20–35 % of TEE). AEE is comprehensive of PPA and NEAT [4]. PPA, or programmed physical activity, is the voluntary physical activity such as sport workouts, while NEAT embraces the energy expended for everything we do that is not sleeping, eating, or sports-like exercise. By the term *other* encompasses all remaining, minor metabolic components such as shiver reflex.

In children and adolescents, we also have to take into account the energy spent for physiological growth.

16.2.4 Estimate Equations

Since the start of the last century, several attempts at BMR prediction have been developed. In particular, predictive equations based on biological variables like weight, height, age, sex, or FFM have been assessed. Predictive equations are developed in healthy subjects by regression analysis of these body independent variables and BMR, the dependent variable measured by the *gold standard* method of direct calorimetry.

The most famous and oldest basal energy expenditure predictive equation was created by Harris and Benedict in 1919 [35] on the basis of weight, height, sex, and age. This equation was tested for the first time on 239 healthy individuals with different BMIs. The population was extended to 337 subjects in 1984, and after almost one century, this equation is still used (Table 16.3).

The Schofield equation with all its variants is another very popular and commonly used predictive equation [36]. The most common variants are the weight-based and the weight–height-based formulas. Its strength rises from the large number of samples used for the creation of the linear regression from which this equation was created: almost 11,000 healthy subjects from a variety of ethnic groups from all over the world. This equation can be considered reliable for normal-weight and overweight individuals [38] (Table 16.3).

Mifflin et al. [37] introduced FFM in their equation as an independent variable, but recent studies have demonstrated that the use of this parameter does not influence the reliability of the equation. Although this equation was not developed on a population as large as Schofield's (498 healthy patients vs. 11,000), the range of BMI used (from 17 to 42) makes it appropriate for obese subjects (Table 16.3).

There are many other predictive equations that essentially differ in the number of subjects used in validation, their ethnic group, age, and BMI (Table 16.3).

As calorimetry, the gold standard technique for measuring BMR, is not feasible in most dietetic settings, it is important to use the most accurate predictive equation to estimate BMR especially in overweight and obese persons.

The choice of the equation is fundamental; the subject analyzed using one of these formulas should have the same features as those used for developing the equation. For example, for obese and overweight German adults, there seem to be no accurate and reliable equations [38].

It is important to keep in mind that these formulas only give a predictive BMR value, which is often not reliable in pathophysiological conditions. In these cases, it is recommended to measure and not estimate the patients' BMR.

Predictive equations also do not take into account individual differences in physical activity level (PPA and NEAT); for example, according to Schofield equation, a professional athlete has the same BMR of a sedentary subject of the same weight and age. So, how can a nutritionist obtain a reliable TEE value from the estimated BMR in order to formulate an efficient diet therapy?

To overcome this gap, Food and Agriculture Organization (FAO) has produced a classification of *physical activity levels* (PALs) (Table 16.4) that, multiplied by BMR, allows to estimate TEE.

Table 16.3 BMR predictive equations

BMR predictive equations		
Harris and Benedict [35]	$n=239$ (136 M, 103 F)	M: $WT \times 13.7516 + HTCM \times 5.0033 - AGE \times 6.755 + 66.473$ F: $WT \times 9.5634 + HTCM \times 1.8496 - AGE \times 4.6756 + 655.0955$
Schofield weight and height [36]	$n=7{,}173$, $n=4814$ 18 years, mean BMI of these 6 groups: 21–24; $n=3{,}388$ Italians (47 %), $n=615$ tropical residents, $n=322$ Indian; 114 published studies, $n=7{,}173$ subjects (11,000 values, includes group mean values); most European and North American subjects (Italian, closed-circuit calorimetry)	M: Age 18–30 years: $0.063 \times WT - 0.042 \times HTM + 2.953$ M: Age 30–60 years: $0.048 \times WT - 0.011 \times HTM + 3.67$ M: Age >60 years: $0.038 \times WT + 4.068 \times HTM - 3.491$ F: Age 18–30 years: $0.057 \times WT + 1.148 \times HTM + 0.411$ F: Age 30–60 years: $0.034 \times WT + 0.006 \times HTM + 3.53$ F: Age >60 years: $0.033 \times WT + 1.917 \times HTM + 0.074$
Mifflin et al. [37]	$n=498$ (251 M, 248 F), $n=264$ normal weight (129 M, 135 F), $n=234$ obese (122 M, 112 F), 19–78 years, BMI 17–42,	$9.99 \times WT + 6.25 \times HTCM - 4.92 \times AGE + 166 \times SEX - 161$
Mifflin et al. (FFM) [37]	$n=498$ (251 M, 248 F), $n=264$ normal weight (129 M, 135 F), $n=234$ obese (122 M, 112 F), 19–78 years, BMI 17–42,	$19.7 \times FFM + 413$

WT weight in kg, *HTCM* height in cm, *HTM* height in meters, *FFM* fat-free mass, *AGE* age in years; *SEX* ($M=1$, $F=0$), *BMR* basal metabolic rate, *M* male, *F* female

Table 16.4 Classification of lifestyles in relation to the intensity of habitual physical activity or PAL [39]

Category	PAL
Sedentary or light-activity lifestyle	1.40–1.69
Active or moderately active lifestyle	1.70–1.99
Vigorous or vigorously active lifestyle	2.00–2.40

A PAL of 2.40 or higher cannot be supported for a long period of time

$$TEE = BMR \times PAL$$

PALs are calculated on the basis of the energy expenditure of various activities, from sleeping (PAL = 1) to intense training (PAL equal to 15 or greater). In validation studies, indirect calorimetry was used as the *gold standard*, and the PAL of each activity was calculated in kcal/kg/h. In order to calculate the final daily PAL value (kcal/kg/day), it is necessary to sum the whole energy expenditure routine of each subject activity in 24 h [39]. PAL values that can be sustained for a long period of time by free-living adult populations range from about 1.40 to 2.40. According to the FAO, PAL values can be divided into three: sedentary, active, and vigorous. So, in the previous example, the final TEE difference between a sedentary subject and an athlete with the same age and weight becomes clear (sedentary TEE = BEE × 1.4 vs. athlete TEE = BEE × 2.4, 42 % TEE variation).

In conclusion, predictive equations corrected for physical activity levels may be suitable for estimating the healthy subject's TEE and for epidemiological studies, but not applicable to all patient categories.

16.2.5 Measurement Methods

Each of the components of TEE (BEE, TEF, AEE) is highly variable, and the total effect of these variances determines the variability in daily TEE among subjects. Measurements of TEE and their application must take into consideration the activity of the subject during the period of measurement in respect to routine daily life, and for this, free-living measurements may be preferred. From an alternative perspective, the measurement of energy expenditure can allow us to assess the relative thermic effects of various foods, nutrient compositions, pharmacological effects, and psychological components. Energy Expenditure can be measured using one of several approaches, including non-calorimetric techniques, direct calorimetry, and indirect calorimetry [40].

16.2.6 Non-calorimetric Approaches

As well as predictive equations, these methods measure or estimate TEE from variables related with energy expenditure. These techniques are often standardized against the calorimetric ones.

Doubly labeled water [41]: this method consists of monitoring carbon dioxide production and energy expenditure through the use of nonradioactive isotopes (D_2O^{18}).

This method is driven by the equilibrium between *body water*, O_2, and expired CO_2:

$$CO_2 + H_2O \leftrightarrow H_2CO_3$$

The body water is traced with isotope O^{18}, and over time, the concentration of marked O_2 in the organism will decrease while CO_2 is expired and body water is lost through urine and respiration.

Both O_2 and H_2 in body water are tagged with known amounts of tracers at the same time. The differences in the elimination rates of the O_2 and H_2 tracers are related to the elimination rate of CO_2. Double-labeled water is given to subjects orally after a sample of urine, saliva, or blood has been collected. A second sample is collected 7–21 days later, and tracer concentrations are determined through mass spectrometry. Body D_2 and O^{18} are measured over time and CO_2 and energy expenditure can be calculated with an error of 6–8 %. The percentage error decreases as the number of samples increases. This method is more indicated for epidemiological and research studies than ambulatory routine, mainly because of the high costs of reagents and the competence required for data analysis; however, it provides a good accuracy and it is applicable to free-living subjects.

Kinematic measurements. These methods are primarily used to estimate individual PPA and NEAT. Some techniques as *cine photography* are specific for confined spaces, while other ones, like *accelerometers* and *pedometers*, are useful for collecting data in *free-living subjects*. In particular, accelerometers detect body displacement electronically with varying degrees of sensitivity: uniaxial accelerometers in one axis and triaxial accelerometers in three axes. Kinematic techniques are generally not sufficient for accurately quantifying TEE, but an acceptable precision can be obtained through triaxial accelerometers [42]; in free-living subjects, data from these devices correlate well with the total daily energy expenditure, measured using doubly labeled water [43]. Triaxial accelerometer is a field method utilizable in ambulatory routine that is allowing us to gain important information about multiple components of a subject's lifestyle (e.g., information about sleep quality) in free-living conditions.

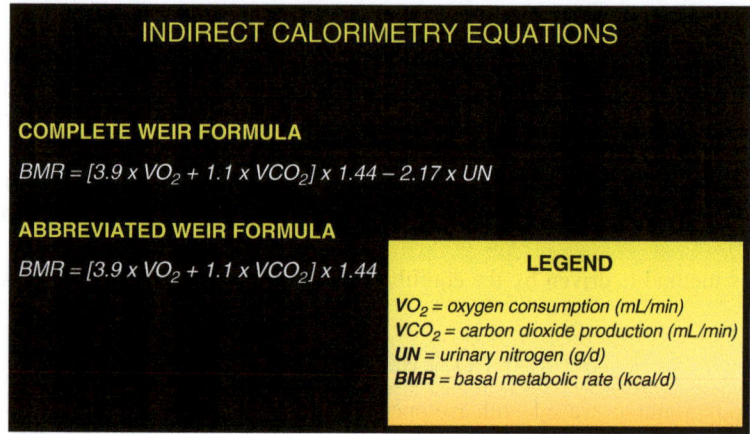

Fig. 16.4 Indirect calorimetry equations [45, 46]

16.2.7 Calorimetry Techniques

Calorimetry techniques are the most accurate methods that allow us to measure energy expenditure with a high rate of accuracy. Energy expenditure can be measured as the sum of work performed on the environment by the organism plus heat released during combustion of food. If the organism is at rest, energy expenditure equals the heat produced by oxidation of energy substrates in foods.

Direct Calorimetry

Direct calorimetry represents the *gold standard method* for energy expenditure measurement [44]. Direct calorimetry is based on the principle that all metabolic processes that occur in the body lead to the production of heat, a process known as thermogenesis.

This technique requires the use of a *metabolic chamber* that allows fine measurement of the heat lost from the human body. It is also suitable to evaluating the thermogenic variations induced by various foods and daily activities. The disadvantages are that the *metabolic chamber* is rather expensive and its use requires a full time technician.

Indirect Calorimetry

Indirect calorimetry is based on the principle that an organism produces energy by the oxidation of energy substrates in foods. The production of energy from these substrates takes place through known stoichiometric reactions in which oxygen is consumed and carbon dioxide produced. From the volume of oxygen consumed (VO_2), the volume of carbon dioxide (VCO_2) produced, and the excretion of urinary nitrogen, the *equation of Weir* [45, 46] (Fig. 16.4) gives the value of energy expenditure. The excretion of urinary nitrogen is often neglected in a simplified version of Weir equation with a minor error (Fig. 16.4). The method thus consists of collecting

Table 16.5 Respiratory quotient of various metabolic substrates

Metabolized substrate	Respiratory quotient (RQ)
Ethanol	0.67
Fat oxidation	0.71
Carbohydrate oxidation	1.0
Protein oxidation	0.82
Lipogenesis	1–1.2
After carbohydrate-based meal	1 ± 0.04
22 h after fatty-acid-based meal	0.71 ± 0.04
After mixed meal	0.86 ± 0.11

This table reports the RQ of various macronutrients. RQ is calculated through indirect calorimetry [46, 50]

expired air using either an airtight rigid structure or a portable flexible bag. There are various types of indirect calorimeters.

The Tissot gasometer [47] is a *rigid total collection system*. In this instrument, the subject has to expire through a mouthpiece and a nonreturn valve into a glass bell suspended over water. The test lasts for about 2 h, and the composition of the air in the bell is periodically analyzed.

Douglas bag [48] represents *a flexible collector system*, in which the patient expires through a mouthpiece into a polyvinyl chloride bag. Again, the volume of expired air is collected and analyzed (e.g., using a mass flow meter), and the concentration of oxygen and carbon dioxide are calculated. This technique is fast (20 min) and relatively cheap compared to other calorimetric methods. However, in order to obtain reliable results, it requires a good instrument maintenance and experienced operator.

Another group of calorimetric techniques is represented by *open-circuit indirect calorimeter systems*, which can be divided into two main groups [40]: *ventilated* open-circuit systems where the patient breaths into a container from which air is drawn and *expiratory collection systems* where a subject inspires from the atmosphere and expires via a nonreturn valve into a measurement unit. In the first case, the air can be collected through the use of mouthpiece, mask, transparent hood, or canopy. The expired air is drawn out through a pump, and the flow rate is accurately measured. The expired air is then mixed using a fan and/or mixing chamber, and a sample of the expired air is dried and analyzed for oxygen and/or carbon dioxide concentrations. This technique allows measurement in a brief lapse of time with a high accuracy rate.

An expiratory collection open-circuit system, on the contrary, has the advantage of being suitable for free-living analysis as many of these devices are portable and allow analysis to be performed over periods as long as 2 days.

Indirect calorimetric techniques can also provide another value: the *respiratory quotient* (RQ).

RQ [49] is calculated from the ratio:

$$RQ = VCO_{2\ eliminated} / VO_{2\ consumed}$$

This value is specific for each metabolized substrate, hence allowing the operator to know which is the nutrient mainly consumed by a subject (Table 16.5). Special care must be taken in interpreting the RQ value since there are many metabolic and nonmetabolic causes that may result in alterations of the physiological range of RQ.

In order to accurately measure the basal metabolic rate, the subject should undergo 8 h of fasting, be awake, and be totally free of stressors. This last aspect is fundamental and takes on particular importance in anxious patients and children where the use of masks or canopies represents an important stressor input which could alter measurement reliability. To ensure patients are adequately relaxed, the experimental environment is therefore extremely important, and even steps such as the use of acoustic supports like classic music may be advisable. Moreover, the operator should also pay attention to the room thermal insulation since RQ is particularly sensible to temperature variations.

Indirect calorimetry represents a useful technique for the customization of a patient's energy requirements and nutrient supply when seeking to improve treatment outcomes in the clinical setting [51] especially in critically ill patients.

With advances in technology, indirect calorimetry has become easier to operate and less expensive, leading to a more widespread use of the instrument.

References

1. Cruz-Jentoft AJ et al (2010) Sarcopenia: European consensus on definition and diagnosis Report of the European Working Group on Sarcopenia in Older People. Age Ageing 39: 412–423
2. Scherzer R et al (2011) Decreased limb muscle and increased central adiposity are associated with 5-year all-cause mortality in HIV infection. AIDS Lond Engl 25:1405–1414
3. El Ghoch M et al (2014) Body composition, eating disorder psychopathology, and psychological distress in anorexia nervosa: a longitudinal study. Am J Clin Nutr 99:771–778
4. Levine JA (2004) Non-exercise activity thermogenesis (NEAT). Nutr Rev 62:S82–S97
5. Dulloo AG, Jacquet J, Montani J-P, Schutz Y (2012) Adaptive thermogenesis in human body weight regulation: more of a concept than a measurable entity? Obes Rev Off J Int Assoc Study Obes 13(Suppl 2):105–121
6. Ouchi N, Parker JL, Lugus JJ, Walsh K (2011) Adipokines in inflammation and metabolic disease. Nat Rev Immunol 11:85–97
7. Ellis KJ (2000) Human body composition: in vivo methods. Physiol Rev 80:649–680
8. Norgan N (2005) Laboratory and field measurements of body composition. Public Health Nutr 8:1108–1122
9. Snyder S et al (1975) Report of the Task Group on reference man: ICRP-23. Pergamon, Oxford
10. Mattsson S, Thomas BJ (2006) Development of methods for body composition studies. Phys Med Biol 51:R203–R228
11. Durnin JV, Womersley J (1974) Body fat assessed from total body density and its estimation from skinfold thickness: measurements on 481 men and women aged from 16 to 72 years. Br J Nutr 32:77–97
12. Jackson AS, Pollock ML (1978) Generalized equations for predicting body density of men. Br J Nutr 40:497–504
13. Jackson AS, Pollock ML, Ward A (1980) Generalized equations for predicting body density of women. Med Sci Sports Exerc 12:175–181

14. Forsyth HL, Sinning WE (1973) The anthropometric estimation of body density and lean body weight of male athletes. Med Sci Sports 5:174–180
15. Siri W (1956) The gross composition of the body. Adv Biol Med Phys 4:239–280.
16. Schoeller D (2005) Hydrometry. In: Heymsfield SB et al. (eds) Human body composition. Second ed. pp 35–50
17. Huxley R, Mendis S, Zheleznyakov E, Reddy S, Chan J (2010) Body mass index, waist circumference and waist:hip ratio as predictors of cardiovascular risk–a review of the literature. Eur J Clin Nutr 64:16–22
18. Allison DB, Zhu SK, Plankey M, Faith MS, Heo M (2002) Differential associations of body mass index and adiposity with all-cause mortality among men in the first and second National Health and Nutrition Examination Surveys (NHANES I and NHANES II) follow-up studies. Int J Obes Relat Metab Disord 26:410–416
19. WHO (2008) Waist circumference and waist–hip ratio: report of a WHO expert consultation. WHO, Geneva, pp 8–11
20. Clinical guidelines on the identification, evaluation, and treatment of overweight and obesity in adults: executive summary. Expert panel on the identification, evaluation, and treatment of overweight in adults (1998). Am J Clin Nutr 68:899–917
21. WHO (2000) Obesity: preventing and managing the global epidemic, vol 894, WHO technical report. WHO, Geneva
22. Westat Inc. (1998) Third National Health and Nutrition Examination Survey (NHANES III), 1988–94. ftp://ftp.cdc.gov/pub/health_statistics/NCHS/nhanes/nhanes3/2A/cff-acc.pdf
23. Ross R et al (2008) Does the relationship between waist circumference, morbidity and mortality depend on measurement protocol for waist circumference? Obes Rev Off J Int Assoc Study Obes 9:312–325
24. Björntorp P (1987) Fat cell distribution and metabolism. Ann N Y Acad Sci 499:66–72
25. Kotler DP et al (1999) Relative influences of sex, race, environment, and HIV infection on body composition in adults. Am J Clin Nutr 69:432–439
26. Heymsfield SB, Wang Z, Visser M, Gallagher D, Pierson RN Jr (1996) Techniques used in the measurement of body composition: an overview with emphasis on bioelectrical impedance analysis. Am J Clin Nutr 64:478S–484S
27. Baumgartner RN et al (1998) Epidemiology of sarcopenia among the elderly in New Mexico. Am J Epidemiol 147:755–763
28. Barthe N, Braillon P, Ducassou D, Basse-Cathalinat B (1997) Comparison of two Hologic DXA systems (QDR 1000 and QDR 4500/A). Br J Radiol 70:728–739
29. Van der Kooy K, Seidell JC (1993) Techniques for the measurement of visceral fat: a practical guide. Int J Obes Relat Metab Disord 17:187–196
30. Mitsiopoulos N et al (1998) Cadaver validation of skeletal muscle measurement by magnetic resonance imaging and computerized tomography. J Appl Physiol Bethesda Md 1985(85): 115–122
31. Fuller NJ et al (1999) Assessment of limb muscle and adipose tissue by dual-energy X-ray absorptiometry using magnetic resonance imaging for comparison. Int J Obes Relat Metab Disord 23:1295–1302
32. Marwan M, Achenbach S (2013) Quantification of epicardial fat by computed tomography: why, when and how? J Cardiovasc Comput Tomogr 7:3–10
33. Lewis CE et al (2000) Weight gain continues in the 1990s: 10-year trends in weight and overweight from the CARDIA study. Coronary artery risk development in young adults. Am J Epidemiol 151:1172–1181
34. Rosenbaum M, Leibel RL (2010) Adaptive thermogenesis in humans. Int J Obes 2005(34 Suppl 1):S47–S55
35. Harris J, Benedict F (1919) A biometric study of basal metabolism in man. Carnegie Institute of Washington, Washington, DC
36. Schofield WN (1985) Predicting basal metabolic rate, new standards and review of previous work. Hum Nutr Clin Nutr 39(Suppl 1):5–41

37. Mifflin MD et al (1990) A new predictive equation for resting energy expenditure in healthy individuals. Am J Clin Nutr 51:241–247
38. Weijs PJM (2008) Validity of predictive equations for resting energy expenditure in US and Dutch overweight and obese class I and II adults aged 18–65 y. Am J Clin Nutr 88:959–970
39. FAO (2001) Human energy requirements, Report of a joint FAO/WHO/UNU expert consultation. Food and nutrition technical report series. Rome, 17–24 Oct 2001
40. Levine JA (2005) Measurement of energy expenditure. Public Health Nutr 8:1123–1132
41. Black AE, Coward WA, Cole TJ, Prentice AM (1996) Human energy expenditure in affluent societies: an analysis of 574 doubly-labelled water measurements. Eur J Clin Nutr 50: 72–92
42. Bouten CV, Westerterp KR, Verduin M, Janssen JD (1994) Assessment of energy expenditure for physical activity using a triaxial accelerometer. Med Sci Sports Exerc 26:1516–1523
43. St-Onge M, Mignault D, Allison DB, Rabasa-Lhoret R (2007) Evaluation of a portable device to measure daily energy expenditure in free-living adults. Am J Clin Nutr 85:742–749
44. Webster JD, Welsh G, Pacy P, Garrow JS (1986) Description of a human direct calorimeter, with a note on the energy cost of clerical work. Br J Nutr 55:1–6
45. de Weir JBV (1949) New methods for calculating metabolic rate with special reference to protein metabolism. J Physiol 109:1–9
46. Matarese L, Fada R (1997) Indirect calorimetry: technical aspects. J Am Diet Assoc 97: S154–S160
47. Tissot J (1904) Nouvelle methode de mesure et d'inscription du debit et des movements respiratories de l'homme et des animaux. J Physiol Pathol Gen 6:688–700
48. De Groot G, Schreurs AW, van Ingen Schenau GJ (1983) A portable lightweight Douglas bag instrument for use during various types of exercise. Int J Sports Med 4:132–134
49. McClave SA et al (2003) Clinical use of the respiratory quotient obtained from indirect calorimetry. JPEN J Parenter Enteral Nutr 27:21–26
50. Compher C, Frankenfield D, Keim N, Roth-Yousey L (2006) Best practice methods to apply to measurement of resting metabolic rate in adults: a systematic review. J Am Diet Assoc 106:881–903
51. Haugen HA, Chan L-N, Li F (2007) Indirect calorimetry: a practical guide for clinicians. Nutr Clin Pract 22:377–388

Psychiatric and Psychological Evaluation

Massimo Cuzzolaro

17.1 Lifestyle Intervention and Counseling (Comprehensive Lifestyle Intervention)

Lifestyle education, provided in individual or group sessions by a trained health worker, is aimed to improve physical activity level, eating behaviors, healthy diet, stress management, and sleep. Therefore, it is a form of psychological intervention for the reason that it involves emotional, cognitive, and behavioral processes, family habits, and social relationships. Furthermore, it requires accurate preliminary assessment pointed to evaluate individual barriers to healthy habits and weight loss and motivational counseling to improve adherence. Electronically delivered programs (web, telephone) are less effective than face-to-face interventions. A recent randomized controlled trial shows that web-based computer-tailored interventions for multiple health behaviors can reach a large number of people at low cost and have a significant public health impact; however, dropout rates were high and effect sizes were modest [1].

Comprehensive lifestyle intervention alone is likely to be more successful in people whose BMI is not too far from the desirable range (<35 kg/m^2). However, it "is foundational to weight loss, regardless of augmentation by medications or bariatric surgery" [2]. An intensive lifestyle intervention on body weight and cardiovascular disease risk factors among severely obese individuals (BMI ≥ 40 kg/m^2) can obtain important results in a significant proportion of patients [3].

Health coaching may be effective in people who suffer from major psychiatric disorders as well [4], but results are controversial [5].

Finally, lifestyle education is ordinarily helpful and often needed after obesity surgery because a considerable proportion of patients are unable to benefit optimally from bariatric surgery in terms of weight loss [6]. As a marginal note, providing

---

M. Cuzzolaro
Eating and Weight Disorders, Editor-in-Chief, Campiglia Marittima, Italy
e-mail: massimo.cuzzolaro@gmail.com; massimo.cuzzolaro@alice.it

information about necessary postoperative lifestyle changes can somewhat reduce the stigma of bariatric surgery [7].

17.2 Obesity and Eating Disorders

Obesity is not classified as a mental disorder per se, and there is no a place for obesity in the DSM-5 [8]. Conversely, in May 2013 binge eating disorder (BED) has become an approved DSM-5 diagnostic category. BED has connected the medical area of obesity with the psychiatric field of eating disorders, and this bridge has attracted increasing attention to the psychological and psychiatric aspects of obesity and contributed to the development of a multidimensional team approach to the assessment and treatment of eating and weight disorders [9].

The core feature of BED is the presence of recurrent episodes of overeating with loss of control and no regular use of inappropriate weight loss behaviors like self-induced vomiting. The frequency cut point for DSM-5 diagnosis is once per week for 3 months.

The results of the National Comorbidity Survey Replication, a face-to-face household study conducted in a large representative sample ($n=9,282$), indicated the following lifetime community prevalence rates of DSM-IV BED in the USA: 3.5 % in women and 2.0 % in men; F to M ratio was 1.75–1.0. Furthermore, lifetime BED was significantly associated with current obesity class III (BMI ≥ 40 kg/m^2) [10].

Obese individuals with binge eating disorder (BED) are at higher risk for developing metabolic syndrome [11]; in particular, there is a significant relationship between BED and type 2 diabetes due to their excess weight and maladaptive eating patterns.

Studies on BED treatment are burdened by several limitations as selection biases (e.g., mostly women and overweight), small samples, high dropout rates, and placebo response [12]. Psychological treatments may be useful, in particular cognitive behavioral therapy, dialectical behavior therapy, and interpersonal psychotherapy. Self-help interventions have a place [13]. A number of psychotropic drugs (in particular antidepressants and anticonvulsants/mood stabilizers like topiramate and zonisamide) may have modest beneficial effects [14].

Binge eating or loss of control eating may be observed in children and adolescents as well, usually associated with overweight/obesity. Binge eating appears independently associated with emotional eating, depression, and anxiety and positively related to parental problems (e.g., underinvolvement, arguments, and depression of family members) and social problems [15].

Other patterns of disordered eating are frequently associated with obesity, especially BED-obesity: picking or nibbling (P&N), night eating (NE), and emotional eating (EE).

Picking or nibbling is an eating behavior characterized by eating in an unplanned and repetitious manner in between meals and snacks [16]. It is highly prevalent across eating disorder diagnoses and seems to be related to poorer weight loss outcomes after bariatric surgery.

Night eating is associated with poorer glycemic control in Type 2 diabetes and disruptions in eating, sleep, and mood [17].

It is well known that eating usually moderates distress (*comfort foods*, typically with high caloric density and palatability). In some people there is a very strong relationship between eating, energy intake, and emotions, above all anger, depression, anxiety, and boredom. EE may be observed in adults, adolescents, and children. Weight loss programs should consider difficulties in the area of affect regulation and stress response. In addition, in the treatment of pediatric obesity, the emotional bond between caregiver and child should be explored as well [18].

The orexigenic hormone ghrelin might play a key role in the relationship between acute and chronic stress and food intake. Its plasma levels are enhanced under conditions of physiological stress, and the ghrelinergic system seems to be a critical factor at the interface of homeostatic control of appetite and reward circuitries, modulating the hedonic aspects of food intake [19]. Perhaps future anti-obesity pharmacotherapies should focus also on the ghrelinergic system to modulate the rewarding properties of food.

17.3 Food Craving and Food Addiction

Food craving has been defined as an intense desire to consume a specific food that is difficult to resist [20]. Despite not necessarily pathological, food craving has been indicated as particularly associated with eating and weight disorders: anorexia nervosa, bulimia nervosa, binge eating disorder, night eating, emotional eating, and obesity.

In recent years, some researchers have asked whether similar behavioral and cognitive changes occur in drug addiction and obesity. At the same time, advances in understanding the overlapping circuits underlying both feeding behaviors and drug addiction may allow us to consider this question from a neurobiological point of view, to complement behavioral perspectives [21]. The strong reinforcing effects of both food and drugs are mediated by rapid dopamine increases in the brain reward centers that, in vulnerable individuals, can override the brain's homeostatic control mechanisms. A functional magnetic resonance imaging study examined the neural correlates of addictive-like eating behavior. Elevated Yale Food Addiction Scale (YFAS) scores [22] were associated with similar patterns of neural activation as substance dependence: elevated activation in reward circuitry in response to food cues (*anticipated receipt*) and reduced activation of inhibitory regions (lateral orbitofrontal cortex) in response to food intake (*receipt*) [23].

One intriguing model considers obesity as an addictive disorder (food addiction), at least in a subgroup of subjects. A recent study [24] found that a subset of 41.5 % of BED patients met the YFAS food addiction cutoff [22]. According to Nora Volkow, both drug addiction and obesity "can be defined as disorders in which the saliency of a specific type of reward (food or drug) becomes exaggerated relative to, and at the expense of others rewards" [25].

From another point of view, a surprising research shows that the food addiction model of obesity does not increase weight bias and could even be helpful in reducing stigma against obese people [26].

The relationships among eating behavior, reward circuitry function, and affect regulation systems represent a fascinating topic, but a detailed understanding of the connections is still lacking. Furthermore, to devise diagnostic criteria based on the above aspects raises multiple difficulties because the phenomena central to this model are basically dimensional.

17.4 Anxiety and Depression

Anxiety and depression often go together with obesity [27].

Data obtained in a cross-sectional survey from 3,361 general practice patients demonstrated a U-shaped relationship between weight and depression, with higher prevalence of depressive symptoms observed among underweight (24 %) and obese individuals (23 %) in comparison with normal-weight (11 %) and overweight (12 %) subjects [28].

Which came first, obesity or depression?

A number of studies suggest a bidirectional relation between obesity and depression. The Nurses' Health Study prospectively followed from 1996 to 2006 65.955 women aged 54–79 years. Depression at the baseline period was associated with an increased risk of obesity at the follow-up period, also in baseline non-obese women. On the other hand, obese women at baseline had a moderately increased risk of depression at the follow-up period compared with baseline normal-weight women, also for new onset of depression [29].

For girls, adolescence is a high-risk period for the development of the comorbidity obesity-depression. A prospective study found that early adolescent-onset depression is associated with elevated risk of later-onset obesity, and obesity, particularly in late adolescence, is associated with increased odds of later depression [30].

17.5 Negative Body Image and Social Stigma

The clinical relevance of studies on body image in subjects with obesity has continued to increase in the years. Such factors as gender, age, degree of obesity, onset age of overweight, ethnicity, social class, history of sexual abuse, teasing and parental criticism about weight, history of weight cycling, and presence of binge eating all show important modulating effects on body uneasiness [31]. Individuals with BED-obesity present greater dissatisfaction and distress about their body appearance than people with non-BED-obesity and may present weight and shape concerns comparable to bulimia nervosa patients and higher than anorexia nervosa patients. Overvaluation of shape/weight in BED should be, but is not yet in DSM-5, a diagnostic specifier for BED [32, 33].

Therefore, assessment and treatment of persons with obesity and BED should consider cognitive as well as behavioral dysfunctional attitudes, and outcome studies should be focused not only on eating behavior but on body image as well.

A circular relationship links together obesity social stigma, internalized stigma, and negative self-image that upset obese persons. Obesity social stigma is pervasive in contemporary societies [34]. Representations of people with obesity as unpleasant, lazy, unintelligent, and with poor self-control are dominant. Prevention programs should take into account this critical problem that contributes to distress, depression, low self-esteem, and disordered eating behaviors.

17.6 Bariatric Surgery Candidates and Psychopathology

A substantial body of level 1 evidence from randomized trials comparing surgical versus nonsurgical approaches to obesity, type 2 diabetes, and other metabolic diseases shows that, at this time, bariatric (or metabolic) surgery is the weight loss treatment of choice for patients with morbid obesity [35]. However, BMI should not be a primary criterion for selection of candidates [36].

A recent review of studies using structured diagnostic interviews [37] shows that the rates of psychopathology in the bariatric surgery candidates are considerably higher than the other two population groups (general population group and non-treatment obese group), in all the samples. Both current and lifetime rates of psychopathology appear high in bariatric surgery candidates: affective disorders are the most common category of *lifetime* Axis I disorders, while anxiety disorders are the most common category of *current* Axis I disorders. Higher rates of psychopathology are associated with female gender, low socioeconomic status, and higher BMI. Bariatric candidates who think that their life will dramatically change after surgery and those with comorbid psychiatric disorders (e.g., severe personality disorder, intense body image disturbance) may show greater difficulties in adapting to the postoperative way of life, and psychological and/or psychiatric treatment, before and after surgery, if surgery is performed, may be necessary [38].

Loss of control is central to psychological disturbance associated with BED. High body uneasiness and feelings of loss of control could drive binge eaters to seek weight loss surgery more often than non-BED obese subjects in an attempt to gain control over both compulsive eating behavior and body shape [39]. Accordingly, the prevalence of BED among bariatric surgery candidates is particularly high, about 10 % [40]. A 2014 study evaluated how many more bariatric surgery candidates met the new, less conservative criteria of DSM-5 for BED: an additional 3.43 % of candidates met the diagnostic threshold for BED when using the DSM-5 criteria. However, they were similar to those meeting the more conservative DSM-IV-TR diagnostic threshold [41]. In obesity surgery candidates, BED is associated with an increased prevalence of psychopathology beyond the already elevated rate observed with obesity class III [42]. Preoperative and postoperative binge eating or grazing has been shown to be associated with poorer weight loss [43]. Nevertheless, BED should not be considered as an absolute contraindication per se. Adequate treatment may help BED patients to obtain positive outcomes from weight loss surgery [44]. These issues should be addressed in the pre- and perioperative period to maximize gains after surgery. That is why, in many hospitals, mental health professionals are a part of the multidimensional process of both the evaluation and treatment of bariatric surgery patients. Some authors speak of *bariatric psychology* [45].

17.7 Weight Regain and Psychopathology After Bariatric Surgery

The operation on its own should be considered as one step in obesity treatment.

Existing literature indicates that, in general, there are improvements in quality of life, sexual functioning, and psychological health after bariatric surgery with peak progresses during the first year of weight loss [46, 47]. The change for the better may be attributed to weight loss and consequential gains in body image and self-concept. Preoperative mental health plays an important role.

However, not all patients report psychological benefits after bariatric surgery. Some patients continue to struggle with weight loss, maintenance and regain, and resulting body image dissatisfaction. Weight recidivism has been observed in a significant proportion of patients after bariatric surgery. A systematic review indicates that the underlying causes leading to weight regain are patient and procedure specific, multifactorial, and overlapping: psychiatric disorders, psychological features, unhealthy lifestyle (physical inactivity and/or dietary noncompliance), endocrine-metabolic diseases, and problems related to surgical procedure [48]. According to the authors of this review, addressing postsurgical weight regain requires a systematic multidisciplinary approach focusing on contributory dietary, psychologic, psychiatric, medical, and surgical factors.

Some patients seem to experience *addiction transfer* [49]: new compulsive behaviors and new addictions may blossom to replace overeating (alcohol, smoking, drugs, gambling, shopping, etc.). In particular, weight loss surgery candidates may have a greater lifetime risk of alcohol use disorders, and after surgery, many patients continue to consume alcohol and not rarely they increase quantities, regardless of greater sensitivity to the intoxicating effects [50].

Eating disorders may emerge after bariatric surgery. In most cases, diagnostic criteria for anorexia nervosa or bulimia nervosa are not satisfied. Segal and coworkers proposed a new category, *postsurgical eating avoidance disorder* [51]. Emotional eating and compulsive grazing are eating patterns that can persist or appear after surgery and negatively affect outcome. The postoperative development of eating disorders in obesity surgery patients seems a quite rare outcome, but it is likely that such symptoms are underreported [52].

17.8 Obesity in People with Serious Mental Illnesses

Persons with mood and anxiety disorders, schizophrenia, post-traumatic stress disorder, personality disorders, etc., are 1.5 to more than three times as likely to be obese as the general population. Overweight/obesity and mental disorders appear frequently together also in children and adolescents. As the prevalence of obesity in people diagnosed as having a mental illness is very high, obesity and obesity-related diseases contribute to the total disability level. In addition, a double social and internalized stigma impairs the quality of life of individuals who are mentally ill and overweight [53].

The interaction of genetic factors, socioeconomic status, lifestyle, and medications likely accounts for the high risk of overweight, metabolic syndrome, and premature mortality in people with serious mental illness. Undoubtedly, most psychotropic drugs – not only antipsychotics but antidepressants and mood stabilizers as well – are associated with the potential to induce weight gain- and obesity-related disorders. When psychiatrists prescribe drugs, they should take into account potential for weight gain, monitor metabolic parameters, and educate their patients and caregivers about the risks and how to prevent them [54].

17.9 Psychometric Instruments

Tests may be helpful to reliably and validly assess specific constructs relevant to eating- and weight-related disorders. From a clinical perspective, an evaluation of single items may offer precious information. Many psychometric instruments exist and new tests emerge continuously. Table 17.1 suggests 20 self-report questionnaires (Q) and interviews (I).

Table 17.1 Eating and weight disorders: 20 psychometric instruments

Name	Type	Target
Beck Depression Inventory [55]	Q	Depression
Binge Eating Scale [56]	Q	Binge eating
Body Uneasiness Test [31]	Q	Body image
Brief Symptom Inventory [57]	Q	Psychopathology
Decisional Balance Inventory [58]	Q	Motivation
Difficulties in Emotion Regulation Scale [59]	Q	Emotion regulation dysregulation
Eating Disorder Examination 16.0D [60]	I	Eating disorders
Eating Disorder Examination Questionnaire 6.0 [61]	Q	Eating disorders
Food craving inventory [20]	Q	Food craving
Impact of Weight on Quality of Life [62]	Q	Quality of life
KINDL-R [63]	Q	Quality of life in children/adolescents
McMaster Family Assessment Device [64]	Q	Family functioning
Rosenberg Self-Esteem Scale [65]	Q	Self-esteem

(continued)

Table 17.1 (continued)

Name	Type	Target
Spielberger State-Trait Anxiety Inventory [66]	Q	Anxiety
State-Trait Anger Expression Inventory [67]	Q	Anger
Symptom Check List [68]	Q	Psychopathology
Temperament and Character 69]	Q	Temperament, character, personality
Three-Factor Eating Questionnaire [70]	Q	Eating behavior
Weight Efficacy Lifestyle questionnaire [71]	Q	Self-efficacy
Yale Food Addiction Scale [22]	Q	Food addiction

References

1. Schulz DN, Kremers SP, Vandelanotte C, van Adrichem MJ, Schneider F, Candel MJ, de Vries H (2014) Effects of a web-based tailored multiple-lifestyle intervention for adults: a two-year randomized controlled trial comparing sequential and simultaneous delivery modes. J Med Internet Res 16:e26
2. Jensen MD, Ryan DH, Apovian CM, Ard JD, Comuzzie AG, Donato KA, Hu FB, Hubbard VS, Jakicic JM, Kushner RF, Loria CM, Millen BE, Nonas CA, Pi-Sunyer FX, Stevens J, Stevens VJ, Wadden TA, Wolfe BM, Yanovski SZ (2014) American College of Cardiology/American Heart Association Task Force on Practice Guidelines, Obesity Society: 2013 AHA/ACC/TOS guideline for the management of overweight and obesity in adults: a report of the American College of Cardiology/American Heart Association Task Force on Practice Guidelines and The Obesity Society. J Am Coll Cardiol, 63:2985–3023
3. Unick JL, Beavers D, Bond DS, Clark JM, Jakicic JM, Kitabchi AE, Knowler WC, Wadden TA, Wagenknecht LE, Wing RR, Look ARG (2013) The long-term effectiveness of a lifestyle intervention in severely obese individuals. Am J Med 126:236–242, 242 e231–232
4. Bonfioli E, Berti L, Goss C, Muraro F, Burti L (2012) Health promotion lifestyle interventions for weight management in psychosis: a systematic review and meta-analysis of randomised controlled trials. BMC Psychiatry 12:78
5. Usher K, Park T, Foster K, Buettner P (2013) A randomized controlled trial undertaken to test a nurse-led weight management and exercise intervention designed for people with serious mental illness who take second generation antipsychotics. J Adv Nurs 69:1539–1548
6. Mechanick JI, Youdim A, Jones DB, Garvey WT, Hurley DL, McMahon MM, Heinberg LJ, Kushner R, Adams TD, Shikora S, Dixon JB, Brethauer S, American Association of Clinical E, Obesity S, American Society for M, Bariatric S (2013) Clinical practice guidelines for the perioperative nutritional, metabolic, and nonsurgical support of the bariatric surgery patient–2013 update: cosponsored by American Association of Clinical Endocrinologists, the Obesity Society, and American Society for Metabolic & Bariatric Surgery. Endocr Pract 19:337–372
7. Vartanian LR, Fardouly J (2014) Reducing the stigma of bariatric surgery: benefits of providing information about necessary lifestyle changes. Obesity (Silver Spring) 22:1233–1237
8. American Psychiatric Association (2013) Diagnostic and statistical manual of mental disorders, DSM-5, 5th edn. American Psychiatric Publishing, Arlington
9. Cuzzolaro M, Vetrone G (2009) Overview of evidence on the underpinnings of binge eating disorder and obesity. In: Dancyger I, Fornari V (eds) Evidence based treatments for eating disorders: children, adolescents and adults. Nova Science Publishers, New York, pp 53–70
10. Hudson JI, Hiripi E, Pope HG Jr, Kessler RC (2007) The prevalence and correlates of eating disorders in the National Comorbidity Survey Replication. Biol Psychiatry 61:348–358

11. Hudson JI, Lalonde JK, Coit CE, Tsuang MT, McElroy SL, Crow SJ, Bulik CM, Hudson MS, Yanovski JA, Rosenthal NR, Pope HG Jr (2010) Longitudinal study of the diagnosis of components of the metabolic syndrome in individuals with binge-eating disorder. Am J Clin Nutr 91:1568–1573
12. Ramacciotti CE, Coli E, Marazziti D, Segura-Garcia C, Brambilla F, Piccinni A, Dell'Osso L (2013) Therapeutic options for binge eating disorder. Eat Weight Disord 18:3–9
13. Beintner I, Jacobi C, Schmidt UH (2014) Participation and outcome in manualized self-help for bulimia nervosa and binge eating disorder – a systematic review and metaregression analysis. Clin Psychol Rev 34:158–176
14. Mitchell JE, Roerig J, Steffen K (2013) Biological therapies for eating disorders. Int J Eat Disord 46:470–477
15. Hartmann AS, Czaja J, Rief W, Hilbert A (2012) Psychosocial risk factors of loss of control eating in primary school children: a retrospective case-control study. Int J Eat Disord 45:751–758
16. Conceicao EM, Crosby R, Mitchell JE, Engel SG, Wonderlich SA, Simonich HK, Peterson CB, Crow SJ, Le Grange D (2013) Picking or nibbling: frequency and associated clinical features in bulimia nervosa, anorexia nervosa, and binge eating disorder. Int J Eat Disord 46:815–818
17. Hood MM, Reutrakul S, Crowley SJ (2014) Night eating in patients with Type 2 diabetes: associations with glycemic control, eating patterns, sleep, and mood. Appetite 79:91–96
18. Vandewalle J, Moens E, Braet C (2014) Comprehending emotional eating in obese youngsters: the role of parental rejection and emotion regulation. Int J Obes (Lond) 38:525–530
19. Schellekens H, Finger BC, Dinan TG, Cryan JF (2012) Ghrelin signalling and obesity: at the interface of stress, mood and food reward. Pharmacol Ther 135:316–326
20. White MA, Whisenhunt BL, Williamson DA, Greenway FL, Netemeyer RG (2002) Development and validation of the food-craving inventory. Obes Res 10:107–114
21. Krashes MJ, Kravitz AV (2014) Optogenetic and chemogenetic insights into the food addiction hypothesis. Front Behav Neurosci 8:57
22. Gearhardt AN, Corbin WR, Brownell KD (2009) Preliminary validation of the Yale Food Addiction Scale. Appetite 52:430–436
23. Gearhardt AN, Yokum S, Orr PT, Stice E, Corbin WR, Brownell KD (2011) Neural correlates of food addiction. Arch Gen Psychiatry 68:808–816
24. Gearhardt AN, White MA, Masheb RM, Grilo CM (2013) An examination of food addiction in a racially diverse sample of obese patients with binge eating disorder in primary care settings. Compr Psychiatry 54:500–505
25. Volkow ND, Wang GJ, Tomasi D, Baler RD (2013) Obesity and addiction: neurobiological overlaps. Obes Rev 14:2–18
26. Latner JD, Puhl RM, Murakami JM, O'Brien KS (2014) Food addiction as a causal model of obesity. Effects on stigma, blame, and perceived psychopathology. Appetite 77C:79–84
27. Brumpton B, Langhammer A, Romundstad P, Chen Y, Mai XM (2013) The associations of anxiety and depression symptoms with weight change and incident obesity: the HUNT study. Int J Obes (Lond) 37:1268–1274
28. Carey M, Small H, Yoong SL, Boyes A, Bisquera A, Sanson-Fisher R (2014) Prevalence of comorbid depression and obesity in general practice: a cross-sectional survey. Br J Gen Pract 64:e122–e127
29. Pan A, Sun Q, Czernichow S, Kivimaki M, Okereke OI, Lucas M, Manson JE, Ascherio A, Hu FB (2012) Bidirectional association between depression and obesity in middle-aged and older women. Int J Obes (Lond) 36:595–602
30. Marmorstein NR, Iacono WG, Legrand L (2014) Obesity and depression in adolescence and beyond: reciprocal risks. Int J Obes (Lond) 38:906–911
31. Marano G, Cuzzolaro M, Vetrone G, Garfinkel PE, Temperilli F, Spera G, Dalle Grave R, Calugi S, Marchesini G (2007) Validating the Body Uneasiness Test (BUT) in obese patients. Eat Weight Disord 12:70–82
32. Cuzzolaro M, Bellini M, Donini L, Santomassimo C (2008) Binge eating disorder and body uneasiness. Psychol Top 17:287–312

33. Grilo CM, White MA, Gueorguieva R, Wilson GT, Masheb RM (2013) Predictive significance of the overvaluation of shape/weight in obese patients with binge eating disorder: findings from a randomized controlled trial with 12-month follow-up. Psychol Med 43:1335–1344
34. De Brun A, McCarthy M, McKenzie K, McGloin A (2014) Weight stigma and narrative resistance evident in online discussions of obesity. Appetite 72:73–81
35. Ribaric G, Buchwald JN, McGlennon TW (2014) Diabetes and weight in comparative studies of bariatric surgery vs conventional medical therapy: a systematic review and meta-analysis. Obes Surg 24:437–455
36. Cummings DE, Cohen RV (2014) Beyond BMI: the need for new guidelines governing the use of bariatric and metabolic surgery. Lancet Diabetes Endocrinol 2:175–181
37. Malik S, Mitchell JE, Engel S, Crosby R, Wonderlich S (2014) Psychopathology in bariatric surgery candidates: a review of studies using structured diagnostic interviews. Compr Psychiatry 55:248–259
38. Kinzl JF (2010) Morbid obesity: significance of psychological treatment after bariatric surgery. Eat Weight Disord 15:e275–e280
39. Colles SL, Dixon JB, O'Brien PE (2008) Loss of control is central to psychological disturbance associated with binge eating disorder. Obesity (Silver Spring) 16:608–614
40. Mitchell JE, Selzer F, Kalarchian MA, Devlin MJ, Strain G, Elder KA, Marcus MD, Wonderlich S, Christian NJ, Yanovski SZ (2012) Psychopathology before surgery in the Longitudinal Assessment of Bariatric Surgery-3 (LABS-3) psychosocial study. Surg Obes Relat Dis 8:533–541
41. Marek RJ, Ben-Porath YS, Ashton K, Heinberg LJ (2014) Impact of using DSM-5 criteria for diagnosing binge eating disorder in bariatric surgery candidates: change in prevalence rate, demographic characteristics, and scores on the Minnesota Multiphasic Personality Inventory – 2 restructured form (MMPI-2-RF). Int J Eat Disord 47:553–557
42. Jones-Corneille LR, Wadden TA, Sarwer DB, Faulconbridge LF, Fabricatore AN, Stack RM, Cottrell FA, Pulcini ME, Webb VL, Williams NN (2012) Axis I psychopathology in bariatric surgery candidates with and without binge eating disorder: results of structured clinical interviews. Obes Surg 22:389–397
43. Conceicao E, Bastos AP, Brandao I, Vaz AR, Ramalho S, Arrojado F, da Costa JM, Machado PP (2014) Loss of control eating and weight outcomes after bariatric surgery: a study with a Portuguese sample. Eat Weight Disord 19:103–109
44. Ashton K, Heinberg L, Windover A, Merrell J (2011) Positive response to binge eating intervention enhances postoperative weight loss. Surg Obes Relat Dis 7:315–320
45. van Hout G, van Heck G (2009) Bariatric psychology, psychological aspects of weight loss surgery. Obes Facts 2:10–15
46. Karlsson J, Taft C, Ryden A, Sjostrom L, Sullivan M (2007) Ten-year trends in health-related quality of life after surgical and conventional treatment for severe obesity: the SOS intervention study. Int J Obes (Lond) 31:1248–1261
47. Sarwer DB, Spitzer JC, Wadden TA, Mitchell JE, Lancaster K, Courcoulas A, Gourash W, Rosen RC, Christian NJ (2014) Changes in sexual functioning and sex hormone levels in women following bariatric surgery. JAMA Surg 149:26–33
48. Karmali S, Brar B, Shi X, Sharma AM, de Gara C, Birch DW (2013) Weight recidivism post-bariatric surgery: a systematic review. Obes Surg 23:1922–1933
49. Reslan S, Saules KK, Greenwald MK, Schuh LM (2014) Substance misuse following Roux-en-Y gastric bypass surgery. Subst Use Misuse 49:405–417
50. Heinberg LJ, Ashton K, Coughlin J (2012) Alcohol and bariatric surgery: review and suggested recommendations for assessment and management. Surg Obes Relat Dis 8:357–363
51. Segal A, Kinoshita Kussunoki D, Larino MA (2004) Post-surgical refusal to eat: anorexia nervosa, bulimia nervosa or a new eating disorder? A case series. Obes Surg 14:353–360
52. Marino JM, Ertelt TW, Lancaster K, Steffen K, Peterson L, de Zwaan M, Mitchell JE (2012) The emergence of eating pathology after bariatric surgery: a rare outcome with important clinical implications. Int J Eat Disord 45:179–184

53. Cuzzolaro M (2013) Obesity. Psychiatric aspects. In: Capodaglio P, Faintuch J, Liuzzi A (eds) Disabling obesity from determinants to health care models. Springer, New York, pp 183–197
54. Hasnain M, Vieweg WV (2013) Weight considerations in psychotropic drug prescribing and switching. Postgrad Med 125:117–129
55. Beck AT, Steer RA, Brown GK (1996) Manual for the Beck Depression Inventory-II, 2nd edn. Psychological Corporation, San Antonio
56. Gormally J, Black S, Daston S, Rardin D (1982) The assessment of binge eating severity among obese persons. Addict Behav 7:47–55
57. Derogatis LR, Melisaratos N (1983) The Brief Symptom Inventory: an introductory report. Psychol Med 13:595–605
58. Ward RM, Velicer WF, Rossi JS, Fava JL, Prochaska JO (2004) Factorial invariance and internal consistency for the Decisional Balance Inventory–Short Form. Addict Behav 29:953–958
59. Gratz KL, Roemer L (2004) Multidimensional assessment of emotion regulation and dysregulation: development, factor structure, and initial validation of the Difficulties in Emotion Regulation Scale. J Psychopathol Behav Assess 26:41–54
60. Fairburn CG, Cooper Z, O'Connor ME (2008) Eating Disorder Examination (Edition 16.0D). In: Fairburn CG (ed) Cognitive behavior therapy and eating disorders. The Guilford Press, New York, pp 265–308
61. Fairburn CG, Beglin SJ (2008) Eating Disorder Examination Questionnaire (EDE-Q 6.0). In: Fairburn CG (ed) Cognitive behavior therapy and eating disorders. The Guilford Press, New York, pp 309–314
62. Kolotkin RL, Head S, Hamilton M, Tse CK (1995) Assessing impact of weight on quality of life. Obes Res 3:49–56
63. Erhart M, Ellert U, Kurth BM, Ravens-Sieberer U (2009) Measuring adolescents' HRQoL via self reports and parent proxy reports: an evaluation of the psychometric properties of both versions of the KINDL-R instrument. Health Qual Life Outcomes 7:77
64. Epstein N, Baldwin L, Bishop D (1983) The McMaster Family Assessment Device. J Marital Fam Ther 9:171–180
65. Schmitt DP, Allik J (2005) Simultaneous administration of the Rosenberg self-esteem scale in 53 nations: exploring the universal and culture-specific features of global self-esteem. J Pers Soc Psychol 89:623–642
66. Kendall PC, Finch AJ Jr, Auerbach SM, Hooke JF, Mikulka PJ (1976) The State-Trait Anxiety Inventory: a systematic evaluation. J Consult Clin Psychol 44:406–412
67. Forgays DG, Forgays DK, Spielberger CD (1997) Factor structure of the State-Trait Anger Expression Inventory. J Pers Assess 69:497–507
68. Derogatis L (1983) SCL90: administration, scoring and procedures manual for the revised version. Clinical Psychometric Research, Baltimore
69. Cloninger CR (2000) A practical way to diagnosis personality disorder: a proposal. J Personal Disord 14:99–108
70. Stunkard A, Messick K (1985) The Three Factor Eating Questionnaire to measure dietary restraint, disinhibition and hunger. J Psychosom Res 29:71–81
71. Clark MM, Abrams DB, Niaura RS, Eaton CA, Rossi JS (1991) Self-efficacy in weight management. J Consult Clin Psychol 59:739–744

Functional Evaluation (Joint and Muscle Problems, Cardiopulmonary Exercise Testing, Disability Evaluation)

18

Gian Pietro Emerenziani, Federico Schena, and Laura Guidetti

18.1 Introduction

Functional evaluation could be interpreted as a set of tests and observations that determine individual functional abilities, strength, skills, and capacity to perform specific daily performance. Therefore, functional evaluation leads us to assess the physical fitness of the subjects providing the baseline data helpful to realize an individualized training program. When performing the functional evaluation, it is important to focus whether the data obtained relates to performance or health. Performance measurements refer to components that contribute to optimal task execution (such as maximal speed, maximal power, etc.), while health measurements refer to components related to health status (such as body composition, bone strength, lipid metabolism, and peak aerobic capacity). The choice to assess performance or health parameters depends on many factors. The assessment of performance parameter is usually more important for athletes or healthy-active subjects than for sedentary, untrained, or subjects with diseases. Obviously, seeing that obesity is associated with an increased risk of heart disease, stroke, hypertension, type II diabetes mellitus, osteoarthritis, and with disability [1–6], the information obtained from functional evaluation should be related to health. Therefore, in obese subjects it is required to assess all components that relate to health. For example, body composition, strength, gait speed, flexibility, peak oxygen consumption, aerobic threshold, and balance. In addition, functional assessment should highlight not only

G.P. Emerenziani • L. Guidetti (✉)
Department of Movement, Human, and Health Sciences,
University of Rome "Foro Italico", Piazza L. De Bosis, 6, Rome 00135, Italy
e-mail: gianpietro.emerenziani@uniroma4.it; laura.guidetti@uniroma4.it

F. Schena
Department of Neurological Sciences and Movement,
University of Verona, Via Casorati 43, Verona 37134, Italy
e-mail: Federico.schena@univr.it

the ability but also the limitations of the subjects. The latter is very important for fitness professionals to realize training programs minimizing the risk of injuries and dropout. We reach the well-known positive effects on health [7–10] by implementing a training program that considers the subjects' abilities and disabilities, in combination with dietary and behavioral modifications.

The test setting for functional assessment in obese subjects includes the physical characteristics to obtain health-related information. For example, in order to assess the peak oxygen capacity, the test protocol should consider the low gait speed and balance capacity typical of obese individuals. Also, muscle problems which could occur during the test performance will influence test results and interpretation. For example, Wright et al. [11] showed that overweight and obese twins were more likely to report low back pain, tension-type or migraine headache, fibromyalgia, abdominal pain, and chronic widespread pain than normal-weight twins after adjustment for age, gender, and depression. These results are also supported by Hitt et al. [12], who affirmed that obese subjects are more likely to experience pain than their normal-weight and underweight counterparts. It is also important to note that disabilities and physical problems themselves may lead to increased risk for obesity. In fact, some disabilities often lead the subjects to have sedentary lifestyle and consequently to have an imbalance between intake and energy expenditure.

18.2 Joint and Muscle Problems

Obesity condition is strongly correlated with joint and muscle problems favoring an increased risk of physical disability [13]. Jensen et al. [13] observed that the relationship between obesity and functional impairment extended in longitudinal follow-up to men and women at a BMI of 35 or greater. It is also important to notice that total fat mass is the body component more strongly associated with increased risk of disability than body fat distribution [14]. Studies have pointed out the relationship between pain and body weight showing that body weight is significantly related with knee, hip, and back pain in older population [15] and with neck and back pain in general population [16]. The prevalence of significant musculoskeletal pain in obese subjects results in a significant negative relationship between obesity and health-related quality of life [17]. These data demonstrate that pain is a strong covariate of obesity, and, therefore, this should be considered in the design and development of obesity treatments. Excess of body fat could cause abnormal posture, both in dynamic [18] and static conditions [19]. This abnormal posture limits the normal joints' physiological range of motion and consequently enhances the risk of musculoskeletal overload [20]. Moreover, increased forces across the joints play a fundamental role in the negative relationship between obesity and weight-bearing joints (back, knees, ankle, and hip), compared to non-weight-bearing joints (shoulder/neck and upper extremities). Therefore, the effects of weight on joints depend on the body regions that are involved. In support of this relation, Shiri et al. [21] analyzed the effects of overweight and obesity on sciatica. The author affirmed that both overweight and obesity conditions are associated with an increasing risk in hospitalization for sciatica and with an increasing risk of surgery for lumbar disk herniation. The increased mechanical loads on knees and the decrease in lower limb flexibility could justify the high incidence of knee osteoarthritis [22] and skeletal alteration in obese subjects [23]. Obesity is also strongly correlated with muscle problems. In fact, a specific feature of obesity called "sarcopenic obesity" has recently become of interest for researchers [24, 25]. This condition emerges when obese subjects have inadequate muscle mass compared to their body size. The imbalance between obesity and muscle function, either defined by small muscle mass or poor muscle strength, is associated with risk of disability. The sarcopenic obesity condition could depend on different factors. First, fat mass increases with the age, whereas muscle mass and strength tend to decline progressively after the age of 40 years. In support of these trends, Droyvold et al. [26] showed that during approximately 10 years, body weight increased in all age groups below 70 years, while Evans et al. [27] analyzed the causes that lead to a loss of skeletal muscle mass during aging. Second, a sedentary lifestyle, typical of obese subjects, speeds on the decrease of skeletal muscle mass and the gain of fat mass. Moreover, more causes of sarcopenic obesity were evaluated such as inflammation, insulin resistance, malnutrition, etc. [24].

18.3 Cardiopulmonary Exercise Testing

Cardiorespiratory fitness, defined as the ability of the body to transport and use oxygen, depends on the integration of cardiac, pulmonary, and musculoskeletal systems. Fitness professionals should be aware that overweight and obese subjects could be poorly conditioned since the aerobic capacity of these subjects has been shown to be low, and in some instances, critically low [28]. De Souza et al. [29] reported that aerobic capacity of severe obese subjects ($44 \leq BMI \leq 54.8$ kg/m^2) ranged from 16.1 to 34.7 ml·min^{-1}kg^{-1}. The poor aerobic capacity must be taken into consideration when determining exercise intensity in deconditioned subjects. Among the parameters to be considered in the exercise program for obese population, intensity has received special attention [10]. Cardiopulmonary exercise test allows the fitness professionals to assess the right intensity of training program. Intensity rate could be described in both absolute and relative terms. Relative terms take into account the exercise capacity of the subjects to perform the activity, while absolute terms only consider the demands of the activity. Cardiopulmonary exercise test provides important data to prescribe the appropriate exercise intensity for overweight and obese subjects in both relative and absolute terms. Commonly, exercise intensity is based on measured, or estimated, peak oxygen uptake ($\dot{V}O_{2peak}$) or maximum heart rate (HR$_{max}$) [30]. However, when a workload is quantified only in relation to $\dot{V}O_{2peak}$ or HR$_{max}$, it can result in different metabolic requirements between subjects. Therefore these variables should be used with caution when prescribing exercise, due to the lower cardiorespiratory fitness of overweight and obese subjects [10].

An alternative approach is to define the exercise intensity in relation to validated physiological break point such as the aerobic/anaerobic threshold. The aerobic threshold marks the upper limit of an almost exclusively aerobic metabolism that permits exercise lasting for ten of minutes at a lactate level of approximately

2 mmol·l^{-1}. The individual aerobic threshold (AerT) represents in general a mild to moderate exercise intensity (31). For these reasons, during the last years, AerT has been used more frequently [31] to prescribe exercise intensity, and it has also been applied in obese population with comorbidity [32]. Considering that the obese population is characterized by a low cardiorespiratory fitness, it can be very important to use threshold concept when exercise intensity has to be chosen. The procedures to determine the AerT [10] during an incremental exercise testing may include protocols based on of blood lactate measurements or on gas exchange analysis. The determination of AerT through gas exchange analysis is a noninvasive practice, and this deserves a special consideration for a simple intensity exercise prescription in overweight and obese subjects. There are different protocols to assess this parameter as described by Emerenziani et al. [10]. One of the suitable methods is the determination of the optimal respiratory efficiency by plotting the ventilatory equivalent ($\dot{V}E/\dot{V}O_2$) as a function of $\dot{V}O_2$ in order to identify the point during exercise where this curve has its minimum value.

18.4 Disability Evaluation

Physical inactivity, a common condition of overweight and obese individuals, is usually associated with low cardiopulmonary values and disabilities. Disability is typically defined as an impairment that limits the capacity of a person to perform daily life activities. Obesity is characterized by a low health-related quality of life due to a disability in strength, gait speed, flexibility, and cardiorespiratory capacity. Disability could be evaluated with different sets of tests, in accordance with the physical capacity to evaluate. Choice of measurement should be limited by practical issues and influenced by functional relevance as well as feasibility. The Medical Outcome Study 36-Item Short Form Health Survey (SF-36) is one of the most used instrument for the evaluation of generic quality of life. It examines eight different items: physical functioning, role limitations due to physical problems, energy/vitality, bodily pain, social functioning, role limitations due to emotional problems, mental health, and general health. Karlsen et al. [33] showed that this tool could be used to evaluate the health-related quality of life in obese population. Moreover, the National Health and Nutrition Examination Survey (NHANES) and the Specific short-form questionnaire for Obesity-related Disabilities (TSD-OC test) could be used to evaluate subjects' well-being [34, 35]. The performance in a specific test such as the 6-min walking test (6MWT) can unveil the limitations in cardiorespiratory and motor functions underlying the obesity-related disability [36]. The 6MWT has been shown to be a reliable and valid test to assess the physical fitness of obese patients [37]. Strength disability could be evaluated by the hand grip strength test or by the lower limb strength test [36]. Spine flexion, together with hip and shoulder flexion, extension, and abduction, could be measured with a standard goniometer [36]. Flexibility could be measured by a sit-and-reach test, in which the subject sits with the knees completely straight and reaches forward slowly using both the hands together [38].

References

1. Atkins JL, Whincup PH, Morris RW, Lennon LT, Papacosta O, Wannamethee SG (2014) Sarcopenic obesity and risk of cardiovascular disease and mortality: a population-based cohort study of older men. J Am Geriatr Soc 62:253–260
2. Irace C, Scavelli F, Carallo C et al (2009) Body mass index, metabolic syndrome and carotid atherosclerosis. Coron Artery Dis 20:94–99
3. Mokdad AH, Ford ES, Bowman BA et al (2001) Prevalence of obesity, diabetes, and obesity-related health risk factors. JAMA 289:76–79
4. Ferraro KF, Su YP, Gretebeck RJ et al (2002) Body mass index and disability in adulthood: a 20-year panel study. Am J Public Health 92:834–840
5. Lippi G, Schena F, Guidi GC (2006) Health benefits of physical activity. CMAJ 175:776–777
6. Drenick EJ, Bale GS, Seltzer F et al (1980) Excessive mortality and causes of death in morbidly obese men. JAMA 243:443–445
7. Donini LM, Cuzzolaro M, Gnessi L et al (2014) Obesity treatment: results after 4 years of a Nutritional and Psycho-Physical Rehabilitation Program in an outpatient setting. Eat Weight Disord 19:249–260
8. Donnelly JE, Blair SN, Jakicic JM et al (2009) American College of Sports Medicine Position Stand. Appropriate physical activity intervention strategies for weight loss and prevention of weight regain for adults. American College of Sports Medicine. Med Sci Sports Exerc 41: 459–471, Erratum in Med Sci Sports Exerc 41:1532
9. Figard-Fabre H, Fabre N, Leonardi A et al (2011) Efficacy of Nordic Walking in obesity management. Int J Sports Med 32:407–414
10. Emerenziani GP, Migliaccio S, Gallotta MC et al (2013) Physical exercise intensity prescription to improve health and fitness in overweight and obese subjects: a review of the literature. Health (Irvine Calif) 5:113–121
11. Wright LJ, Schur E, Noonan C et al (2010) Chronic pain, overweight, and obesity: findings from a community-based twin registry. J Pain 11:628–635
12. Hitt HC, McMillen RC et al (2007) Comorbidity of obesity and pain in a general population: results from the Southern Pain Prevalence Study. J Pain 8:430–436
13. Jensen GL, Friedmann JM (2002) Obesity is associated with functional decline in community-dwelling rural older persons. J Am Geriatr Soc 50:918–923
14. Visser M, Marris TB, Langlois J et al (1998) Body fat and skeletal muscle mass in relation to physical disability in very old men and women of the Framingham Heart Study. J Gerontol A Biol Sci Med Sci 53:214–221
15. Anderson RE, Crespo CJ, Bartlett SJ et al (2003) Relationship between body weight gain and significant knee, hip, and back pain in older Americans. Obes Res 11:1159–1162
16. Webb R, Brammah T, Lunt M et al (2003) Prevalence and predictors of intense, chronic, and disabling neck and back pain in the UK general population. Spine 28:1195–1202
17. Sach TH, Barton GR, Doherty M et al (2007) The relationship between body mass index and health-related quality of life: comparing the EQ-5D, Euro-Qol VAS and SF-6D. Int J Obes 31:189–196
18. Mignardot JB, Olivier I, Promayon E et al (2013) Origins of balance disorders during a daily living movement in obese: can biomechanical factors explain everything? PLoS One 8:e60491
19. Park W, Singh DP, Levy MS et al (2009) Obesity effect on perceived postural stress during static posture maintenance tasks. Ergonomics 52:1169–1182
20. Viester L, Verhagen EA, Oude Hengel KM et al (2013) The relation between body mass index and musculoskeletal symptoms in the working population. BMC Musculoskelet Disord 14:238
21. Shiri R, Lallukka T, Karppinen J et al (2014) Obesity as a risk factor for sciatica: a meta-analysis. Am J Epidemiol 179:929–937
22. Menegoni F, Galli M, Tacchini E et al (2009) Gender-specific effect of obesity on balance. Obesity (Silver Spring) 17:1951–1956
23. Migliaccio S, Greco EA, Fornari R et al (2013) Skeletal alterations in women affected by obesity. Aging Clin Exp Res 25(Suppl 1):35–37

24. Stenholm S, Harris TB, Rantanen T et al (2008) Sarcopenic obesity: definition, cause and consequences. Curr Opin Clin Nutr Metab Care 11:693–700, Review
25. Donini LM, Savina C, Coletti C et al (2010) Obesity in the elderly. Ann Ig 22:499–511
26. Droyvold WB, Nilsen TI, Kruger O et al (2006) Change in height, weight and body mass index: longitudinal data from the HUNT study in Norway. Int J Obes 30:935–939
27. Evans WJ (2010) Skeletal muscle loss: cachexia, sarcopenia, and inactivity. Am J Clin Nutr 91:1123S–1127S
28. Mollaoglu H, Ucok K, Kaplan A et al (2012) Association analyses of depression, anxiety, and physical fitness parameters in Turkish obese adults. J Back Musculoskelet Rehabil 25:253–260
29. de Souza SA, Faintuch J, Sant'anna AF (2010) Effect of weight loss on aerobic capacity in patients with severe obesity before and after bariatric surgery. Obes Surg 20:871–875
30. Pinet BM, Prud'homme D, Gallant CA et al (2008) Exercise intensity prescription in obese individuals. Obesity 16:2088–2095
31. Meyer T, Lucía A, Earnest CP et al (2005) A conceptual framework for performance diagnosis and training prescription from submaximal gas exchange parameters-theory and application. Int J Sports Med 26:S38–S48, Review
32. Kunitomi M, Takahashi K, Wada J et al (2007) Re-evaluation of exercise prescription for Japanese type 2 diabetic patients by ventilatory threshold. Diabetes Res Clin Pract 50:109–115
33. Karlsen TI, Tveitå EK, Natvig GK et al (2011) Validity of the SF-36 in patients with morbid obesity. Obes Facts 4:346–351
34. Cui W, Zack MM, Wethington H (2014) Health-related quality of life and body mass index among US adolescents. Qual Life Res 23:2139–2150
35. Donini LM, Brunani A, Sirtori A et al (2011) SIOSISDCA task force: assessing disability in morbidly obese individuals: the Italian Society of Obesity test for obesity-related disabilities. Disabil Rehabil 33:2509–2518
36. Donini LM, Poggiogalle E, Mosca V et al (2013) Disability affects the 6-minute walking distance in obese subjects (BMI>40 kg/m(2)). PLoS One 8:e75491
37. Beriault K, Carpentier AC, Gagnon C et al (2009) Reproducibility of the 6-minute walk test in obese adults. Int J Sports Med 30:725–727
38. Kim JW, Seo DI, Swearingin B et al (2013) Association between obesity and various parameters of physical fitness in Korean students. Obes Res Clin Pract 7:67–74

Impairment of Quality of Life in Obesity

19

Carlo M. Rotella and Barbara Cresci

19.1 Which Quality of Life?

The complications of obesity possibly determining premature mortality include cardiovascular diseases, diabetes mellitus, dyslipidemia, sleep apnea and respiratory failure, osteoarthritis, infertility, some forms of cancer (colon, breast, prostate, endometrium), depression, and impairment of health-related quality of life [1]. Improvement of quality of life is recognized as a relevant measure of treatment outcome in obese patients, both in medically and surgically treated cases [2]. There is an open discussion about the meaning of quality of life and what issues are really important for patient well-being. The concept of quality of life is a major point when discussing measures aimed at defining the impact of diseases (obesity in this case) on functional status and well-being. The quality of life concept is multifaceted and can be approached from different perspectives. Many terms have been used interchangeably: quality of life, health status, and health-related quality of life (HRQL). Anyway, quality of life refers not only to health status but also to environmental and economic factors that can obviously affect well-being. HRQL is the functional effect of a medical condition and/or its therapy on a patient. Therefore, HRQL is subjective and multidimensional, including physical and occupational function, psychological state, social interaction, and somatic sensations [3].

C.M. Rotella, MD (✉)
Department of Biomedical and Experimental Sciences,
Obesity Agency, Careggi University Hospital, Florence, Italy

Department of Biomedical, Experimental and Clinical Sciences,
University of Florence, Viale Pieraccini 6, Florence 50134, Italy
e-mail: carlomaria.rotella@unifi.it

B. Cresci
Endocrinology Unit, Careggi University Hospital,
Viale Pieraccini 6, Florence 50134, Italy
e-mail: b.cresci@dfc.unifi.it

© Springer International Publishing Switzerland 2015
A. Lenzi et al. (eds.), *Multidisciplinary Approach to Obesity: From Assessment to Treatment*, DOI 10.1007/978-3-319-09045-0_19

Therefore, we can imagine how difficult it is to try and measure someone's quality of life. As a result, for a long time, hundreds of tests have been designed to measure different aspects of quality of life [4].

19.2 Why Do We Need to Assess Quality of Life?

First, HRQL assessments are commonly administered initially to assess the overall impact of a particular condition on functioning and well-being. This provides additional information beyond those offered by traditional medical and clinical measures; this can help to understand the wide variability in individual responses to similar conditions [5]. Second, HRQL measures can be used as an outcome esteem to evaluate the effects of treatment. HRQL can also be used to assess the efficacy and cost-effectiveness of treatment interventions [6, 7]. Finally, on a wider perspective, information on quality of life may also influence the development of clinical pathways, healthcare expenditures, and public health policy.

19.3 Measuring Quality of Life: Instruments

HRQL can be measured by either generic or obesity-specific instruments.

19.3.1 Generic HRQL Instruments

Generic instruments are designed to measure broad aspects of quality of life. These instruments are not designed to assess quality of life relative to a particular medical condition but rather provide a generalized assessment.

The SF-36 Health Survey3 is the most widely used and validated HRQL instrument [8]. The scores are standardized from 0 for poor health to 100 for good health. Scores from the SF-36 Health Survey can be compared with established scores of healthy persons in the USA (US norms). There are eight health domains within the SF-36: physical functioning (measures the limitation in performance of physical activities), role-physical (measures the limitation in daily activities as a result of physical health), role-emotional (measures limitation in daily activities as a result of emotional problems), bodily pain (measures the pain-related functional limitations), vitality (measures the energy level), mental health (measures the presence and degree of depression and anxiety), social functioning (measures the limitations in social functioning), and general health (measures an individual's perception of his/her health).

Other generic instruments have been used with obese patients [9], such as the Satisfaction with Life Scale, the Extended Satisfaction with Life Scale and the Quality of Life Inventory, the Nottingham Health Profile (38 questions), and the Sickness Impact Profile (136 items).

The major advantage of generic measures is that they allow for comparisons of HRQL across a variety of medical conditions. Moreover, generic instruments can be administered to different populations to examine the impact of various healthcare/therapeutic programs on HRQL. On the other hand, the major limitation of generic HRQL instruments is that they do not assess potential condition-specific domains of HRQL. Because of this, they may not be sufficiently sensitive to detect subtle treatment effects. [10].

19.3.2 Specific Instruments

The second approach to HRQL assessment involves the use of instruments that are specific to a disease, population, or specific clinical problems. Measures designed for specific diseases or populations will probably be more sensitive and therefore have greater relevance in medical practice. A commonly used specific tool is the Obesity-Related Well-Being (ORWELL 97) questionnaire [11], which has been developed and validated by our group. The ORWELL 97 is a self-reported measure of obesity-related, perceived, quality of life, measuring obesity-related domains such as social activities, self-esteem, and sexual attractiveness. The novelty of the ORWELL 97 questionnaire is that it takes into consideration not only the intensity but also the subjective relevance of physical and psychosocial distress. In fact, a group of obese patients was asked to describe the effects of being overweight in their everyday life and to indicate the most distressing physical and psychological symptoms; on the basis of the most commonly voiced concerns, the authors identified 18 items.

The Impact of Weight on Quality of Life (IWQOL) scale [12] and the Health State Preference (HSP) scale in persons with obesity [13] are other examples of obesity-specific HRQL instruments. The IWQOL is a 74-item measure that assesses the effect of weight along eight domains of functioning: health, social/interpersonal, work, mobility, self-esteem, sexual life, activities of daily living, and comfort with food.

Other obesity-specific instruments are the Moorehead-Ardelt Quality of Life Questionnaire (5 questions) [14], the Obesity-Specific Quality of Life questionnaire (11 questions) [15], and the Quality of Well-Being Scale (50 questions) [16]. In particular, the Moorehead-Ardelt QoL Questionnaire is a simple bariatric-specific questionnaire, used effectively as part of the Bariatric Analysis and Reporting Outcome System (BAROS). The Moorehead-Ardelt Quality of Life Questionnaire assesses self-esteem, physical activity, social life, work conditions, and sexual activity/interest. Points are added for positive changes and subtracted for negative changes.

Even if disease-specific instruments probably provide a better assessment of HRQL than generic instruments, the major variable is based on the goals and aims of the research. In fact, it has been shown that disease-specific instruments are more powerful in detecting treatment effects than generic instruments [17]. Moreover, it has also been demonstrated that obesity-specific measures of psychological distress correlate more highly with relative body weight than general measures of psychological distress [18].

The "fair" consensus reached among quality of life researchers is that both generic and disease-specific instruments should be used to provide the most comprehensive assessment of HRQL possible, even if this could be of more difficult management for the patient (patient burden) and also for the inquirer (data management, discrepancies between the results, etc.).

19.4 Obesity and HRQL

It is widely known that obesity adversely affects HRQL [19]. Therefore, HRQL is now considered a priority in the treatment of chronic diseases and may be selected as a clinical-relevant outcome in treatment programs. Nevertheless, several review articles and meta-analyses have found an inconsistent relation between obesity and psychological outcomes, including psychological well-being and quality of life [20]. The QUOVADIS study [21] showed that psychopathological disturbances are the most relevant factors associated with poor HRQL in obese patients, affecting not only psychosocial but also physical domains, largely independent of the severity of obesity. Moreover, mixed evidence has been shown for body image and self-esteem as predictors of weight control [22]. The real problem is probably that the majority of studies have been restricted to the evaluation of the role of obesity on the prevalence of selected chronic diseases or mortality and a few empirical studies have estimated the influence of obesity on HRQL [10]. Undoubtedly, there are many variables that should be taken into account, such as comorbidities, BMI, age and sex of the patients, and also the presence of eating disorders.

Substantial HRQL impairments are known to occur in the severely obese patients, even if the independent impact that weight itself has on quality of life is generally small [23, 24]. Anyway, it has been demonstrated that, in comparison with a normal BMI, obesity is associated with a lower HRQL, even after controlling for patient characteristics and comorbidity [25]. A quite recent work has shown that women probably suffer a disproportionately large share of the disease burden of overweight and obesity, which is not due solely to differences in medical comorbidity. The possibility that aspects of emotional well-being may mediate the association between obesity and physical health functioning warrants further attention in this regard. These findings therefore indicate the need to stratify data by gender [26].

The association between age and weight-related quality of life in overweight/obese individuals has also been investigated. Weight-related quality of life seems to be more impaired with increasing age for physical function, sexual life, and work. However, increasing age was associated with less impairment for self-esteem and public distress [27]. It has also been demonstrated that in postmenopausal women, depressed mood may amplify the negative impact of obesity on physical HRQL [28].

The impairment of HRQL in obese patients is increased by the presence of eating disorders [29]. Moreover, obese individuals with BED have impaired functioning on psychosocial aspects of HRQL in addition to poorer physical functioning associated with obesity [30]. These psychological factors should therefore be thoroughly assessed and taken into account in global strategies aiming to improve the well-being of obese patients.

Another major point in assessing HRQL in obese patients is the impact of the possible various comorbidities. According to different studies, morbid obesity clearly contributes to the impairment of health-related quality of life [31]. In this view, it could be of interest to understand the independent impact of specific comorbidities on HRQL and how this might vary across the different HRQL instruments. Very recently, a cross-sectional analysis of 500 severely obese subjects performed using several validated (specific and generic) instruments has shown that the clinical impact of BMI on physical and general HRQL was small and mental health scores were not associated with BMI. On the contrary, chronic pain, depression, and sleep apnea were consistently associated with lower HRQL [32].

References

1. Brown WV, Fujioka K, Wilson PW et al (2009) Obesity: why be concerned? Am J Med 4(1):S4–S11
2. Karlsson J, Taft C, Ryden A et al (2007) Ten-year trends in health-related quality of life after surgical and conventional treatment for severe obesity: the SOS intervention study. Int J Obes (Lond) 31(8):1248–1261
3. Ahmed S, Berzon RA, Revicki DA, International Society for Quality of Life Research et al (2012) The use of Patient-reported Outcomes (PRO) within comparative effectiveness research: implications for clinical practice and health care policy. Med Care 50:1060–1070. doi:10.1097/MLR.0b013e318268aaff
4. Fallowfield LJ (1996) Quality of quality of life data. Lancet 348:42110
5. Katz DA, McHorney CA, Atkinson RL (2000) Impact of obesity on health-related quality of life in patients with chronic illness. J Gen Intern Med 15(11):789–796
6. Jhingran P, Cady RK, Rubino J et al (1996) Improvements in health related quality of life with sumatriptan treatment for migraine. J Fam Pract 42:36–42
7. Ware JE, Bayliss MS, Rogers WH et al (1996) Differences in 4-year health outcomes for elderly and poor, chronically ill patients treated in HMO and fee-for-service systems. JAMA 276:1039–1047
8. Ware JE, Snow KK, Kosinski M et al (1993) SF-36 health survey: manual and interpretation guide. New England Medical Center, Boston
9. Alfonso VC (1995) Measures of quality of life, subjective well-being, and satisfaction with life. In: Allison DB (ed) Handbook of assessment methods for eating behaviors and weight-related problems: measures, theory, and research. Sage Publications, Thousand Oaks, pp 23–57
10. Fontaine KR, Barofsky I (2001) Obesity and health-related quality of life. Obes Rev 2:173–182
11. Mannucci E, Ricca V, Barciulli E et al (1999) Quality of life and overweight: the obesity related well-being (Orwell 97) questionnaire. Addict Behav 24:345–357
12. Kolotkin RL, Head S, Hamilton MJ et al (1995) Assessing impact of weight on quality of life. Obes Res 3:49–56
13. Barajas GMA, Robledo ME, Garcia TN et al (1998) Quality of life in relation to health and obesity in a primary care center. Rev Esp Salud Publica 72:221–231
14. Fontaine KR, Cheskin LJ, Barofsky I (1996) Health-related quality of life in obese persons seeking treatment. J Fam Pract 43:265–2705
15. Oria HE, Moorehead MK (1998) Bariatric Analysis and Reporting Outcome System (BAROS). Obes Surg 8:487–499

16. Le Pen C, Levy E, Loos F et al (1998) "Specific" scale compared with "generic" scale: a double measurement of the quality of life in a French community sample of obese subjects. J Epidemiol Community Health 52:445–450
17. Nguyen N, Varela EJ, Nguyen T et al (2006) Quality of life assessment in the morbidly obese. Obes Surg 16:531–533
18. Laupacis A, Wong C, Churchill D (1991) The use of generic and specific quality of life measures in hemodialysis patients treated with erythropoietin. Con Clin Trials 12:168S–179S
19. Klesges RC, Klem ML, Klesges LM (1992) The relationship between changes in body weight and changes in psychological functioning. Appetite 19:145–153
20. McElroy SL, Kotwal R, Malhotra S et al (2004) Are mood disorders and obesity related? A review for the mental health professional. J Clin Psychiatry 65:634–651
21. Mannucci E, Petroni ML, Villanova N, QUOVADIS Study Group et al (2010) Clinical and psychological correlates of health-related quality of life in obese patients. Health Qual Life Outcomes 8:90–99
22. Teixeira PJ, Going SB, Sardinha LB et al (2005) A review of psychosocial pre-treatment predictors of weight control. Obes Rev 6:43–65
23. de Zwaan M, Petersen I, Kaerber M et al (2009) Obesity and quality of life: a controlled study of normal-weight and obese individuals. Psychosomatics 50:474–482
24. Dolan P, Kavetsos G (2012) Educational interventions are unlikely to work because obese people aren't unhappy enough to lose weight. BMJ 345:e848
25. Sach T, Barton GR, Doherty M et al (2007) The relationship between body mass index and health-related quality of life: comparing the EQ-5D, EuroQol VAS and SF-6D. Int J Ob 31:189–196
26. Mond JM, Baune BT (2009) Overweight, medical comorbidity and health-related quality of life in a community sample of women and men. Obesity 17:1627–1634
27. Zabelina DL, Erickson AL, Kolotkin RL et al (2009) The effect of age on weight-related quality of life in overweight and obese individuals. Obesity 17:1410–1413
28. Heidelberg DA, Holle R, Lacruz ME et al (2011) Do diabetes and depressed mood affect associations between obesity and quality of life in postmenopause? Results of the KORA-F3 Augsburg population study. Health Qual Life Outcomes 9:97
29. Folope V, Pharm CC, Grigioni S et al (2012) Impact of eating disorders and psychological distress on the quality of life of obese people. Nutrition 28:e7–e13
30. Rieger E, Wilfley DE, Stein RI et al (2005) A comparison of quality of life in obese individuals with and without binge eating disorder. Int J Eat Disord 37:234–240
31. Duval K, Marceau P, Lescelleur O et al (2006) Health-related quality of life in morbid obesity. Obes Surg 16:574–579
32. Warkentin LM, Majumdar SR, Johnson JA et al (2014) Predictors of health-related quality of life in 500 severely obese patients. Obesity. doi:10.1002/oby.20694

Part IV
Therapeutic Approach

Therapeutic Education and Psychotherapy

20

Giovanni Gravina, Monica Palla, Carla Piccione, and Grazia Nebbiai

20.1 Introduction

Psychological issues play significant roles in both the development and consequences of obesity. Studies have found that some people eat more when affected by depression, anxiety, or other emotional disorders. Being overweight and obese is often the cause of these psychological disorders. It is a vicious cycle whereby the greater the emotional conflicts and difficulties, the greater the incidence of unhealthy eating and obesity.

A multidisciplinary approach that addresses psychological, social, environmental, and biological factors of obesity is critical to ensure comprehensive care, as well as best practices and outcomes. The importance of dealing with the psychological aspects in the treatment of obesity has become more explicit over the last two decades. Not only is the role of a psychologist important for treatment of obesity and pre-surgical psychological assessment, but also following weight loss to help the patient to adjust the subsequent emotional, behavioural, and social changes that often occur. The achievement of substantial weight loss from bariatric surgical or nonsurgical approaches is significantly related to one's ability to make permanent changes in one's lifestyle that involves not only adherence to more appropriate nutritional intake and exercise but also improved management of stress and emotional states with decreased reliance on eating as a coping mechanism.

G. Gravina (✉) • M. Palla • C. Piccione • G. Nebbiai
Centro per i Disturbi Alimentari – Casa di Cura San Rossore, Pisa, Italia

Center for Eating Disorders - Casa di Cura San Rossore, Pisa, Italy
e-mail: gravina@sanrossorecura.it

20.2 Physician Communication Style

The weight loss programmes, based on diet and physical activity, require also learned cognitions about food and eating and changes in lifestyle, habits, and behaviour. Obese people experience many difficulties to start losing weight and to maintain weight loss. Psychological factors play a relevant role to determine these problems. In obese individuals there are frequent mood alterations, low self-esteem, negative body image, emotional discomforts, and interpersonal relationship difficulties. Various comorbidities and functional limitations associated with obesity can adversely affect physical quality of life. Poor health and employment-related as well as other forms of social discrimination can add to the psychological distress in obese individuals [1].

On this basis, treating obesity, the first aspect to consider is the physician's and health worker's competence to deal with psychological issues and to manage the relationship with the patient [2].

Patients suffering from obesity need a multidimensional evaluation intended to design an individualized treatment plan applying different procedures and therapeutic strategies.

Integrating several competences in team-based approach demands specific education, skills, training, and expertise [3] also with regard to the psychological aspects of the disease.

Particular attention must be given to patient-centred care, working alliance, effective communication, and empathy. These dimensions of care are useful in the approach to many diseases, but they represent necessary characteristics of the doctor–patient relationship in the treatment of obesity [4].

Providers approach the "patient as person" (rather than patient as disease or organ), taking into account the meaning of the illness to the patient in his or her broader life context [5]. Patient-centred communication is responsive to the patients' emotional state and concerns and encourages patients to participate in decision making [6, 7].

Working alliance includes cognitive and emotional components of the patient–physician relationship, promotes patient's self-efficacy, and is associated with patient adherence to the treatment [8].

Effective communication has the potential to regulate patient's emotions, facilitate comprehension of medical information, and allow for better identification of patient's needs, perceptions, and expectations.

Communication strategies for building better relationships with patients are nonverbal and verbal strategies, shared decision making, and motivational intervention.

Empathy is the core element of the relationship, representing the competence of a physician to understand the patient's situation, perspective, and feelings; to communicate that understanding and check its accuracy; and to act on that understanding in a helpful therapeutic way. Empathy can therefore be defined at three levels: as an attitude (affective level), as a competency (cognitive level), and as an action (behavioural level). Empathy in patient–physician encounters was associated with patient's behaviour change [9], decrease in patient's anxiety and distress, and better clinical outcomes [10].

20.3 Therapeutic Education

In addition to the skills concerning the relationship and the effective communication style, to better address the psychological issues of patients, physicians can use a more structured approach defined as therapeutic patient education (TPE).

TPE is a systemic, patient-centred learning process, useful in the treatment of chronic diseases, primarily in diabetes and obesity also [11, 12].

TPE is an integral part of treatment and care focused on patients' needs, resources, and values.

TPE allows patients to be active participants improving their knowledge and skills not only concerning their illness but also their treatment.

In order to be properly accomplished, TPE involves an open-minded professional approach and a strong availability to inter-professional as well as interdisciplinary network, including physicians, nurses, dietitians, physiotherapists, psychiatrists, psychologists, and social workers.

According to a definition of a World Health Organization working group, therapeutic patient education is "designed to enable a patient (or a group of patients and families) to manage the treatment of their condition and prevent avoidable complications, while maintaining or improving quality of life".

It takes into account coping with the disease, locus of control, health beliefs, and sociocultural perceptions; subjective and objective needs of patients, whether expressed or not.

TPE is a continuous process, which has to be adapted to the course of the disease and to the patient and the patient's way of life. Health-care providers should be able to adapt their professional behaviour to patients and their disease, communicate empathetically with patients, recognize the needs of patients, help patients learn, and take account of the patients' emotional state, their experience, and their representations of the disease and its treatment.

TPE is designed therefore to train patients in the skills of self-managing or adapting treatment to their particular chronic disease and in coping processes and skills. It should also contribute to reduce the cost of long-term care for patients and society.

20.4 Psychological Factors and Obesity

Psychological factors contribute to the onset and maintenance of overweight and obesity in children, adolescents, and adults, also playing a significant role in determining difficulties for the treatment of obesity. Furthermore some obesity phenotypes appear to be related with specific psychological states and traits. Negative body image, low self-esteem, mood disorders, and social and family factors affect individuals in different ways and contribute to weight gain and failure in weight loss management. Assessment of these mental health factors and treatment by one of several mental health treatment models may not only improve self-worth but also weight loss and maintenance.

Research on personality and obesity reveals a complex relationship. Individual personality traits are related to a dynamic combination of weight status, treatment-seeking behaviour, comorbidities, and intervention success [13].

Statistically significant personality differences have been identified between obese and nonobese populations, but such data does not permit to determine an obese personality profile [13].

On the other hand, some studies show that obese individuals tend to be more impulsive, addictive, anxious, and novelty seeking than healthy-weight counterparts even after controlling for treatment-seeking behaviour and binge eating [14, 15].

Many studies agree in pointing out a deficiency in the emotional component of obese subjects. Indeed, a cofactor in some obese individuals is assumed to be immature affect regulation, which has its roots in the interaction with the primary caregivers and is related to early attachment experiences.

Attachment theory assumes that humans have a biologically predisposed attachment system [16] responsible for the strong emotional mother–child (primary caregiver–child) relationship. This system is activated as soon as an outer or inner danger arises that cannot be overcome by the child himself and thus has a survival-ensuring function.

A child's feelings, expectations, and behavioural strategies are integrated into this attachment relationship, which develops during the first year of life. In its basic structure, it is stable over time and forms an emotional basis throughout life, although change in different directions is possible through emotional experiences in new relationships or through psychotherapy. Attachment styles are currently differentiated as secure and insecure (preoccupied, dismissing, fearful–avoidant, and unresolved), and it is likely that children's relationships with adults other than the mother, such as father, grandparents, teachers, or care providers, also influence children's attachment security.

Some interesting studies noted an association between attachment and obesity based on maternal–child interaction such as maternal responsiveness, child engagement, and child negativity [17].

Another essential indication, derived from the original studies of H. Bruch, points up that obese individuals are not able to distinguish feeling of hunger from other physical needs or from emotional tension and psychological stress.

Some authors highlight that there is evidence that obesity and the metabolic syndrome can result from physiologic and behavioural responses to psychological stress [18–20].

The physiologic mechanisms appear to be related to neuroendocrine pathways, such as those involving cortisol, insulin, leptin, and neuropeptide Y [21].

Empirical observations support the possibility that children with a secure pattern of attachment are more easily comforted in stressful situations and are better able to regulate negative emotions; these behaviours are reflected in healthier patterns of physiologic responses to stress [22].

The stress response behavioural mechanisms may include eating to cope with negative emotions [23]. Secure attachment could reduce the risk for childhood obesity by preventing frequent or exaggerated stress responses from disrupting the normal functioning and development of physiologic systems that affect energy balance, body weight, and fat distribution.

Securely attached children who are better able to regulate their emotions may be less likely to eat in response to emotional distress in early childhood when the systems in the limbic brain that regulate both emotion and appetite are developing concurrently [21].

All of these elements may be determinant not only in promoting obesity but also in causing difficulties for physicians taking in charge patients in adult life and in influencing the outcome of treatment.

Concerning the therapy of obese subjects, the relationship with the therapist plays a decisive role. These relationships depend especially on earlier experiences and the attachment style of the patient.

Moreover patient–therapist relationship is assessed to be more positive in secure compared to insecure participants. This corresponds to observations indicating that securely attached individuals have better access to their emotions and eating habits, can therefore better perceive, understand and name them, and thus also have better prerequisites for successful weight reduction [24]. Individuals with an insecure attachment style are more likely to have problems with these issues; in the case of emotional entanglement, for example, preoccupied attached individuals do not perceive eating as an attempt to compensate. Dismissively attached individuals tend to have difficulties in experiencing emotions and thus compensate by eating [25].

On this basis, over time, to deal the psychological issues associated with obesity, different psychotherapy-related approaches have been used in the treatment [26].

20.5 Behaviour Therapy

The lifestyle modification programmes combining diet, physical activity, and behaviour therapy were well formulated in the Diabetes Prevention Program and Look AHEAD research studies [27, 28].

Behavioural treatments appear to work primarily by enhancing dietary restraint by providing adaptive dietary strategies and by discouraging maladaptive dietary practices, and by increasing motivation to be more physically active. Therapy aims to provide the individual with coping skills to handle various cues of overeating and to manage lapses in diet and physical activity when they occur.

Therapeutic techniques derived from behavioural psychology include stimulus control (remove triggers for excessive eating and increase positive cues for exercising), goal setting (patients are educated to plan specific and quantifiable weekly goals, which should be realistic and moderately challenging), and self-monitoring (patients are educated to write down the time, amount, type, and calorie content of foods and beverages they are going to consume in a monitoring record and then to check in "real time", while eating, if they respect what they had planned) [29].

Behaviour therapy (BT) may be held as the first line of intervention for overweight and obese individuals. Behavioural treatments have demonstrated effectiveness in the treatment of obesity, improving weight loss also in combination with other approaches for lifestyle modification [30].

In spite of this evidence, BT does not allow effective results in many cases, especially with regard to the maintenance of acquired weight loss. Behaviour therapy and lifestyle modification approaches result, on the average, in a short-term weight loss of 10 %, but long-term effects of such programmes are disappointing, in fact in most cases 30–50 % of the weight lost is regained within the first year after the end of the programme and continues to steadily increase until stabilizing near baseline weight in 5 years after treatment [31].

20.6 Motivational Interview

A substantial body of researches confirm the poor maintenance of weight loss in obese individuals following treatment by lifestyle modification programmes combining diet, physical activity, and behaviour therapy [32].

Remarkably difficult stages in the treatment of obesity are the initiation of changes, the compliance with therapeutic advice as well as the maintenance of the achieved weight loss. In these phases of the treatment, a key problem appears to be the resistance to change, based on psychological issues.

For these reasons regarding the need to address resistance to change, at the beginning and in the course of a treatment of obesity, it may be useful to evaluate the readiness to change of obese individuals which is possible by means of a structured test, so-called TRE-MORE test, recently validated for the clinical practice [33].

Concerning the approach to the obese patient's resistance, motivational interview (MI) may be of particular interest [34].

Referring to the transtheoretical model of behaviour change [35], MI is an intervention that derives from a social cognitive theoretical framework and is designed to favour an individual's motivation to change problematic behaviours. MI is a patient-centred approach that emphasizes individual autonomy and a collaborative relationship between patient and provider. This approach takes the form of psychotherapy and differs from a traditional patient education-based intervention, which mostly tends to provide advice and information [36, 37].

MI strives to help patients move towards behaviour change by assisting them in the process of identifying, articulating, and strengthening personally relevant reasons for change, eliciting personal goals, problem-solving barriers to change by highlighting benefits of change and reducing the perceived costs of change, and addressing ambivalence about the change. This approach uses an emphatic, interactive style that supports self-determination, enhances self-efficacy, and underscores individual control for behaviour change [38].

Despite the efficacy of MI techniques to influence readiness for behaviour change [39, 40], there are still few data in the literature concerning this approach outside of the domain of substance and alcohol addiction. Many studies suggest that MI strategies used alone or in combination with other behavioural interventions have led to increased exercise in different types of diseases. Studies using MI combined with various diet and exercise strategies have demonstrated improved weight loss and treatment adherence in obese and diabetic patients [41].

An interesting study on a group of obese patients who failed to lose sufficient weight during a lifestyle modification programme shows that the patients who later received MI sessions subsequently lost significantly more weight and engaged in significantly more weekly exercise than those who did not receive the intervention [42]. Moreover emerging research concerning the efficacy of MI for the maintenance of weight loss and improved psychosocial functioning of obese adults [43] and isolating the unique contributions of MI to weight loss treatment suggests that this approach has utility as part of a comprehensive multicomponent obesity intervention [44].

On this basis, the use of MI, if confirmed by further investigation with larger patient samples, seems to promise interesting results in the treatment of obesity [45].

In recent years some studies have shown that high-fat/high-sugar food and drugs that cause addiction act similarly on brain reward pathways [46], and there is growing evidence on brain reward dysfunction in both obesity and binge-eating disorder [47–49]. Such brain abnormalities may be linked with behavioural problems, including high impulsivity and the inability to delay gratification. In addition, overabundance of high-fat/high-sugar food in the environment may place individuals with genetic, neurological, and/or cognitive–behavioural vulnerabilities at increased risk of development of food addiction in binge eating and obesity.

Therefore, in light of the demonstrated effectiveness of MI in the treatment of addictions to alcohol and drugs, it is possible that this psychotherapeutic approach has additional reasons for its application in the treatment of obesity.

20.7 Cognitive–Behavioural Therapy

Cognitive–behavioural therapy (CBT) for the treatment of obesity has been applied over the years assuming that cognitions influence both feelings and behaviours. A new form of CBT was designed to enhance acceptance of their shape in obese individuals and encourage their implementation of weight maintenance behaviour. When cognitive techniques are added to BT, they appear to improve programme success, reduce weight regain, and increase psychological well-being [50].

The CBT approach helps manage problems in a more positive way, examining how your actions can affect how you think and feel. CBT works by helping make sense of overwhelming problems by breaking them down into smaller parts. Thoughts, feelings, physical sensations, and actions are interconnected, often trapping one in a negative spiral. CBT helps stop these negative cycles. It aims to break down factors that are making one feel wrong, anxious, or scared so that they are more manageable. It can show how to change these negative patterns to improve the way one feels.

CBT is utilized in the treatment of obesity as a way to help individuals change their negative eating behaviours and incorporate healthy lifestyle changes. The CBT interventions are self-monitoring techniques (e.g. food and exercise journals), stress management, stimulus control (e.g. eating only at the kitchen table), social support, problem-solving, and cognitive restructuring (e.g. to have more realistic weight loss goals, avoidance and challenging of self-defeating beliefs).

These strategies are aimed at identifying and modifying aversive thinking patterns and mood states to facilitate weight loss [51].

The addition of cognitive therapy to a standard dietetic treatment for obesity might not only be effective in reducing weight and related concerns, depressed mood, and low self-esteem, but might also prevent relapse and have an enduring effect that lasts beyond the end of treatment. Moreover some authors have shown that incorporating additional cognitive components into the cognitive–behavioural treatment of obesity can improve both short- and long-term outcomes [52, 53].

CBT showed efficacy also in the treatment of BED [54] in which it is necessary to modify the highly dysfunctional eating habits even before the start of a programme for weight loss. The most important therapeutic goals of the CBT programme are normalization of eating habits and stopping the binge-eating episodes; promoting physical activity and a positive body experience; learning specific skills such as assertiveness; installing a functional self-evaluation system; learning to identify, tolerate, and express negative emotions; promoting self-esteem; and prevention of relapse [55].

Interesting studies regarding the effectiveness of CBT interventions for the treatment of obesity in a group show that results are not inferior to a similar programme applied in individual setting, and it may enhance weight loss in the short term [56, 57].

Other studies have shown that CBT is well suited to treating obesity in children and adolescent, given the emphasis on breaking negative behaviour cycles and recommending to extend therapy beyond the individual treatment milieu to include the family, peer network, and community domains to promote behaviour change, minimize relapse, and support healthy long-term behaviour maintenance [58].

Finally, even in combination with bariatric surgery, CBT has demonstrated effectiveness in improving the results of treatment and keeping them. In fact psychological factors play a substantial role also with regard to the surgical treatment of obesity [59]. Moreover in obese patients looking for bariatric surgery, the prevalence of psychiatric and personality disorders is higher than that in obese individuals from the community [60].

Psychological assessment with a focus on special factors that could affect the bariatric surgery outcomes (depression, anxiety, eating disorders, self-esteem, personality disorders, quality of life) is recommended, and it has been introduced over 20 years.

Psychological factors such as current substance abuse or dependence, current acute or inadequately managed mental illness, or lack of comprehension of risks, benefits, expected outcomes, alternatives and lifestyle changes required with bariatric surgery, and unwillingness to comply with postsurgical protocol, can be considered as factors to deny or defer surgery.

Data about psychological disorders in obese patients before and after bariatric surgery as well as the assessment and impact of these factors on post-surgery outcomes highlighted the usefulness of psychological treatment to enhance the results. Recent studies have shown the efficacy of CBT programmes to prevent weight regain in morbid obese individuals treated with bariatric surgery; moreover combining bariatric surgery with CBT weight loss programme after surgery might help weight control [61, 62].

Despite increasing positive experience, some studies lead to different conclusions on the greater effectiveness of CBT in the treatment of obesity, suggesting that the differences between standard behaviour therapy and cognitive–behavioural therapy of obesity lie more in their underlying theories than in their implementation [63].

Another study, comparing short- and longer-term effects of a new form of CBT with BT and with a minimal intervention, a form of guided self-help (GSH), shows that the great majority of the participants lost weight and then regained it; even if the weight loss was greater for the CBT compared to BT and CBT was also successful at achieving change in participants' acceptance of shape, CBT was no better than BT to prevent posttreatment weight regain, and only a low proportion of patients in both treatment conditions were able to maintain either a 5 or 10 % weight loss throughout follow-up [31].

20.8 Interpersonal Psychotherapy

Interpersonal psychotherapy (IPT) has been particularly applied to the treatment of BED based on a strong body of evidence demonstrating a consistent relationship between poor interpersonal functioning and eating disorders in adults and adolescents [64–66].

Binge eating is the most common eating pattern seen in obesity, and BED is now included among the structured forms of eating disorder (DSM V). With respect to obesity, BED is reliably associated with a higher BMI, presents greater functional impairment and lower quality of life, and shows significantly greater levels of psychiatric disturbances.

The interpersonal model posits that social problems create an environment in which binge eating develops and is maintained as a coping mechanism, serving to reduce negative affect in response to unfulfilling social interactions. Binge eating may, in turn, worsen interpersonal problems by increasing social isolation and impeding on fulfilling relationships, thereby maintaining the eating disorder [67].

Suppressed affect is often present in people with BED; so, instead of expressing negative affect, they eat to cope. IPT helps individuals acknowledge and express this painful affect so that they can better manage negative feelings without turning to food.

IPT also seeks to reduce binge-eating pathology by supporting the development of healthy interpersonal skills that can replace maladaptive behaviours and promote a positive self-image.

Finally IPT is the only treatment that has shown comparable long-term outcomes to CBT. Moreover IPT has shown greater efficacy for patients with more severe eating pathology and lower self-esteem and thus may be a more appropriate first-line treatment for such individuals [68].

20.9 Dialectical Behaviour Therapy

Efficacy in the treatment of BED was found by using the dialectical behaviour therapy (DBT) [69, 70]. DBT has been structured by Marsha Linehan for the treatment of women with borderline personality disorder; the focus of the treatment is to restore the ability to identify, accept, and regulate their emotions.

The modification of DBT for BED is based on the affect regulation model of binge eating, which posits that binge eating occurs in response to intolerable emotional experiences when more adaptive coping mechanisms are not accessible.

20.10 Other Psychotherapeutic Approaches

Since systematic reviews or controlled studies on humanistic and psychodynamic therapies in treatment of obesity are not available [71], and considering the limitations and inadequacies of the approaches discussed above, alternative psychotherapeutic treatments have been tested.

A small number of studies on psychotherapy-related approaches, e.g. relaxation therapy or hypnotherapy, failed to demonstrate any decisive positive outcomes.

Combination therapies involving behavioural and biological therapies, especially mind–body interventions, have been proposed. Two mind–body modalities, energy psychology and mindfulness meditation, are reviewed for their potential in treating weight loss, stress, and behaviour modification related to binge-eating disorder. Mindfulness meditation and practices show compelling evidence and exhibit initially promising outcomes but require further evidence-based trials [72, 73].

Finally, according to some authors, it should be noted that, for the large prevalence of obesity, individual- or small-group-based interventions are insufficient to serve the population masses requiring treatment. On this basis, the proposed manualized self-help programmes, such as guided self-help CBT, may be helpful, at least for individuals with low level of additional psychological problems [31, 74]; the development of community or Web-based programmes and community-development tactics to increase healthy lifestyles may also be useful [75].

> **Conclusions**
>
> Assessment and treatment of the patient's psychological traits are extremely important for the positive outcome in the therapy of obesity.
>
> Physicians and health workers must have the expertise to deal with psychological issues and to manage the relationship with obese patients.
>
> The behavioural, cognitive, and emotional factors (especially the ability to identify, accept, and regulate emotions) should always be taken into consideration and managed with psychological treatment, together with standard interventions on diet, exercise, and, when indicated, surgical therapy.
>
> Despite all efforts, therapeutic success of obesity treatment is often lacking. Therapeutic approaches discussed above, effective in some cases, do not always achieve the expected result. This may be the case especially for those cases of

obesity that occur with morbid characteristics or more dysfunctional eating pattern.

Thus treatment of obesity remains a challenge even more difficult when presented with significant psychopathological aspects such as a strong deficiency in emotional regulation or binge-eating disorder.

Nevertheless people who are overweight or obese benefit from psychological interventions to enhance weight reduction, even if it is necessary to continue research and to implement it in effective treatments of obesity.

Among the psychotherapies of obesity, BT and CBT, as well as IPT and DBT especially for BED, have evidence of effectiveness; MI and other psychotherapeutic approaches can enhance the possibilities of treatment.

Recent research has increased knowledge of different phenotypes of obesity and indicated that certain psychological treatment models are more effective than others for specific subset of patients showing different behaviours and psychological characteristics. Incorporating such knowledge in treatment planning should help to individuate the model of psychotherapy most effective depending on the specific type of obesity.

Thus, notwithstanding the usefulness of psychotherapy in the treatment of obesity, the effectiveness of different psychotherapeutic approaches must be better assessed with further study and confirmation.

References

1. Katz DA, McHorney CA, Atkinson RL (2000) Impact of obesity on health-related quality of life in patients with chronic illness. J Gen Intern Med 15:789–796
2. Fairburn CG, Cooper Z (2011) Therapist competence, therapy quality, and therapist training. Behav Res Ther 49(6–7):373–378
3. Donini LM, Cuzzolaro M, Spera G et al (2010) Obesity and eating disorders. Indications for the different levels of care. An Italian expert consensus document. Eat Weight Disord 15:1–31
4. Larson EB, Yao X (2005) Clinical empathy as emotional labor in the patient-physician relationship. JAMA 293(9):1100–1106
5. Mead N, Bower P (2000) Patient-centredness: a conceptual framework and review of the empirical literature. Soc Sci Med 51(7):1087–1110
6. Roter D (2000) The enduring and evolving nature of the patient-physician relationship. Patient Educ Couns 39:5–15
7. Roter D, Frankel RM, Hall JA et al (2006) The expression of emotions through nonverbal behavior in medical visits. J Gen Intern Med 21:S28–S34
8. Fuertes JN, Mislowack A, Bennett J et al (2007) The physicians-patient working alliance. Patient Educ Couns 66(1):29–36
9. Cox ME, Yancy WS Jr, Coffman CJ et al (2011) Effects of counseling techniques on patient's weight-related attitudes and behaviors in a primary care clinic. Patient Educ Couns 85(3):363–368
10. Derksen F, Bensing J, Lagro-Janssen A (2013) Effectiveness of empathy in general practice: a systematic review. Br J Gen Pract 63:76–84
11. Golay A, Lagger G, Chambouleyron M et al (2008) Therapeutic education of diabetic patients. Diabetes Metab Res Rev 24(3):192–196
12. Lagger G, Pataky Z, Golay A (2010) Efficacy of therapeutic patient education in chronic diseases and obesity. Patient Educ Couns 79(3):283–286

13. Ryden A, Sullivan M, Torgerson JS et al (2004) A comparative study of personality in severe obesity: a 2 year follow-up after intervention. Int J Obes 28:1485–1493
14. Davis C, Levitan RD, Carter J et al (2008) Personality and eating behaviors: a case control study of binge eating disorder. Int J Eat Disord 41:243–250
15. Sullivan S, Cloninger CR, Przybeck TR (2007) Personality characteristics in obesity and relationship with successful weight loss. Int J Obes 31:669–674
16. Bowlby J (1969) Attachment and loss, vol 1, Attachment. The Hogarth Press and the Institute of Psycho-Analysis, London
17. Anderson S, Whitaker R (2011) Attachment security and obesity in US preschool-aged children. Arch Pediatr Adolesc Med 165(3):235–242
18. De Vriendt T, Moreno LA, De Henauw S et al (2009) Chronic stress and obesity in adolescents: scientific evidence and methodological issues for epidemiological research. Nutr Metab Cardiovasc Dis 19(7):511–519
19. Tsigos C, Chrousos GP (2000) Stress, obesity, and the metabolic syndrome: soul and metabolism. Ann N Y Acad Sci 1083:11–13
20. Bjorntorp P, Rosmond R (2000) The metabolic syndrome-a neuroendocrine disorder? Br J Nutr 83(Suppl 1):49–57
21. Warne JP (2009) Shaping the stress response: interplay of palatable food choices, glucocorticoids, insulin and abdominal obesity. Mol Cell Endocrinol 300(1–2):137–146
22. Schore AN (2005) Attachment, affect regulation, and the developing right brain: linking developmental neuroscience to pediatrics. Pediatr Rev 26(6):204–217
23. Macht M (2008) How emotions affect eating: a five-way model. Appetite 50(1):1–11
24. Kiesewetter S, Köpsel A, Köpp W et al (2010) Psychodynamic mechanism and weight reduction in obesity group therapy – first observations with different attachment styles. Psychosoc Med 31:7
25. Kiesewetter S, Köpsel A, Mai K et al (2012) Attachment style contributes to the outcome of a multimodal lifestyle intervention. Biopsycho Soc Med 6(1):3
26. Shaw K, O'Rourke P, Del Mar C et al (2005) Psychological interventions for overweight and obesity (Review). Cochrane Database Syst Rev;2:CD003818
27. Diabetes Prevention Program (DPP) Research Group (2002) The diabetes prevention program (DPP): description of lifestyle intervention. Diabetes Care 25:2165–2171
28. The Look AHEAD Research Group (2006) The look AHEAD study: a description of the lifestyle intervention and the evidence supporting it. Obesity 14:737–752
29. Dalla Grave R, Centis E, Marzocchi R et al (2013) Major factors for facilitating change in behavioral strategies to reduce obesity. Psychol Res Behav Manag 6:101–110
30. Butryn ML, Webb V, Thomas A et al (2011) Behavioural treatment of obesity. Psychiatr Clin N Am 34(4):841–859
31. Cooper Z, Doll HA, Hawker DM et al (2010) Testing a new cognitive behavioural treatment for obesity: a randomized controlled trial with three-year follow-up. Behav Res Ther 48: 706–713
32. Fabricatore A, Wadden TA (2006) Obesity. Annu Rev Clin Psychol 2:357–377
33. Cresci B, Castellini G, Pala L et al (2011) Motivational readiness for treatment in weight control programs: the TREatment MOtivation and REadiness (TRE-MORE) test. J Endocrinol Invest 34(3):70–77
34. Miller WR, Rollnick S (eds) (2002) Motivational interviewing: preparing people for change, 2nd edn. Guilford Press, New York
35. Prochaska JO, DiClemente CC (1992) Stages of change in the modification of problem behaviors. Prog Behav Modif 28:183–218
36. Britt E, Hudson SM, Blampied NM (2004) Motivational interviewing in health settings: a review. Patient Educ Couns 53:147–155
37. Rubak S, Sandbaek A, Lauritzen T et al (2005) Motivational interviewing: a systematic review and meta-analysis. Br J Gen Pract 55:305–312
38. Smith DE, Heckemeyer CM, Kratt PP et al (1997) Motivational interviewing to improve adherence to a behavioral weight-control program for older obese women with NIDDM. Diabetes Care 20(1):52–54

39. Burke BL, Arkowitz H, Menchola M (2003) The efficacy of motivational interviewing: a meta-analysis of controlled clinical trials. J Consult Clin Psychol 71:843–861
40. Hettema J, Steele J, Miller WR (2005) Motivational interviewing. Ann Rev Clin Psychol 1:91–111
41. Van Dorsten B (2007) The use of motivational interviewing in weight loss. Curr Diab Rep 7:386–390
42. Carels RA, Darby L, Cacciapaglia HM et al (2007) Using motivational interviewing as a supplement to obesity treatment: a stepped care approach. Health Psychol 26:369–374
43. Rieger E, Dean HY, Steinbeck KS et al (2009) The use of motivational enhancement strategies for the maintenance of weight loss among obese individuals: a preliminary investigation. Diab Ob Metab 11:637–640
44. Armstrong M, Mottershead TA, Ronksley PE et al (2011) Motivational interviewing to improve weight loss in overweight and/or obese patients: a systematic review and meta-analysis of randomized controlled trials. Obes Rev 12:709–723
45. DiLillo V, West DS (2011) Motivational interviewing for weight loss. Psychiatr Clin N Am 34:861–869
46. Volkow ND, Wang GJ, Fowler JS et al (2008) Overlapping neuronal circuits in addiction and obesity: evidence of systems pathology. Philos Trans R Soc Lond B Biol Sci 363:3191–3200
47. Berthoud H-R, Lenard NR, Shin AC (2011) Food reward, hyperphagia, and obesity. Am J Physiol Regul Integr Comp Physiol 300(6):R1266–R1277
48. Epstein LH, Salvy SJ, Carr KA et al (2011) Food reinforcement, delay discounting and obesity. Physiol Behav 100(5):438–445
49. Gearhardt AN, White MA, Potenza MN (2011) Binge eating disorder and food addiction. Curr Drug Abuse Rev 4(3):201–207
50. Cooper Z, Fairburn CG (2001) Testing a new cognitive behavioural treatment for obesity: a randomized controlled trial with three-year follow-up. Behav Res Ther 39(5):499–511
51. Fairburn CG (2008) Cognitive behavior therapy and eating disorders. Guilford Press, New York
52. Werrij MQ, Janssen A, Mulkens S et al (2009) Adding cognitive therapy to dietetic treatment is associated with less relapse in obesity. J Psychosom Res 67(4):315–324
53. Van Dorsten B, Lindley E (2011) Cognitive and behavioral approaches in the treatment of obesity. Med Clin N Am 95:971–988
54. Iacovino JM, Gredysa DM, Altman M et al (2012) Psychological treatments for binge eating disorder. Curr Psychiatry Rep 14(4):432–446
55. Adriaens A, Pieters G, Campfort V et al (2008) A cognitive-behavioural program (one day a week) for patients with obesity and binge eating disorder: short-term follow-up data. Psychol Top 17(2):361–371
56. Cresci B, Tesi F, La Ferlita T et al (2007) Group versus individual cognitive-behavioral treatment for obesity: results after 36 months. Eat Weight Disord 12:147–153
57. Minniti A, Bissoli L, Di Francesco V et al (2007) Individual versus group therapy for obesity: comparison of dropout rate and treatment outcome. Eat Weight Disord 12(4):161–167
58. Wilfley D, Kolko RP, Kass AE (2011) Cognitive behavioral therapy for weight management and eating disorders in children and adolescents. Child Adolesc Psychiatr Clin N Am 20:271–285
59. Greenberg I, Sogg S, Perna FM (2009) Behavioral and psychological care in weight loss surgery: best practice update. Obesity 17:880–884
60. Kalarchian MA, Marcus MD, Levine MD et al (2007) Psychiatric disorders among bariatric surgery candidates: relationship to obesity and functional health status. Am J Psychiatry 164:328–334
61. Pataky Z, Carrard I, Golay A et al (2011) Psychological factors and weight loss in bariatric surgery. Curr Opin Gastroenterol 27:167–173
62. Odom J, Zalesin KC, Washington TL et al (2010) Behavioral predictors of weight regain after bariatric surgery. Obes Surg 20:349–356
63. Fabricatore A (2007) Behavior therapy and cognitive-behavioral therapy of obesity: is there a difference? J Am Diet Ass 107:92–99

64. Almeida L, Savoy S, Boxer P (2011) The role of weight stigmatization in cumulative risk for binge eating. J Clin Psychol 67(3):278–292
65. Striegel-Moore RH, Fairburn CG, Wilfley DE et al (2005) Toward an understanding of risk factors for binge-eating disorder in black and white women: a community based case-control study. Psychol Med 35:6
66. Tanofsky-Kraff M, Wilfley DE, Young JF et al (2007) Preventing excessive weight gain in adolescents: interpersonal psychotherapy for binge eating. Obesity 15(6):1345–1355
67. Rieger E, Van Buren DJ, Bishop M et al (2010) An eating disorder-specific model of interpersonal psychotherapy (IPT-ED): causal pathways and treatment implications. Clin Psychol Rev 30:400–410
68. Wilson GT, Wilfley DE, Agras WS et al (2010) Psychological treatments of binge eating disorder. Arch Gen Psychiatry 67:94–101
69. Safer DL, Robinson AH, Jo (2010) Outcome from a randomized controlled trial of group therapy for binge-eating disorder; comparing dialectical behavior therapy adapted for binge eating to an active comparison group therapy. Behav Ther 41:106–120
70. Telch CF, Agras WS, Linehan MM (2001) Dialectical behavior therapy for binge eating disorder. J Consult Clin Psychol 69:1061–1065
71. Becker S, Rapps N, Zipfel S (2007) Psychotherapy in obesity-a systematic review. Psychother Psychosom Med Psychol 57(11):420–427
72. Sojcher R, Gould Fogerite S, Perlman A (2012) Evidence and potential mechanisms for mindfulness practices and energy psychology for obesity and binge-eating disorder. Explore (NY) 8(5):271–276
73. Lacaille J, Ly J, Zacchia N (2014) The effects of three mindfulness skills on chocolate cravings. Appetite 76:101–112
74. Wilson GT, Zandberg LJ (2012) Cognitive-behavioral guided self-help for eating disorders: effectiveness and scalability. Clin Psychol Rev 32:343–357
75. De Zwaan M, Herpertz F, Zipfel S et al (2012) INTERBED: internet-based guided self-help for overweight and obese patients with full or subsyndromal binge eating disorder. A multicenter randomized controlled trial. Trials 13:220

Dietary Intervention and Nutritional Counseling

21

Alessandro Pinto, Lucia Toselli, and Edda Cava

21.1 Introduction

The best dietary approach, recommended by health organizations such as the National Institutes of Health (NIH) and the American Heart Association (AHA), is a low-fat diet providing 20–30 % of energy as fats, 55–70 % as carbohydrates and 15–20 % as proteins. This approach is in accord with the population Dietary Reference Values (DRVs) that advise 20–35 % as Reference Intake (RI) range for lipids. Despite this recommendation, the poor efficacy of the traditional dietary treatment together with the high prevalence of *overweight* and *obesity* allowed the growing number of alternative dietary proposals, with some differences in energy percentage as macronutrients, not always in agree with the RI or supported by scientific evidences [1–5].

Several systematic reviews and meta-analysis comparing the different dietary models have been published but, considering the variability in study design, including sample size, duration, population, and macronutrient composition, there is no conclusive evidence especially in regard to a long-lasting *weight loss* and comorbidity improvement. Conversely, there is increasing evidence that the treatment of overweight or obesity should be a multidisciplinary approach, joining together caloric restriction, exercise, and behavior modification [6].

Scientific literature deals with dietary models usually defined "high protein" when the proteins provide ≥25 E% of total daily energy intake (TDEI); "low fat" if fats provide ≤30 E% or "high fat" >30 E%; and "low-carbohydrate diets" when CHOs intake is ≤45 E%; different combinations of these models are also described. According to *Freedman M.R.* et al. [7], a comprehensive comparison of different dietary models should include a careful analysis of the results on the following

---

A. Pinto (✉) • L. Toselli • E. Cava
Food Science and Human Research Unit, Medical Pathophysiology, Food Science and Endocrinology Section, Experimental Medicine Department, "Sapienza" University of Rome, P.le Aldo Moro, 5, Rome CAP 00141 RM, Italy
e-mail: alessandro.pinto@uniroma1.it; lucia.toselli@uniroma1.it; eddaka@yahoo.it

© Springer International Publishing Switzerland 2015
A. Lenzi et al. (eds.), *Multidisciplinary Approach to Obesity*:
From Assessment to Treatment, DOI 10.1007/978-3-319-09045-0_21

outcomes: size and composition of weight loss (loss of body fat, BF, and lean body mass, LBM), long-term maintenance, nutritional quality of a *diet* (vitamin and mineral adequacy), metabolic parameters (e.g., blood glucose, insulin sensitivity, lipid levels, uric acid, and ketone bodies), influence on hunger, appetite, and subsequent food intake, psychological well-being, risk for chronic disease, and changes in long-term hormonal regulators of energy intake and expenditure (e.g., insulin and leptin). Specific relevant topics for the definition of general criteria to develop a suitable dietary protocol will be discussed hereinafter.

21.2 High-Protein Versus Standard-Protein Diets for Weight Loss: The Issue of Adequate Protein Intake

High-protein diets (*HPD*) (protein intake ≥ 25 E%) are among the most popular diets, although there is no consensus about the long-term efficacy and the potential harms. Compared to isocaloric standard-protein (SPD) and to low-fat diets (LFD), HPDs provide a limited advantage in reduction of body weight (BW), BF, and triacylglycerols (TAG) and in mitigating the loss of *LBM* and basal metabolic rate (BMR), but there are no significant differences in total cholesterol (TC), LDL cholesterol (LDL-C), HDL cholesterol (HDL-C), blood pressure (BP), fasting plasma insulin, and glucose [8, 9]. It is difficult to provide the evidence whether the effects of HPD are due to the increased dietary proteins or to the mutual variation of CHOs and/or fat intake [10]. Several hypotheses have been suggested to explain the HPD results: a greater satiety effect, a higher dietary-induced thermogenesis (DIT), the *ketone* synthesis (in low CHOs-HPD) which improves the LBM preservation by a hypothesized anabolic effect on the muscle protein metabolism, and a higher sensitivity of the central nervous system to leptin [11, 12]. However, the *USDA/ARS* [13] review concludes that BW loss is not directly related to the macronutrients proportion in the diet when energy intake is reduced. As regards to the potential adverse effects induced by a too-high protein intake, acute adverse effects have been reported for protein intakes ≥ 45 E%, but not up to 35 E%, and the European Food Safety Authority (EFSA) suggests that an intake of twice the population reference intake (PRI) is safe in adults [10].

Beyond the size of BW loss, the preservation of LBM is another issue of the HPD, but this hypothesis has not been yet unequivocally demonstrated. Physiologically, the total BW loss is made up of about 75 % BF and 25 % LBM [14]. A daily protein intake of 0.8–1.2 g/kg/day should be sufficient to sustain satiety, BMR, and LBM, regardless of dietary CHO content with a greater effect in studies of >3 months [15, 16]. Several observations should be carried out about the protein intake cutoff to distinguish HPD and SPD. First, the "safe level of protein intake" (PRI) is 0.83 g/kg BW per day [17, 10]; as a result any protein intake lower than the PRI cannot be considered adequate even if results are between 10 and 15 % of the TDEI. Second, the caloric restriction results in a significant decrease in *nitrogen* balance [18]. Protein: energy ratio should be an essential issue to evaluate the adequacy of protein intake during low-calorie diets to satisfy protein metabolism and avoid the metabolic shift of protein to gluconeogenesis or ATP synthesis. Analyzing studies on nitrogen balance in adults has been established that 1 mg nitrogen/kg/day is gained per extra intake of 1 kcal/kg/day [19]. Third point, obesity is associated with a chronic low-grade inflammation, which induces insulin resistance. Insulin resistance, inflammation, and oxidative stress could have a role in the obesity-related impairment in protein metabolism and turnover, as they are associated not only with increased BF but also with low muscle mass and muscle strength (sarcopenia) [20].

Westerterp-Plantenga MS et al. [21] reviewed the effects of relatively HPD during BW loss and maintenance and concluded that an intake of 1.2 g/kg BW is beneficial to body composition, improves BP, and reduces the risk of BW regain, and no kidney problems occur in healthy subjects. Contradictory results are described for the effects of HPD on insulin sensitivity and glucose tolerance [10].

Concluding, these observations support an average *protein* intake ≈1.2 g/ kg ideal BW per day during caloric restriction [21–24] and underline the need to define the individual adequate protein intake as absolute amount (g/kg of ideal BW), rather than as percentage of TDEI. This issue must be taken into account running meta-analyses or systematic reviews of literature comparing HPD with well-balanced standard diets, especially regarding the preservation of LBM.

21.3 Low Versus Standard Carbohydrate Diets for Weight Loss: The Matter of Glycemic Index/Load in Weight Management

Commonly, *low-carbohydrate diets* (*LChoDs*) are considered to contain <100 g/day or <30 % of energy from CHOs. Since LChoDs usually contain a relatively increased proportion of the other macronutrients, these diets are often "high protein" or "high fat." LChoDs rule out or significantly reduce the intake of some foods, such as cereals and fruits, resulting in a low fiber intake and increase the assumption of animal foods to achieve an adequate protein and energy intake. However, LChoDs do not have a fixed cutoff for CHOs intake or macronutrients ratio and not necessarily are high in protein or fat, depending on the level of caloric restriction and the food sources [25]. Several studies report that LChoDs result in a more rapid short-term BW loss and in greater improvements in TAG and HDL-C, but not in TC and LDL-C, than conventional low-calorie diets at 3 and 6 months, with no differences observed after 12 months [26–29]. Conversely, a recent meta-analysis [30] reported persistent although small effects of LCho-HPD on BW, BF, and fasting TAG also after 12 months; moreover, the effect on fasting insulin was small and probably related to the decreasing BF rather than macronutrient intake differences; no differences were observed in other plasma *lipids*, glucose, and LBM. Therefore, the apparent preservation of *LBM* in the short term [15] should be lost during BW regain in the follow-up period when the subjects having a normal protein intake regain the LBM lost. Furthermore, a systematic review of *LChoDs* found that the BW loss is associated with the length of the diet and the energy restriction rather than the CHO restriction [31]. There are some concerns about potential adverse effects, and there is a need for long-term studies to measure changes in nutritional status and body composition during the LChoD and to assess fasting and postprandial cardiovascular risk factors and adverse effects. Without these informations LChoD cannot be recommended [26, 32]. Conversely, many studies demonstrated the beneficial effects of the *Mediterranean diet*, characterized by a balanced intake of macronutrient, albeit the CHO intake is at the lower tail of the RI and the fat intake, with monounsaturated fatty acids (MUFA) as the main source, at the higher tail of the RI; it was effective in reducing adiposity and other metabolic features of the metabolic syndrome [33, 34]. Unlike the LChoD but yet related to the dietary intake of CHOs, the role of *low glycemic index or load diets* (*LGIDs*) has been recently proposed as useful tool in BW management. It has been suggested that LGID may promote a greater loss of BW and BF and a better improvement in lipid profile (TC and LDL-C) than other dietary models [35]. The mechanisms involved in BW management might include the ability to promote satiety and delay hunger, reducing fluctuations in glycemia and insulinemia, promoting higher rates of fat oxidation and minimizing decreases in metabolic rate during energy restriction, and at last increasing the intake of whole grains with greater food volume [36].

Schwingshackl L. and Hoffmann G. [37], in a systematic review and meta-analysis, provided evidence about beneficial effects of long-term interventions with a LGID in regard to fasting *insulin* and proinflammatory markers, such as C-reactive protein as primary prevention of obesity-associated diseases; no significant changes were observed for blood lipids, anthropometric measures, HbA1c, and fasting glucose, while the decrease in LBM was significantly higher in LGID. This result could be explained assuming that a key requisite of a diet aimed to preserve LBM could be the CHOs to proteins ratio. An increasing proportion of protein to CHOs (in particularly an 1:2 protein/CHO ratio) in BW loss diet is more feasible and satiating, and it is associated to a better improvement in BF%, WC, and waist/hip ratio, plus it supports the preservation of LBM compared with the other diets and may be more effective in reducing long-term chronic disease risk improving blood lipids and glucose homeostasis [38, 39]. Therefore, it could be concluded that LGID is not more effective than traditional low-fat diet for BW loss or BW maintenance in general but may be beneficial for patients with certain risk factors such as insulin resistance [26].

21.4 Low-Fat Diet or Normal-Fat Diet: One or More Reference Model for Weight Loss?

The NIH clinical guidelines [14] provide a strong and consistent evidence that an average BW loss of 8 % of initial BW, with a decrease in abdominal fat, can be obtained over 3–12 months by an individually planned *low calorie diet* (*LCD*), creating a deficit of 500–1,000 kcal/day, aimed at achieving a BW loss of 0.5–1 kg/week. The NIH panel highlights that reducing fats as part of an LCD is a practical way to reduce calories and, in addition, *lower-fat diets* (*LFDs*), low in saturated fatty acids (SFA), reduce serum cholesterol levels and consequently the cardiovascular risk (CVR). The RCTs selected in NIH review tested the effects of LFD ranging from 20 to 30 % of calories from fat and between 1,200 and 2,300 cal. These studies, taken together, show how LFD can contribute to lower the caloric intake even when caloric reduction is not the focus of the intervention, and if LCD is low in fat contribution, better BW loss is achieved. However, there is little evidence that LFDs, per se, cause BW loss independently from caloric reduction.

Beyond the NIH statement evidence [14], some remarks have to be expressed. *Schwingshackl L.* et al. [40] compared in a systematic review and meta-regression analysis the long-term (≥ 12 months) effects of LFD (lipid intake ≤ 30 % of TDEI) versus high-fat diets (HFD, lipid intake >30 % of TDEI) on blood lipid levels in overweight and obese patients. The results of the meta-regressions support the hypothesis that the heterogeneity in TC and HDL-C outcomes might be explained by a wide range in total *fat* (>30–60 %) and mainly in the percentage distributions of SFA, MUFA, and polyunsaturated fatty acids (PUFA): increases in TC levels were associated with higher SFA and lower PUFA, whereas a rise in HDL-C level was related to higher amounts of total fat especially in MUFA content, such as in the *Mediterranean diet*. A meta-analysis of short-term studies suggested that LFD results in higher TAG levels and lower HDL-C levels compared to diets in which SFA are completely replaced by unsaturated fatty acids. No significant differences in the BW change were observed between LFD and HFD, but this observation was no longer valid if only trials adopting a LCD were selected. The authors underline that BW loss might represent a potential confounder in the interpretation of blood lipid levels variation, indeed, and there was a significantly greater decrease in BW in the HFD compared with the LFD counterparts; this may explain the seeming observation that LFDs do not exert any beneficial effects on TC and LDL-C levels in studies aiming at BW loss (in contrast to the observations made when all studies were included in the meta-analyses). Supporting these findings, *Dattilo AM* et al. [41] demonstrated that 1Kg of BW loss is associated with a 1.93 mg/dL decrease in TC and a 0.77 mg/dL decrease in LDL-C level, respectively. It must be remarked that a diet high in MUFA, as the Mediterranean-style diet, compared with LFD improves more CVR factors, markers of vascular inflammation, and glycemic control [40, 42] without significant differences in glucose or insulin concentrations during the OGTT, in the Matsudas index, in BW, or in body composition [43].

21.4.1 The Very-Low-Energy Diets (VLED) and the Ketogenic Diet

According to NIH clinical guidelines [14], diets are categorized on the energy intake basis as:

- *Low-calorie diet* (*LCD*): a calorie restriction ranging between about 800 and 1,500 cal (approximately 12–15 kcal/kg BW) per day
- *Very-low-calorie diet* (*VLCD*): a diet of 800 or fewer calories (approximately 6–10 kcal/kg BW) per day

The VLCD are designed for subjects with a BMI ≥ 30 kg/m^2, with increased CVR, amendable by BW loss. These diets should only be used for a short time, about 12 weeks, and the patients should be monitored by a physician every 2 weeks during the period of rapid BW loss (e.g., 1.5–2.5 kg/week). The *side effects* are usually mild and easily managed: cholelithiasis, cold intolerance, hair loss, headache, fatigue, dizziness, dehydration with electrolyte abnormalities, muscle cramps, nausea, constipation, or diarrhea. The risk of cholelithiasis can be decreased by ursodeoxycholic acid, including a moderate amount of fat in the diet and limiting the rate of BW loss to 1.5 kg/week. The majority of the side effects, including death, occurred when dieters consumed products that contained low-quality protein (e.g., hydrolyzed collagen) and were deficient in vitamins and minerals. Presently VLCD are considered safe and effective using high-quality proteins (e.g., milk, egg, or soy) or VLCD formulas, designed to provide all the nutrients needed and in appropriately selected individuals dieting for 8 weeks or fewer under careful medical supervision [43, 45]. The NIH clinical guidelines [14] report the results of studies that compared the amount of BW loss obtained by VLCD versus LCD in short (end of VLCD active phase: 12–16 weeks) and long term (24 weeks–5 years) concluding that VLCD produce greater initial BW loss than LCD; in the long term (>1 year), on the other hand, no significant differences are observed because a rapid BW reduction does not allow a gradual acquisition of changes in eating behavior and hence more BW is usually regained later on. Indeed a rapid BW regain between 6 and 12 months is observed if a maintenance program (dietary and behavioral support with increased physical activity) is not included [26, 47]. A significant improvement in BP, WC, and lipid profile is also reported but the results are more likely to be associated with the extent of BW loss, rather than the dietary model. More recent studies have confirmed this observation highlighting the high risk of nutritional inadequacies unless VLCD are supplemented with vitamins and minerals and hypothesizing an increased risk of BED (binge eating disorder) following the "yo-yo" effect of rapid BW loss and regain. The long-term evidence remains unclear; however, the intermittent VLCD use does not seem to be associated to any detrimental effect on metabolic parameters such as BMR, fasting insulin, insulin resistance, leptin, inflammatory markers, lipids, or BP [44, 46]. Formerly, *Fricker J.* et al. [47] studied the changes in LBM during the VLCD by nitrogen balance, demonstrating that the BMR-LBM ratio quickly decreases of about 15 % during the first week of a VLCD and this decrease persists but tapers off in the following weeks. This result suggests a metabolic adaptation of obese women to a VLCD, which leads to an increase in LBM energy metabolism efficiency, and it concurs with the decrease in the BMR-LBM ratio found in lean healthy men after 24 weeks of an LCD and in chronic human malnutrition.

The use of *ketogenic diets (KD)* as BW-loss therapy is an old proposal and became popular in the 1970s with the "Atkins Diet" in particular [48, 49]. Moreover the treatment of the epilepsy resistant to pharmacological therapy with KD has been well established, but in the last years an increasing amount of evidences suggests that KDs could have a therapeutic role in several diseases. It should be stated that not all *VLCD* are ketogenic, and the degree of CHOs restriction required to achieve ketosis remains unclear [25], although the term "ketogenic diet" is usually referred to diets containing ≤50 g/day CHOs with a relative increase in the proportions of protein and fat [50]. Increasing serum or urinary ketones is reported in subjects on daily intakes of CHOs >50 g, and conversely, not everyone assuming ≤50 g of CHOs has urinary ketone levels on trace or greater. The *macronutrient* composition of the diet is an important determinant of ketosis, e.g., LChoD high in protein may not cause ketosis, as up to 57 g glucose can be produced from 100 g of dietary protein, and KD used in the treatment of pediatric epilepsy typically restricts protein as well as CHOs (using a ratio of fat to CHO and protein of 3:1 or 4:1, respectively). According to *Stock AL and Yudkin J* [51], ketosis will occur when fat intake exceeds twice the CHOs intake plus half the protein intake. Together, data indicate that CHO restriction is a more important determinant of ketosis than restriction of total calories. *Ketones* are normally present in small amounts in the blood of healthy individuals following an overnight fasting or prolonged exercise, with plasma levels reported in the ranges of 0.2–0.5 mM [52]. Circulating ketone levels can increase up to 50-fold during periods of caloric deprivation, with β-hydroxybutyrate levels reported to be 4–5 mM in the blood following a 5–8 day fast. An excess of circulating ketones, which are strong organic acids that fully dissociate at physiological pH and overload the buffering capacity of serum and tissues, may result in metabolic acidosis, a potentially life-threatening condition. Moreover, increased ketone levels may affect the brain microvascular endothelium permeability and cerebral edema has been associated with diabetic ketoacidosis. However, such effects are observed only when ketones overreach physiological levels (10–20 mM or higher) during pathological states [53]. About the short-term safety, serious adverse events are reported to occur in adults on a low-calorie ketogenic diet (LCKD), including acute pancreatitis, exacerbation of panic disorder, severe metabolic acidosis, dehydration, severe electrolyte impairments, and hypokalemia, possibly associated with sudden cardiac death. Very few studies examined the effects of LCKD for periods longer than 12 months in adults: the risk of nutritional inadequacy depends on several factors, including the overall composition of the diet, nutrient sources, degree of CHOs restriction, and diet duration. Since dietary CHO restriction often results in increased protein intake, it is difficult to separate the renal and bone effects of *LCKD* from the effects of increased dietary protein. Therefore, the long-term effects of LCKD on renal and bone health are unknown [25, 54]; nonetheless, examining body composition, studies have generally found a reduction in BF with preservation of *LBM* [25]. There are contrasting theories regarding the mechanisms LCKDs work on, and, anyway, some of the initial BW loss is due to increased diuresis (renal sodium and water loss), both as a result of glycogen depletion and ketonuria. *Paoli A* et al. [50] summarized and listed in order of importance and available evidence the hypothesized effects of VLCKDs:

1. Reduction in appetite due to higher *satiety* effect of proteins, effects on appetite control hormones, and to a possible direct appetite-suppressant action of the KBs, although there is conflicting evidence regarding this issue in the published literature
2. Reduction in lipogenesis and increased *lipolysis*
3. Reduction in the resting respiratory quotient (RRQ) and, therefore, greater metabolic efficiency in consuming fats
4. Increased metabolic costs of gluconeogenesis and thermic effect of proteins

It has also been hypothesized an up-regulation of mitochondrial uncoupling proteins with a resultant wasting of ATP as heat [25].

However, the US Department of Agriculture concludes that diets, reducing calories, will result in effective BW loss independent of the macronutrient composition, which is considered less important or even irrelevant [50], and the studies evaluating long-term outcomes of LCKD found a greater BW loss at 3–6 months, with no difference at 12 months. In studies comparing LCKDs and LFDs, the LCKDs are significantly associated with a greater reduction in TAG and an increase (or less of a decrease) in HDL, although this result seems to be explained by differences in BW loss. Conversely, LFDs generally have a more beneficial effect on LDL levels than LCKD. Despite their unfavorable effect on total LDL levels, several studies have found a beneficial effect of LCKD on certain *lipoprotein* subclasses, with a reduction in VLDL, an increase in large LDL, and a reduction in small LDL particles [25]. In conclusion, the classic LCKD containing high fat, low CHOs, and low protein are difficult to manage, are unpalatable, and may present an increased atherogenic risk as serum levels of cholesterol and triglycerides are often elevated [55].

21.5 Criteria for the Formulation of a Balanced Diet in Obese Patient

It is clear that any low-calorie *diet* resulting in a negative energy balance produces BW loss in the short term (3–12 months); nevertheless, the optimal macronutrient composition of the diets continues to be controversial and object of ongoing researches.

A useful algorithm to develop a well-balanced dietary plan involves the following steps:

1. Setting the energy intake to obtain a suitable BW loss
2. Setting the protein intake
3. Splitting the nonprotein kcal (NP-kcal) between CHOs and lipids
4. Verifying the adequacy of micronutrients (vitamins and minerals) and fiber intake
5. Scheduling meals

The first step must take into account the broad interindividual variability (15 % on average) of the *BMR* normalized to the LBM in subjects of same sex, age, BW, and body size. Regarding the 24 h-energy expenditure (24-EE), this variability reaches 30 %, related to the individual energy expenditure for any physical activities (affected by muscle tone, ergonomic efficacy, intensity, etc.) [56]. It should be stressed that in obese subjects the BMR is higher than in lean subjects, since both LBM and BF are increased [57].

In clinical practice the BMR is calculated by predictive regression equations using sex, age, BW, and height (e.g., Harris-Benedict equation or Schofield et al., quoted in FAO/WHO/ONU report, 1985) with an average standard error of 10 % in the single subject and 2 % in population groups [56]. More recent predictive equations give slightly lower errors in overweight subjects [58], e.g., the Mifflin St. Jeor equation or the Livingston equation, which are useful to predict the BMR in adults of various BMI levels, although the accuracy is lower in obese than nonobese people [59, 60].

A higher accuracy in estimating the BMR can be reached taking into account the *LBM*, by means of prediction equations such as the J. Cunningham equation [61]. Obviously it is critical an accurate assessment of the BC to avoid a source of bias. Several limits are embedded to the usual inexpensive and noninvasive methods in the outpatient practice (anthropometrics and Biolectrical Impedance Analysis, BIA), that are only partly overtaken by dual energy x-ray absorptiometry (DEXA). Evaluating BC allows to identify the "desirable BW," essential to establish the individual adequate energy and protein intake, indeed:

1. In a "*normative* approach" aimed to BW loss, BMR must be esteemed using "desirable BW," while a "*conservative* approach" uses the subject actual weigh.
2. "Desirable BW" is in accord to an optimal ratio between BF and LBM, taking into account that these are physiologically increased in obese subjects and assuming that the *exceeding BW* consist of BF 75 % and LBM 25 %.
3. LBM is the mean factor affecting BMR, therefore, predicting equations that include LBM have higher accuracy; in order to preserve the LBM, energy intake should not be lower than BMR −10 E%.
4. Protein PRI is about 1 g/kg or better 1.2 g/kg of "desirable BW" in agreement with the findings of the literature previously reported; in calculating the "desirable BW" it is essential to take into account the 25 % of the exceeding BW as LBM, in order to preserve the LBM during the BW loss; likewise, the LBM loss should not exceed the 25 % of the BW loss, when it occurs [14].

When it is not possible to assess the BC, "desirable BW" could be esteemed adding a 25 % of the exceeding BW (as hypothetical LBM) to the "ideal BW" resulting by the common literature equations.

Afterwards, *physical activity level (PAL)* should be assessed. Subject must collect a record of any activity performed in a 24 h period (sleeping, eating, walking, working, all other activity such as personal hygiene, sport, hobbies, etc.). Alternatively but less accurately, it is possible to carry out a physical activity recall [56, 62]. A specific energetic value is assigned to every activity and the PAL is calculated through a factorial procedure as weighted average of all these activity, adjusted for the time dedicated to each [63, 64]. Finally, to calculate the 24 h-EE in Kcal/day, BMR is multiplied by the PAL esteemed (Table 21.1). It is possible to simplify this procedure, with a satisfying accuracy, using average PAL values codified by lifestyle ranges as "light," "moderate," or "heavy" (Fig. 21.1) [56, 62].

To lose 1 kg/week of BF, it is necessary a daily negative energy balance of about 1,000 kcal, and the guidelines usually suggest a moderate reduction of the TDEI, around 500–1,000 kcal/die cut down from the estimated *24 h-EE* or from the usual TDEI, whether the subject's BW is steady and anyway never going below the BMR more than 10 %; this is aimed to a gradual and long-lasting weight loss: losing 3–5 kg

Table 21.1 Criteria for the formulation of a dietary plan

Parameters	Determinant factors		
Desirable weight	Body composition: lean body mass (LBM)/fatty mass (FM)		
Basal metabolic rate (BMR)	Sex	Conservative approach	Normative approach
	Age		
	Height	BMR is calculated utilizing the actual weight	BMR is calculated utilizing the desirable weight
	Weight		
	LBM		
Physical activity level (PAL)	Frequency, intensity, and duration of the different activities during the 24 h, included the sleeping time	Physical activity energy expenditure is affected by the actual weight	
Daily energy expenditure (24 h-EE)	BMR × PAL		

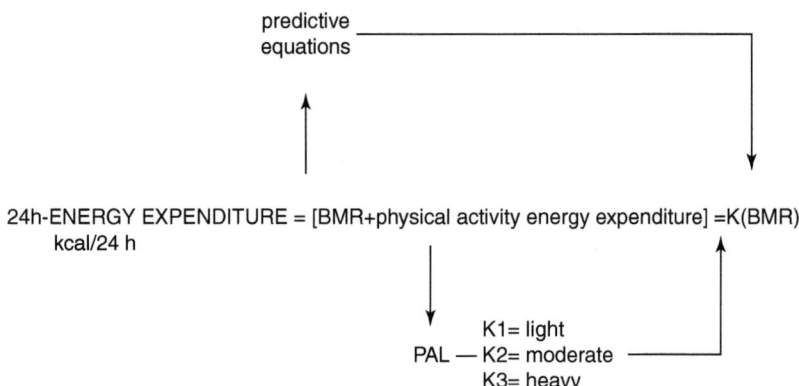

Fig. 21.1 Algorithm to calculate the 24 h-daily expenditure

of BW is an excellent achievement, allowing to preserve the LBM and prevent the dehydration, without raising the risk of eating disorders. Cognitive-behavioral therapy together with physical activity program gives the best and long-lasting results [14, 65].

To define an adequate dietary energy intake, it is also necessary to take into account the patient's eating habit (quality and quantity of food consumption, meals planning, and eating disorders suspected by psychodynamic tests). Food surveys could be retrospective, with the use of memory such as the 24/48 h recall, food frequency, dietary history, or perspective by recording the weight or the estimated quantity of the foods consumed.

Usually, food frequency questionnaire, dietary history, and food diary allow to collect all the data required. Then, the calculated 24 h-EE can be compared to the actual TDEI taking into account the BW changes. Energy balance is the difference between food intake and energy expenditure [*24 h-EE* = BMR + DIT (diet-induced thermogenesis) + PA (physical activity)]. This balance is positive in obese subjects actively gaining BW; instead, if the BW is steady, the TDEI is equivalent to 24 h-EE and the subject is in energetic balance with a TDEI not necessarily too high.

Established the most adequate energy intake to obtain a healthy BW loss, it should be set the *protein* intake level as above stated (1–1.2 g/kg "desirable BW") and the protein-kcal must be apart from the NP-kcal which, in the end, have to be split between CHOs and lipids, pointing out that proteins and *CHOs* provide 4 kcal/g while lipids 9 kcal/g. Fifty percent of protein intake should come from animal source and the other 50 % from plant to avoid a high intake of animal *lipids* and meanwhile providing an adequate intake of vegetable protective factors (phytochemicals). Assuming the *nitrogen (N)* content of the proteins to be on average 16 %, it is easy to state that 6.25 g of proteins are equivalent to 1 g of N. It must be emphasized that in order to achieve an efficient protein synthesis, 100–150 nonprotein kcal (NP-kcal) are needed for every intake of 1 g N or 6.25 g proteins. In a dietary plan providing for the actual energy expenditure, protein amount could not be higher than 13–15 % of the TDEI, but in formulating a low-calorie diet, protein requirements must be counted in grams/kg of "desirable BW" to meet the proteins need [66].

Once satisfied the protein requirement, NP-kcal should be split as CHOs, 65–70 E%, and lipids, 30–35 E%. The distribution of NP-kcal requires a careful screening of comorbidities: this is a critical issue for the metabolic effects of the dietary models described above, to avoid the possible adverse effects or in order to exploit their metabolic properties. Total CHOs should be composed between complex, 80 %, and simple, 20 %. The amount of fats should consist of SFAs (1/3), MUFAs (1/2), n PUFAs (1/6), and the RI of EFAs (essential fatty acids) and of the liposoluble vitamins (α-tocopherol, β-carotene, vitamin D) have to be assured; to respect this proportion, it is sufficient to have an intake of 30 % as animal fats and 70 % as vegetable fats. Animal fats, indeed, consist of 2/3 SFAs and 1/3 MUFA with a low PUFA content, and instead plant source are made up of 1/3 SFA and 2/3 MUFA and PUFA [67] (Fig. 21.2). With respect to the TDEI, total CHOs intake should provide 45–60 % of TDEI, with maximum 15 % of simple sugar, while fats should provide 20–35 % of TDEI [67]. The highest values of the range (RI) should be considered only in the low-carbohydrate diets, when required. In other cases, the intake of total lipids must be ≤30 %, SFAs 7–10 %, and trans-fatty acids ≤1 % of TDEI [26, 67]. On the other hand, a too-low-fat diet has poor organoleptic properties, resulting bland and tasteless. Olive oil should not be removed since its composition in MUFA helps to keep an adequate HDL cholesterol level. To achieve a good level of ω-3-fatty acids, 150 g of any kind of fish twice a week are enough, better if chosen among *anchovy, sardine, mackerel*, or similar. In the end, an eating plan well balanced and consistent with dietary guidelines endorses to consume at least five servings of fruits and vegetables per day, emphasizing the use of whole grains, with a daily *fiber* intake of 35 g or more. BW-loss diet that excludes one or more foods or food groups and/or substantially restrict macronutrients intake below the PRI could produce nutrient deficiencies and increase health risks. The *micronutrient* intake level should be evaluated on a weekly basis or on a longer term for liposoluble

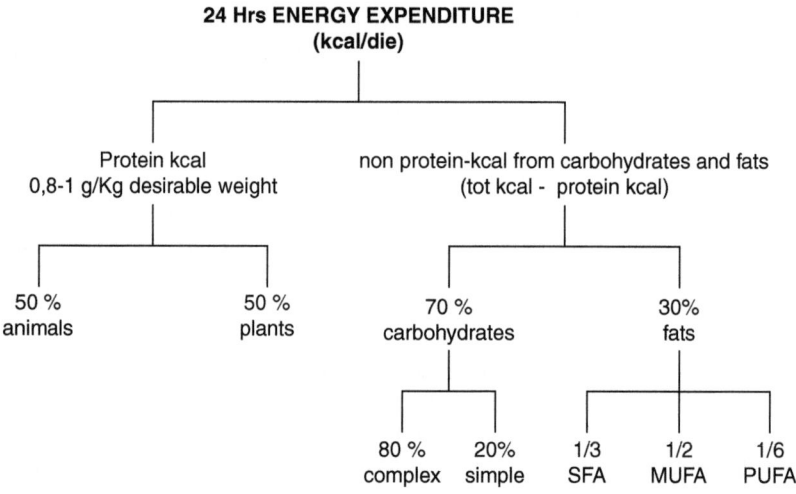

Fig. 21.2 Flow chart to allocate the macronutrients in a balanced diet

vitamins and β-carotene; in a moderate low-calorie diet, it is possible to meet PRI by the weekly consumption of the different food groups as suggested by the guidelines for a healthy diet [67]. The supply of essential fatty acids, minerals, vitamins, and fiber has to be checked in relation to the DRVs (Table 21.2).

21.6 Nutritional Counseling and Conclusion

The World Health Organization defined obesity as a serious chronic disease, largely preventable through lifestyle changes [75]. This definition means that although the weight loss is essential for reducing the risk of obesity-associated comorbidities and mortality, the acquisition of a healthy lifestyle should be the main objective of the whole therapeutic intervention. Dietary treatment should instruct patients on how to modify their diets in order to lower the caloric intake, obtaining a slow and progressive BW loss, reducing CVR, and other comorbidities. It was described an inverse relation between adherence to a *Mediterranean* dietary pattern and the prevalence of obesity in a free-eating, population-based sample of men and women, irrespective of various potential confounders [68]; several studies support the evidence that promoting eating habits consistent with Mediterranean diet (MD) nutrients pattern may be a useful and safe strategy for the treatment of obesity [69]. The MD features were recently revised by Bach-Faig A et al. [72]: the MD is rich in plant foods (cereals, fruits, vegetables, legumes, tree nuts, seeds, and olives), with olive oil as the principal source of added fat, along with high-to-moderate intakes of fish and seafood; moderate consumption of eggs, poultry, and dairy products (cheese and yogurt); low consumption of red meat; and a moderate intake of alcohol (mainly wine during meals) [70].

Table 21.2 Criteria to develop a balanced diet in obese subjects

Criteria			Parameters
1	Intake energy	Energy intake: reducing 500–1,000 kcal from the usual intake and anyway never < BMR −10 %	Estimate basal metabolic rate (BMR)
			Estimate 24 h energy expenditure (24 h-EE)
		Aim: ↓ 3–5 Kg/month	Assessing nutritional habits (usual energetic intake)
			Body weight changes in the last month (steady state or dynamic)
2	Protein intake	1 g protein/Kg desirable weight	Desirable weight
		100–150 kcal nonprotein/g nitrogen intake	Metabolic impairments and/or pathological conditions, e.g., kidney failure, microalbuminuria of nephrotic syndrome, etc.)
3	Nonprotein kcal Allocation (carbohydrates and lipids)	Total fats: 20–35 % total kcal	Dietary reference intakes
		Saturated fatty acids: ≤ 7–10 % tot. kcal trans-fatty acid ≤1 % tot. kcal	Nutritional status assessment
			Metabolic impairments (dyslipidemia, diabetes, etc.)
		Monounsaturated fatty acids: ≤15 % tot kcal	
		Polyunsaturated fatty acids: ≤10 % tot. kcal Essential fatty acids: ω-6 = 2 % and ω-3 = 0,5 % tot kcal	
		Cholesterol: ≤300 mg/die	
		Carbohydrates: ≥ 45 % tot kcal; ≥100 g/die	
		Simple sugars: ≤15 % tot. kcal	
		Calcium: 1,000–1,500 mg/die	
		NaCl: ≤6 g o Na 2,4 g/die	
4	Verifying fiber and micronutrients intake (minerals and vitamins)	Evaluation of the need to use nutritional supplements	Dietary reference intakes
		Fiber: 35 g	Nutritional status assessment
			Energy intake of the diet
5	Meal scheduling	Frequency complying with recommended requirements in guidelines	Usual day schedule
			Meal consumption modalities
		Food choices variety	Nutritional habits
		Regular meals	Limits (family, socials, working, food preferences, etc.)

Corbalán MD et al. [69] assert that "although there is no all-inclusive diet for the treatment of *obesity* and metabolic syndrome, a Mediterranean-style diet has most of the desired attributes, including lower refined carbohydrate content, high fiber content, moderate fat content (mostly unsaturated), and moderate to high vegetable protein content." According to the recommendations of the Spanish Society of Community Nutrition, the distribution of macronutrient components in MD is: 35 % fat (<10 % SFA and 20 % MUFA), 50 % CHOs, and 15–20 % protein [69].

Educational efforts should highlight the following topics as reported NIH clinical *guidelines* [14]:

- Energy value of different foods
- Food composition: fats, CHOs (including dietary fiber), and proteins
- Reading nutrition labels to determine caloric content and food composition
- New habits of purchasing with preference to low calorie foods
- Food preparation avoiding adding high-calorie ingredients during cooking (e.g., spreads and oils)
- Avoiding overconsumption of high-calorie foods (both high-fat and high-CHO foods)
- Maintaining adequate water intake
- Reducing portion sizes
- Limiting alcohol consumption

Whatever else is reported by healthy eating guidelines and effectively depicted in the *diet* pyramid or "eatwell plate" showing the proportions of food groups that should be eaten daily in a well-balanced diet completes these topics.

However, a successful BW loss is more likely to occur when patients' food preferences are considered to tailor an individual diet, adapted to the specific realities of different countries and to the variations in the dietary pattern related to geographical, socio-economic, and cultural contexts, taking into account the traditional, local, eco-friendly, and biodiverse products, thereby contributing to a higher and long-term sustainable compliance.

In the traditional framework, the patient is in a state of almost total dependence by the physician, and hence this model has been defined prescriptive, directive, paternalistic, or authoritarian. On the other side, the obese patients live in a dichotomous relationship with food, friend, or foe, and they think that the diet is not a means to improve their health status but a way to prove their willpower. In this perspective, when the patient transgresses the diet, he experiences a failure resulting in reduced self-esteem. Conversely, the nutritional *counseling* aims to "enable" the patient to make a decision about personal choices or problems or issues directly concerning themselves. The counseling procedure emphasizes the importance of the self-perception, self-determination, and self-control, taking the shape of helping a relationship finalize to return to autonomy, a greater sense of dignity and self-esteem to the person [70]. As in all chronic diseases, the objective is not the full recovery, but in the case of *obesity* can represent a way aimed at not only the weight loss but also in the ability to self-manage risk situations, to develop active lifestyle, and knowing how to choose what is really important to live fully their own existence and thus enhance the quality of life. The aim should be not only to improve the knowledge of the patients but especially their skills, know-how, and their ability to master events, known as how to be. The main tools at the basis of nutritional *counseling* are common with the cognitive behavioral therapy: therapeutic alliance, therapeutic adherence, motivation, problem solving, empowerment, and narrative medicine. The latest experience bears the *cognitive behavioral therapy* (*CBT*) as a key tool to achieve a lifestyle change and thus a long-lasting and stable BW loss. It has been designed to improve diet and physical activity compliance in the patients combining the behavioral method of influencing and reinforcing a positive behavior to the cognitive approach of conditioning emotions and human behavior by thoughts [71].

In summary, dietary intervention should respect physiological and metabolic bases. Any exception should take in account coexistent metabolic impairments and is allowed only if supported by clinical scientific evidences. The effectiveness of the dietary *therapy* should be evaluated in risk reduction for mortality and morbidity and in the ability of maintaining the results achieved rather than considering the BW loss only. The dietary intervention must follow a thorough *multidimensional* assessment of the biological (nutritional status), psychological, and social indices that could affect the BW gain and the unhealthy food habits. Since among the "dieters" there is a dropout rate of 40 % after 12 months [72], while a long-term success occurs only in ≤15 % [73], it is necessary to promote an active involvement of the patients, planning realistic solutions and goals to comply with, and trying to avoid unreachable achievements. Although the basis to formulate a balanced diet is strict scientific evidence, a high degree of *flexibility* is required to reach a good compliance of the patient [74, 75]. A good experience and knowledge by the professional operators can turn the dietary prescription into a guideline for a nutritional "reeducational" intervention.

References

Introduction

1. Wing RR, Phelan S (2005) Long-term weight loss maintenance. Am J Clin Nutr 82(1 Suppl):222S–225S. Review. PubMed PMID: 16002825
2. Elte JW, Castro Cabezas M, Vrijland WW, Ruseler CH, Groen M, Mannaerts GH (2008) Proposal for a multidisciplinary approach to the patient with morbid obesity: the St. Franciscus Hospital morbid obesity program. Eur J Intern Med 19(2):92–98. doi:10.1016/j.ejim.2007.06.015. Epub 2008 Jan 11. Review. PubMed PMID: 18249303
3. World Health Organisation (2004) Global strategy on diet, physical activity and health. WHO, Geneva, 700
4. Veerman JL, Barendregt JJ, van Beeck EF, Seidell JC, Mackenbach JP (2007) Stemming the obesity epidemic: a tantalizing prospect. Obesity (Silver Spring) 15(9):2365–2370. PubMed PMID: 17890506
5. Waters E, de Silva-Sanigorski A, Hall BJ, Brown T, Campbell KJ, Gao Y, Armstrong R, Prosser L, Summerbell CD (2011) Interventions for preventing obesity in children. Cochrane Database Syst Rev (12):CD001871. doi:10.1002/14651858.CD001871.pub3. Review. PubMed PMID: 22161367
6. Clifton PM (2008) Dietary treatment for obesity. Nat Clin Pract Gastroenterol Hepatol 5(12):672–681. doi:10.1038/ncpgasthep1283. Epub 2008 Oct 14. Review. PubMed PMID: 18852729
7. Freedman MR, King J, Kennedy E (2001) Popular diets: a scientific review. Obes Res 9(Suppl 1):1S–40S. Review. PubMed PMID: 11374180

High Protein Versus Standard Protein Diets for Weight Loss: The Issue of Adequate Protein Intake

8. Wycherley TP, Moran LJ, Clifton PM, Noakes M, Brinkworth GD (2012) Effects of energy-restricted high-protein, low-fat compared with standard-protein, low-fat diets: a meta-analysis of randomized controlled trials. Am J Clin Nutr 96(6):1281–1298. doi:10.3945/ajcn.112.044321. Epub 2012 Oct 24. Review. PubMed PMID: 23097268
9. Santesso N, Akl EA, Bianchi M, Mente A, Mustafa R, Heels-Ansdell D, Schünemann HJ (2012) Effects of higher- versus lower-protein diets on health outcomes: a systematic review and meta-analysis. Eur J Clin Nutr 66(7):780–788. doi:10.1038/ejcn.2012.37. Epub 2012 Apr 18. Review. PubMed PMID: 22510792; PubMed Central PMCID: PMC3392894
10. EFSA Panel on Dietetic Products, Nutrition and Allergies (NDA)(2012) Scientific opinion on dietary reference values for protein. EFSA Journal 10(2):2557 [66 pp.]. doi:10.2903/j.efsa.2012. 2557. Available online: www.efsa.europa.eu/efsajournal
11. Weigle DS, Breen PA, Matthys CC, Callahan HS, Meeuws KE, Burden VR, Purnell JQ (2005) A high-protein diet induces sustained reductions in appetite, ad libitum caloric intake, and body weight despite compensatory changes in diurnal plasma leptin and ghrelin concentrations. Am J Clin Nutr 82(1):41–48. PubMed PMID: 16002798
12. Paddon-Jones D, Westman E, Mattes RD, Wolfe RR, Astrup A, Westerterp-Plantenga M (2008) Protein, weight management, and satiety. Am J Clin Nutr 87(Suppl):S1558–S1561
13. USDA/ARS (United States Department of Agriculture Agricultural Research Service) (2009) USDA National Nutrient Database for Standard Reference, Release 22. Nutrient Data Laboratory Home Page. Available from: http://www.ars.usda.gov/ba/bhnrc/ndl
14. National Heart, Lung, and Blood Institute in cooperation with The National Institute of Diabetes and Digestive and Kidney Diseases (1998) Clinical guidelines on the identification, evaluation, and treatment of overweight and obesity in adults. The evidence report. NIH publication no. 98-4083 National Institutes of Health
15. Krieger JW, Sitren HS, Daniels MJ, Langkamp-Henken B (2006) Effects of variation in protein and carbohydrate intake on body mass and composition during energy restriction: a meta-regression 1. Am J Clin Nutr 83(2):260–274. PubMed PMID: 1646998
16. Martens EA, Westerterp-Plantenga MS (2014) Protein diets, body weight loss and weight maintenance. Curr Opin Clin Nutr Metab Care 17(1):75–79. doi:10.1097/MCO.0000000000000006. PubMed PMID: 24310056
17. WHO/FAO/UNU (World Health Organization/Food and Agriculture Organization of the United Nations/United Nations University) (2007) Protein and amino acid requirements in human nutrition. Report of a joint WHO/FAO/UNU expert consultation. WHO technical report series, no 935, 284 pp
18. Smith WJ, Underwood LE, Clemmons DR (1995) Effects of caloric or protein restriction on insulin-like growth factor-I (IGF-I) and IGF-binding proteins in children and adults. J Clin Endocrinol Metab 80(2):443–449. PubMed PMID: 7531712
19. Pellett PL, Young VR (1992) The effects of different levels of energy intake on protein metabolism and of different levels of protein intake on energy metabolism: a statistical evaluation from the published literature. In: Scrimshaw NS, Schürch B (eds) Protein energy interactions. International Dietary Energy Consultancy Group Switzerland, Lausanne, pp 81–136
20. Guillet C, Masgrau A, Walrand S, Boirie Y (2012) Impaired protein metabolism: interlinks between obesity, insulin resistance and inflammation. Obes Rev 13(Suppl 2):51–57. doi:10.1111/j.1467-789X.2012.01037.x
21. Westerterp-Plantenga MS, Lemmens SG, Westerterp KR (2012) Dietary protein – its role in satiety, energetics, weight loss and health. Br J Nutr 108(Suppl 2):S105–S112. doi:10.1017/S0007114512002589. Review. PubMed PMID: 23107521
22. Pasiakos SM, Cao JJ, Margolis LM, Sauter ER, Whigham LD, McClung JP, Rood JC, Carbone JW, Combs GF Jr, Young AJ (2013) Effects of high-protein diets on fat-free mass and muscle protein synthesis following weight loss: a randomized controlled trial. FASEB J 27(9):3837–3847. doi:10.1096/fj.13-230227. Epub 5. PubMed PMID: 23739654

23. Tang M, Armstrong CL, Leidy HJ, Campbell WW (2013) Normal vs. high-protein weight loss diets in men: effects on body composition and indices of metabolic syndrome. Obesity (Silver Spring) 21(3):E204–E210. doi:10.1002/oby.20078. PubMed PMID: 23592676
24. Soenen S, Martens EA, Hochstenbach-Waelen A, Lemmens SG, Westerterp-Plantenga MS (2013) Normal protein intake is required for body weight loss and weight maintenance, and elevated protein intake for additional preservation of resting energy expenditure and fat free mass. J Nutr 143(5):591–596. doi:10.3945/jn.112.167593. Epub 2013 Feb 27. PubMed PMID: 23446962

Low Versus Standard Carbohydrate Diets for Weight Loss: The Matter of Glycemic Index/Load in Weight Management

25. Sumithran P, Proietto J (2007) Ketogenic diets for weight loss: a review of their principles, safety and efficacy. Obes Res Clin Pract. 2008;2(1):I–II. doi: 10.1016/j.orcp.11.003. PubMed PMID: 24351673
26. Fitch A, Everling L, Fox C, Goldberg J, Heim C, Johnson K, Kaufman T, Kennedy E, Kestenbaun C, Lano M, Leslie D, Newell T, O'Connor P, Slusarek B, Spaniol A, Stovitz S, Webb B (2013) Institute for Clinical Systems Improvement. Prevention and management of obesity for adults. Updated. https://www.healthpartners.com/ucm/groups/public/@hp/@public/documents/documents/cntrb_037112.pdf
27. Tian H, Mills KT, Yao L, Demanelis K, Eloustaz M, Yancy WS, Jr TN, Kelly JH, Bazzano LA (2012) Effects of low-carbohydrate diets versus low-fat diets on metabolic risk factors: a meta-analysis of randomized controlled clinical trials. Am J Epidemiol 176(Suppl):S44–S54
28. Focster GD, Wyatt HR, Hill JO, McGuckin BG, Brill C, Mohammed BS, Szapary PO, Rader DJ, Edman JS, Klein S (2003) A randomized trial of a low-carbohydrate diet for obesity. N Engl J Med 348(21):2082–2090. PubMed PMID: 12761365
29. Stern L, Iqbal N, Seshadri P, Chicano KL, Daily DA, McGrory J, Williams M, Gracely EJ, Samaha FF (2004) The effects of low-carbohydrate versus conventional weight loss diets in severely obese adults: one-year follow-up of a randomized trial. Ann Intern Med 140(10):778–785. PubMed PMID: 15148064
30. Clifton PM, Condo D, Keogh JB (2014) Long term weight maintenance after advice to consume low carbohydrate, higher protein diets – a systematic review and metaanalysis. Nutr Metab Cardiovasc Dis 24(3):224–235. doi:10.1016/j.numecd.2013.11.006. Epub 20. PubMed PMID: 24472635
31. Saris WH (2003) Sugars, energy metabolism, and body weight control. Am J Clin Nutr 78(4):850S–857S. Review. PubMed PMID: 14522749
32. Astrup A, Meinert Larsen T, Harper A (2004) Atkins and other low-carbohydrate diets: hoax or an effective tool for weight loss? Lancet 364(9437):897–899. Review. PubMed PMID: 15351198
33. Mobbs CV, Mastaitis J, Yen K, Schwartz J, Mohan V, Poplawski M, Isoda F (2007) Low-carbohydrate diets cause obesity, low-carbohydrate diets reverse obesity: a metabolic mechanism resolving the paradox. Appetite 48(2):135–138. Epub 2006 Dec 1. Review. PubMed PMID: 17141367; PubMed Central PMCID: PMC2714161
34. Schröder H, Marrugat J, Vila J, Covas MI, Elosua R (2004) Adherence to the traditional mediterranean diet is inversely associated with body mass index and obesity in a spanish population. J Nutr 134(12):3355–3361. PubMed PMID: 15570037
35. Thomas DE, Elliott EJ, Baur L (2007) Low glycaemic index or low glycaemic load diets for overweight and obesity. Cochrane Database Syst Rev (3):CD005105. Review. PubMed PMID: 17636786
36. McMillan-Price J, Brand-Miller J (2006) Low-glycaemic index diets and body weight regulation. Int J Obes 30(Suppl 3):S40–S46
37. Schwingshackl L, Hoffmann G (2013) Long-term effects of low glycemic index/load vs. high glycemic index/load diets on parameters of obesity and obesity-associated risks: a systematic review and meta-analysis. Nutr Metab Cardiovasc Dis 23(8):699–706. doi:10.1016/j.numecd.2013.04.008. Epub 2013 Jun 17. Review. PubMed PMID: 23786819

38. Layman DK, Boileau RA, Erickson DJ, Painter JE, Shiue H, Sather C, Christou DD (2003) A reduced ratio of dietary carbohydrate to protein improves body composition and blood lipid profiles during weight loss in adult women. J Nutr 133(2):411–417. PubMed PMID: 12566476
39. Campbell DD, Meckling KA (2012) Effect of the protein: carbohydrate ratio in hypoenergetic diets on metabolic syndrome risk factors in exercising overweight and obese women. Br J Nutr 108(9):1658–1671. doi:10.1017/S0007114511007215. PubMed PMID: 22243943

Low Fat Diet or Normal Fat Diet: One or more Reference Model for Weight Loss?

40. Schwingshackl L, Hoffmann G (2013) Comparison of effects of long-term low-fat vs high-fat diets on blood lipid levels in overweight or obese patients: a systematic review and meta-analysis. J Acad Nutr Diet 113:1640–1661 (B)
41. Dattilo AM, Kris-Etherton PM (1992) Effects of weight reduction on blood lipids and lipoproteins: a meta-analysis. Am J Clin Nutr 56(2):320–328. PubMed PMID:1386186
42. Shai I, Schwarzfuchs D, Henkin Y, Shahar DR, Witkow S, Greenberg I, Golan R, Fraser D, Bolotin A, Vardi H, Tangi-Rozental O, Zuk-Ramot R, Sarusi B, Brickner D, Schwartz Z, Sheiner E, Marko R, Katorza E, Thiery J, Fiedler GM, Blüher M, Stumvoll M, Stampfer MJ, Dietary Intervention Randomized Controlled Trial (DIRECT) Group (2009) Weight loss with a low-carbohydrate, Mediterranean, or low-fat diet. N Engl J Med 359(3):229–241. doi:10.1056/NEJMoa0708681; Erratum in: N Engl J Med. 31;361(27):2681. PubMed PMID: 18635428
43. Due A, Larsen TM, Hermansen K, Stender S, Holst JJ, Toubro S, Martinussen T, Astrup A (2008) Comparison of the effects on insulin resistance and glucose tolerance of 6-mo high-monounsaturated-fat, low-fat, and control diets. Am J Clin Nutr 87(4):855–862. PubMed PMID: 18400707

The Very-Low-Energy Diets (VLED) and the Ketogenic Diet

44. Tsai AG, Wadden TA (2006) The evolution of very-low-calorie diets: an update and meta-analysis. Obesity (Silver Spring) 14(8):1283–1293. Review. PubMed PMID: 1698807
45. U.S. Department of Health and Human Services (August 2008 Updated December 2012) Very low-calorie diets. WIN Weight-control Information Network. NIH publication no. 03–3894
46. Mulholland Y, Nicokavoura E, Broom J, Rolland C (2012) Very-low-energy diets and morbidity: a systematic review of longer-term evidence. Br J Nutr 108(5):832–851. doi:10.1017/S0007114512001924. Epub 2012 Jul 17. Review. PubMed PMID: 22800763
47. Fricker J, Rozen R, Melchior JC, Apfelbaum M (1991) Energy-metabolism adaptation in obese adults on a very-low-calorie diet. Am J Clin Nutr 53(4):826–830. PubMed PMID: 2008860
48. Yang MU, Van Itallie TB (1976) Composition of weight lost during short-term weight reduction. Metabolic responses of obese subjects to starvation and low-calorie ketogenic and nonketogenic diets. J Clin Invest 58(3):722–730. PubMed PMID: 956398; PubMed Central PMCID: PMC333231
49. Bistrian BR (1978) Recent developments in the treatment of obesity with particular reference to semistarvation ketogenic regimens. Diabetes Care 1(6):379–384. PubMed PMID: 729452
50. Paoli A, Rubini A, Volek JS, Grimaldi KA (2013) Beyond weight loss: a review of the therapeutic uses of very-low-carbohydrate (ketogenic) diets. Eur J Clin Nutr 67(8):789–796.

doi:10.1038/ejcn.2013.116. Epub 2013 Jun 26. Review. PubMed PMID: 23801097, PubMed Central PMCID: PMC3826507
51. Stock AL, Yudkin J (1970) Nutrient intake of subjects on low carbohydrate diet used in treatment of obesity. Am J Clin Nutr 23(7):948–952. PubMed PMID: 5455557
52. Laffel L (1999) Ketone bodies: a review of physiology, pathophysiology and application of monitoring to diabetes. Diabetes Metab Res Rev 15(6):412–426. Review. PubMed PMID: 10634967
53. Clarke K, Tchabanenko K, Pawlosky R, Carter E, Todd King M, Musa-Veloso K, Ho M, Roberts A, Robertson J, Vanitallie TB, Veech RL (2012) Kinetics, safety and tolerability of (R)-3-hydroxybutyl (R)-3-hydroxybutyrate in healthy adult subjects. Regul Toxicol Pharmacol 63(3):401–408. doi:10.1016/j.yrtph.2012.04.008. Epub 2012
54. Bergqvist AG, Schall JI, Stallings VA, Zemel BS (2008) Progressive bone mineral content loss in children with intractable epilepsy treated with the ketogenic diet. Am J Clin Nutr 88(6):1678–1684. doi:10.3945/ajcn.2008.26099. PubMed PMID: 19064531
55. McPherson PA, McEneny J (2012) The biochemistry of ketogenesis and its role in weight management, neurological disease and oxidative stress. J Physiol Biochem 68(1):141–151. doi:10.1007/s13105-011-0112-4. Epub 2011 Oct 8. Review.PubMed PMID: 21983804

Criteria for the Formulation of a Balanced Diet in Obese Patient

56. Società Italiana di Nutrizione Umana (S.I.N.U.) (2000) Livelli di assunzione raccomandati di energia e nutrienti per la popolazione italiana. LARN. Revisione 1996. Ed. EDRA, Milano
57. Elia M (1992) Organ and tissue contribution to metabolic rate. In: Kinney JM, Tucker HN (eds) Energy metabolism. Tissue determinants and cellular corollarie. Raven Press, New York, pp 61–79
58. Mifflin MD, St Jeor ST, Hill LA, Scott BJ, Daugherty SA, Koh YO (1990) A new predictive equation for resting expenditure in healthy individuals. Am J Clin Nutr 51:241–247
59. Frankenfield D, Roth-Yousey L, Compher C (2005) Comparison of predictive equations for resting metabolic rate in healthy nonobese and obese adults: a systematic review. J Am Diet Assoc 105(5):775–789. Review. PubMed PMID: 15883556
60. Frankenfield DC (2013) Bias and accuracy of resting metabolic rate equations in non-obese and obese adults. Clin Nutr 32(6):976–982. doi:10.1016/j.clnu.2013.03.022. Epub. PubMed PMID: 23631843
61. Cunningham J (1980) A reanalysis of the factor influencing basal metabolism rate in normal adults. Am J Clin Nutr 33:2372–2374
62. Polito A, Ferro Luzzi A (2006) Energia: misura e bisogni. In: Costantini MA, Cannella C, Tomassi G. Il Pensiero scientifico editore, Rome (2nd eds): pp 215–250
63. Report of a Joint FAO/WHO/UNU expert consultation on energy and protein requirements. WHO technical report series 724, Geneva 1985 – ISBN 92 4 120724 8, Reprinted 1987, 1991
64. Ainsworth BE, Haskell WL, Herrmann SD, Meckes N, Bassett DR Jr, Tudor-Locke C, Greer JL, Vezina J, Whitt-Glover MC, Leon AS (2011) Compendium of physical activities: a second update of codes and MET values. Med Sci Sports Exerc 43(8):1575–1581. doi:10.1249/MSS.0b013e31821ece12. PubMed PMID: 21681120
65. Committee to develop criteria for evaluating the outcomes of approaches to prevent and treat obesity, food and nutrition board, institute of medicine, National Academy of Sciences. Weighting the options: criteria for evaluating weight-management programs. Edizione italiana a cura della Task Force Obesità Italia (TFOI). ed. Pendragon, 1998
66. Donini LM, Pinto A, Cannella C (2004) Diete iperproteiche ed obesità. Ann Ital Med Int 19:36–42
67. Società Italiana di Nutrizione Umana (S.I.N.U.) (2012) LARN – Livelli di Assunzione di Riferimento di Nutrienti ed energia per la popolazione italiana. Revisione 2012. http://www.sinu.it/documenti/20121016_LARN_bologna_sintesi_prefinale.pdf

Nutritional Counseling and Conclusion

68. Panagiotakos DB, Chrysohoou C, Pitsavos C, Stefanadis C (2006) Association between the prevalence of obesity and adherence to the Mediterranean diet: the ATTICA study. Nutrition 22(5):449–456. Epub 2006 Feb 2. PubMed PMID: 16457990
69. Corbalán MD, Morales EM, Canteras M, Espallardo A, Hernández T, Garaulet M (2009) Effectiveness of cognitive-behavioral therapy based on the Mediterranean diet for the treatment of obesity. Nutrition 25(7–8):861–869. doi:10.1016/j.nut.2009.02.013. PubMed PMID: 19539176
70. Mucchielli R. Apprendere il counseling (2001) Manuale di autoformazione al colloquio d'aiuto. Erickson, Trento. ISBN: 88-7946-053-6
71. Società Italiana dell'obesità (SIO)– Associazione Italiana di Dietetica e Nutrizione Clinica (ADI) (2012/2013) Standard Italiani per la cura dell'obesità. http://www.sio-obesita.org/Standard.pdf
72. Bach-Faig A, Berry EM, Lairon D, Reguant J, Trichopoulou A, Dernini S, Medina FX, Battino M, Belahsen R, Miranda G, Serra-Majem L, Mediterranean Diet Foundation Expert Group (2011) Mediterranean diet pyramid today. Science and cultural updates. Public Health Nutr 14(12A):2274–2284. doi:10.1017/S1368980011002515. Review. PubMed PMID: 22166184
73. Dansinger ML, Gleason JA, Griffith JL, Selker HP, Schaefer EJ (2005) Comparison of the atkins, ornish, weight watchers, and zone diets for weight loss and heart disease risk reduction: a randomized trial. JAMA 293:43–53
74. Ayyad C, Andersen T (2000) Long-term efficacy of dietary treatment of obesity: a systematic review of studies published between 1931 and 1999. Obes Rev 1:113–119
75. World Health Organization (WHO) (2000) Obesity: preventing and managing the global epidemic, WHO technical report series, no 894. Consultation on obesity, Geneva, 3–5 June 1997 (Switzerland), 252 p. ISBN 9241208945. Languages: English (reprinted 2004), French (2003)

Physical Activity and Training Prescription

22

Cosme F. Buzzachera, Marco Meucci, and Carlo Baldari

Overweight and obesity are defined by a body mass index (BMI) of 25–29.9 $kg.m^{-2}$ and 30 $kg.m^{-2}$ or greater, respectively. It is known that the prevalence rates of overweight and obesity are rising alarmingly among adults in both developed and developing countries [1]. The increasing rates of overweight and obesity are of concern because of the demonstrated association of excessive body weight with numerous chronic conditions like cardiovascular disease, type 2 diabetes, osteoarthritis, asthma, and certain cancers. The development and implementation of effective interventions for the treatment of excessive body weight and the limitation of obesity-related long-term comorbidities are considered an important public health initiative [2]. Of those who are overweight and/or obese in the USA, nearly 74 % of women and 60 % of men report using one or more weight management strategy [3]. However, it should be noted that even if they achieve weight loss by using management strategies, most of them will experience weight regain over time [4]. This low success rate of lifestyle interventions for overweight and obese adults presents a significant public health challenge.

This chapter describes the interplay among daily physical activity, exercise, and dietary regimens and illustrates how an understanding of exercise prescription can be helpful for the development of effective interventions for the treatment of

---

C.F. Buzzachera
Department of Physical Education, North University of Parana
Avenida Marselha, 591, Londrina, Parana 86041-120, Brazil
e-mail: cosme.buzzachera@unopar.br

M. Meucci
Department of Health and Exercise Science, Appalachian State University,
111 Rivers Street, Boone, NC 28608-2071, USA
e-mail: meuccim@appstate.edu

C. Baldari (✉)
Department of Movement, Human, and Health Sciences,
University of Rome "Foro Italico", Piazza L. De Bosis, 6, Rome 00135, Italy
e-mail: carlo.baldari@uniroma4.it

excessive body weight in adults. First, we will discuss about the key role of physical activity in the prevention of weight gain. Second, we will examine how we can maximize weight control by using an adequate dose of exercise and/or dietary regimen. Third, we will describe how physical activity can promote health benefits for overweight adults independent of body weight. Throughout the chapter, physical activity is defined as any bodily movement produced by skeletal muscles requiring a considerable increase of energy expenditure as compared to a resting phase. Physical activity in daily life may include occupational, conditioning, sports, household, or other activities. Otherwise, exercise is defined as a subset of physical activity that is planned, structured, and repetitive with final or intermediate objectives of the improvement or maintenance of physical fitness.

22.1 Energy Balance and the Role of Physical Activity

As previously noted by Hill and colleagues, obesity is often considered to be a result of assuming too many calories and not getting enough physical activity [5]. This debate about the role of physical activity and/or dietary regimens is often emphasized in the literature [6, 7]; however, it seems clear that this discussion has not yet produced effective or innovative solutions. From a theoretical perspective, the key to managing body weight is related to energy balance. Specifically, a body weight is maintained, over a specified time, if energy intake and energy expenditure are equal. This energy balance is the goal for the prevention of initial weight gain or weight regain after weight loss. Otherwise, body weight can change only when energy intake is not equal to energy expenditure over a given period of time. This energy imbalance is necessary to elicit an energy deficit and promote weight loss in overweight and obese adults [5]. Physical activity, defined as any bodily movement produced by skeletal muscles that requires energy expenditure, is considered a key strategy to the creation of energy deficit in weight loss programs. It should be noted that daily physical activity is the most variable component of energy expenditure and consists of the amount of physical activity performed multiplied by the energy cost of that activity, aside from the energy expended through the resting metabolic rate and the thermic effect of food. However, although physical activity in terms of structured exercise is an essential component of weight loss programs, health professionals are strongly encouraged to understand the magnitude of the contribution of physical activity to weight loss in adults in excess of body weight [8].

Previous research has emphasized the importance of physical activity in terms of structured exercise in the prevention and management of obesity [5, 8], and generic guidelines originally developed for the wider population have been adapted for these specific populations. In fact, physical activity is recommended as an important part of weight management by all public health agencies and scientific organizations, including Centers for Disease Control [9], American Heart Association [10], and American College of Sports Medicine [11]. However, previous studies have found that greater changes in body weight are caused by reductions in energy intake (e.g., diet) [7, 12]. For example, Hagan and colleagues [7] observed that after

3 months, of a dietary restriction of 945 kcal for obese women and 1,705 kcal a day for obese men, body weight decreased by 5.5 and 8.4 kg, respectively. Conversely, performing an exercise training program that included 30 min of walk or jog activities for 5 days a week, obese women and men spent 190 and 255 kcal per session, resulted in a marginal weight loss of 0.6 and 0.3 kg, respectively. Conflicting evidences have been reported also by other authors who used structured, weight loss programs to increase energy expenditure via exercise. Using short-term intervention protocols lasting up to 6 months, they demonstrated that exercise training could be as effective as weight loss programs using energy restriction [6, 13, 14]. Another study conducted by Ross and colleagues [13] on 52 obese men reported a 7.5 kg (3 %) weight loss after 3 months of intervention aiming to reduce obesity and related comorbidities through a dietary restriction of 700 kcal a day or increasing energy expenditure through exercise. These results may confirm that when the energy deficits imposed by diet only and diet plus exercise interventions are similar, weight loss and percent change in body weight are similar. However, most overweight and obese adults are not able to engage in sufficient levels of exercise to produce the magnitude of weight loss typically found with energy restrictions [8]. For example, a 90 kg person would need to perform about 115 min a day of brisk walking to expend 700 kcal a day in exercise to produce this magnitude of weight loss, which is clearly an unrealistic situation for an individual who is engaging in a physical activity program.

22.2 Physical Activity to Improve Body Control

22.2.1 Mode of Exercise

Physical activity in terms of exercise in the prevention and management of obesity should focus on endurance (or cardiovascular/aerobic) modes of exercise. Specifically, this mode of exercise may lead individuals to expend a considerable amount of energy in a given period of time, which in turn may be useful for achieving the target of 2,000 kcal per week. In general, endurance training has been categorized as either weight bearing or non-weight bearing. For example, walking is classified as a weight-bearing activity and is currently considered one of the best modes of exercise for several reasons, including experience of all individuals with the activity and safety. Walking is also available to most individuals and does not require special facilities [15]. However, it should be noted that some people have preexisting musculoskeletal conditions that could prevent certain modes of weight-bearing activities. These conditions are often related to pain in the lower back, hip, knee, and ankle joints that may be chronic. In this case, non-weight-bearing activities, such as stationary cycling, recumbent cycling, upper-body ergometry, water activities, and others, should be selected. These activities are useful at any time but are particularly useful for those with joint injury or pain. In summary, health professionals are encouraged to include endurance training as an important part of their physical activity programs for overweight and obese adults.

Recent guidelines on exercise for weight loss and weight maintenance include resistance training as part of the exercise prescription. However, researchers have noted that resistance training alone is ineffective in promoting weight loss and maintenance in overweight and obese adults but it leads to significant reductions in body weight and fat mass when combined to endurance training [16–18]. Furthermore, interventions that combined dietary energy restrictions with resistance exercise have shown no weight loss advantages in comparison with energy restrictions plus other forms of exercise [17]. However, resistance training as well as endurance plus resistance training can increase lean body mass more than endurance training alone. These results suggest that although the energy expenditure associated with resistance training is not large, resistance training may increase muscle mass which may in turn increase 24 h energy expenditure. These benefits of resistance training on muscle structure and function may be advantageous for improving the ability to perform activities of daily living in overweight and obese adults, which in turn results in improvements in quality of life. Thus the addition of resistance training may promote benefits for adults in excess of body weight for reasons other than the impact of this form of exercise and weight loss.

22.2.2 Duration

In order to obtain valuable benefits from an exercise training program on weight loss, individuals need to participate in adequate levels of physical activity. Although there are current recommendations with respect to the amount of physical activity useful for weight management in sedentary individuals [10, 11], research has demonstrated that large amounts may be needed for most of the overweight individuals. In fact, a considerable amount of cross-sectional studies indicated an inverse relationship between body weight or body mass index and physical activity [19, 20] highlighting a dose-response relationship between body weight or body mass index and physical activity levels. For example, Mctiernan and collaborators [21] observed that a group of 40–75-year-old men and women lost 1.8 and 1.4 kg of body weight and 3.0 and 1.9 % of body fat, respectively, after 12 months of an exercise program designed to promote 300 min of moderate physical activity a week, in comparison with a sedentary counterpart. Importantly, a significant dose-effect relationship in weight loss was observed when physical activity is performed for more than 250 min a week. These data are similar from those found in previous studies and indicate that greater amounts of physical activity resulted in greater amounts of weight loss. For example, in two separate studies, Jakicic and colleagues [22, 23] have found that long-term weight loss was improved in overweight and obese women with the addition of 200–300 min a week of physical activity. Taken together, these studies highlight that moderate-to-vigorous physical activity of 150–250 min a week with an energy equivalent of about 1,200–2,000 kcal a week may be enough to prevent a weight gain greater than 3 % in most adults.

22.2.3 Intensity

When prescribing an exercise session, intensity component could be described in absolute or relative terms. Relative intensity takes into consideration the exercise capacity of the individual to perform the activity, while absolute intensity only considers the demands of the activity [24]. Health benefits of physical activity can be promoted performing exercise with low intensity (predominantly aerobic) and long duration or exercise with high intensity (predominantly anaerobic) and short duration. However, intensity and duration components must be regulated so that the intensity is low enough to allow suitable durations and expends the recommended caloric energy. For most of the overweight adults engaging in an exercise program, the sustainable intensity will not be sufficient to cause improvements in cardiorespiratory fitness, because the initial focus should be on weight loss and maintenance increasing energy expenditure [11]. As the exercise program progresses and the individual is able to better tolerate the exercise session, higher-intensity activities above the 60 % heart rate reserve (maximum heart rate minus resting heart rate) should be prescribed by health professionals. However, exercise intensities between 40 and 59 % heart rate reserve are encouraged to initial exercisers, even if lower intensities must be prescribed for very deconditioned patients [25]. It should be noted that exercise intensity is inversely related to exercise adherence [26]; thus, health professionals are encouraged to "push up" their overweight patients in order to avoid a premature dropout. With regard to exercise adherence, it should be noted that prescribed intensities are considered less pleasant than preferred intensities in sedentary, overweight adults [27, 28]. Thus self-paced protocols where individuals are encouraged to choose their intensity must be reinforced by health professionals to ensure a more positive affective response during exercise, which in turn may prevent dropout [29, 30]. Taken together, these data suggest that health professionals should focus not only on "physiological" prescription but also on "behavioral" prescription to ensure future exercise participation.

22.3 Body Weight Control and Health Benefits for Overweight Adults

Research has emphasized that physical activity may lead to health benefits whether weight is lost and perhaps even if weight is gained [31, 32]. This may indicate that overweight and obese adults may realize improvements in health-related outcomes independent of weight loss. Data from longitudinal studies such as the CARDIA study demonstrate that adults maintain a stable body mass index minimized the undesirable changes in cardiovascular disease risk factors occurring with aging [31]. Similarly, Wei and colleagues [33] found that cardiorespiratory fitness, a health-related component directly associated with physical activity participation (see Chap. 18), is a strong and independent predictor of cardiovascular disease and of all-cause mortality in adults, regardless of variations in body mass index. More importantly, the reduction of chronic health risks is seen even with minimal weight loss of less than 3 % [34]. Taken together, these findings support the importance of physical activity and exercise participation of adults in excess of body weight.

References

1. World Health Organization Western Pacific Region (2000) Redefining obesity and its treatment. Health communications Australia, Melbourne
2. Ness-Abramof R, Apovian CM (2006) Diet modification for treatment and prevention of obesity. Endocrine 29:5–9
3. Yaemsiri S, Slining MM, Agarwal SK (2010) Perceived weight status, overweight diagnosis, and weight control among US adults: the NHANES 2003–2008 Study. Int J Obes 35:1063–1070
4. Tsai AG, Wadden TA (2005) Systematic review: an evaluation of major commercial weight loss programs in the United States. Ann Intern Med 142:56–66
5. Hill JO, Wyatt HR, Peters JC (2012) Energy balance and obesity. Circulation 126:126–132
6. Donini LM, Cuzzolaro M, Gnessi L et al (2014) Obesity treatment: results after 4 years of a nutritional and psycho-physical rehabilitation program in an outpatient setting. Eat Weight Disord. doi:10.1007/s40519-014-0107-6
7. Hagan RD, Upon SJ, Wong L et al (1986) The effects of aerobic conditioning and/or calorie restriction in overweight men and women. Med Sci Sports Exerc 18:87–94
8. Jakicic JM, Otto AD (2005) Physical activity considerations for the treatment and prevention of obesity. Am J Clin Nutr 82:226S–229S
9. Expert Panel on the Identification, Evaluation, and Treatment of Overweight in Adults (1998) Clinical guidelines on the identification, evaluation, and treatment of overweight and obesity in adults: executive summary (1-3). Am J Clin Nutr 68:899–917
10. Haskell WL, Lee IM, Pate RR et al (2007) Physical activity and health: updated recommendation for adults from the American College of Sports Medicine and the American Heart Association. Med Sci Sports Exerc 39:1423–1434
11. Donnelly JE, Blair SN, Jakicic JM et al (2009) Appropriate physical activity intervention strategies for weight loss and prevention of weight regain for adults. Med Sci Sport Exerc 41:459–471
12. Garrow JS, Summerbell CD (1995) Meta-analysis: effect of exercise, with or without dieting, on the body composition of overweight subjects. Eur J Clin Nutr 49:1–10
13. Ross R, Dagnone D, Jones PJH et al (2000) Reduction in obesity and related comorbid conditions after diet-induced weight loss or exercise-induced weight loss in men and women. Ann Inter Med 133:92–103
14. Wood PD, Stephanick ML, Dreon DM et al (1988) Changes in plasma lipids and lipoproteins in overweight men during weight loss through dieting as compared with exercise. N Engl J Med 319:1173–1179
15. Lee C, Ory MG, Yoon J et al (2013) Neighborhood walking among overweight and obese adults: age variations in barriers and motivators. J Community Health 38:12–22
16. Fencki S, Sarsan A, Rota S et al (2006) Effects of resistance or aerobic exercises on metabolic parameters in obese women who are not on a diet. Adv Ther 23:404–413
17. Wadden TA, Vogt RA, Andersen RE (1997) Exercise in the treatment of obesity: effects of four interventions on body composition, resting energy expenditure, appetite, and mood. J Consult Clin Psychol 65(269–277):1831–1837
18. Willis LH, Slentz CA, Baterman LA et al (2012) Effects of aerobic and/or resistance training on body mass and fat mass in overweight or obese adults. J Appl Physiol 12:1381–1387
19. Ball K, Owen N, Salmon J et al (2001) Associations of physical activity with body weight and fat in men and women. Int J Obes 25:914–919
20. Martinez JA, Kearney JM, Kafatos A et al (1999) Variables independently associated with self-reported obesity in the European Union. Public Health Nutr 2:125–133

21. McTiernan A, Sorensen B, Irwin ML et al (1997) Exercise effect on weight and body fat in men and women. Obesity 15:1496–1512
22. Jakicic JM, Marcus BH, Gallagher KL et al (2003) Effect of exercise duration and intensity on weight loss in overweight, sedentary women. JAMA 290:1323–1330
23. Jakicic JM, Marcus BH, Lang W et al (2008) Effect of exercise on 24-month weight loss maintenance in overweight women. Arch Intern Med 168:1550–1559
24. Emerenziani GP, Migliaccio S, Gallotta MC et al (2013) Physical exercise intensity prescription to improve health and fitness in overweight and obese subjects: a review of the literature. Health 5:113–121
25. Pinet GM, Prud'Homme D, Gallant CA et al (2008) Exercise intensity prescription in obese individuals. Obesity 16:2088–2095
26. Williams DM, Dunsiger S, Ciccolo JT et al (2008) Acute affective response to a moderate-intensity exercise stimulus predicts physical activity participation 6 and 12 months later. Psychol Sport Exerc 9:231–245
27. Ekkekakis P, Lind E (2006) Exercise does not feel the same when you are overweight: the impact of self-selected and imposed intensity on affect and exertion. Int J Obes 30:652–660
28. Parfitt G, Rose EA, Burgess WM (2006) The psychological and physiological responses of sedentary individuals to prescribed and preferred intensity exercise. Br J Health Psychol 11:39–53
29. DaSilva SG, Guidetti L, Buzzachera CF et al (2011) Psychophysiological responses to self-paced treadmill and overground exercise. Med Sci Sports Exerc 43:1114–1124
30. DaSilva SG, Guidetti L, Buzzachera CF et al (2009) The influence of adiposity on physiological, perceptual, and affective responses during walking at a self-selected pace. Percept Mot Skills 109:41–60
31. Lloyd-Jones DM, Liu K, Colangelo LA et al (2007) Consistently stable or decreased body mass index in young adulthood and longitudinal changes in metabolic syndrome components: the Coronary Artery Risk Development in Young Adults Study. Circulation 115:1004–1011
32. Norman JE, Bild D, Liu K et al (2003) The impact of weight change on cardiovascular disease risk factors in young black and white adults: the CARDIA study. Int J Obes 27:369–376
33. Wei M, Kampert J, Barlow CE et al (1999) Relationship between low cardiorespiratory fitness and mortality in normal weight, overweight, and obese men. JAMA 282:1547–1553
34. Donnelly JE, Jacobsen DJ, Snyder Heelan KA et al (2000) The effects of 18 month of intermittent vs continuous exercise on aerobic capacity, body weight and composition, and metabolic fitness in previously sedentary, moderately obese females. Int J Obes 24:566–572

Prescription Medications for the Treatment of Obesity

23

Valentina Lo Preiato, Elena Daniela Serban, Renato Pasquali, and Uberto Pagotto

23.1 Introduction

Modifications in lifestyle remain the most important aid to effectively tackle obesity, but the low rate of success in most obese subjects and the need for continued intervention, not always accessible due to elevated health care costs, have limited the efficacy of this approach. On the other hand, bariatric surgery represents an alternative remedy with a high rate of stable and significant success in body weight reduction and consequent cardiometabolic parameter amelioration. However, it is hard to hypothesize that this option could be applied on a large scale due to the high costs, the inherent surgical risks, and the maladaptive postoperative compliance from some patients [1].

Taking into account the limitations provided by lifestyle changes and bariatric surgery mentioned above, one might conclude that there could be some room for the pharmacological approach to obesity. However, the last 30 years have produced poor results and limited success in generating drugs devoid of important side effects to tackle obesity and its comorbidities. This has caused pharmaceutical companies to substantially reduce investments in research and development in this field.

V.L. Preiato • E.D. Serban • R. Pasquali • U. Pagotto (✉)
Division of Endocrinology, Department of Medical and Surgical Science, Centre for Applied Biomedical Research (C.R.B.A.), S. Orsola-Malpighi Hospital, University of Bologna, Via Massarenti 9, 40138 Bologna, Italy

Division of Endocrinology, Department of Medical and Surgical Science, S. Orsola-Malpighi Hospital, University Alma Mater Studiorum, Via Massarenti 9, 40138 Bologna, Italy
e-mail: va_lopreiato@libero.it; danna_es@yahoo.com; renato.pasquali@unibo.it; uberto.pagotto@unibo.it

© Springer International Publishing Switzerland 2015
A. Lenzi et al. (eds.), *Multidisciplinary Approach to Obesity: From Assessment to Treatment*, DOI 10.1007/978-3-319-09045-0_23

23.2 The Pharmacotherapy of Obesity Between Guidelines and Regulatory Agencies

Recently, new guidelines for the management of overweight and obesity in adults have been approved in the USA [1]. The concept has been reinforced that all patients for whom weight loss is recommended should be offered or referred for comprehensive lifestyle intervention. It has also been reestablished that if a patient presents with a body mass index (BMI) ≥30 or ≥27 with comorbidities and is unable to lose weight or to sustain weight loss with comprehensive lifestyle intervention, pharmacological therapy should be taken into account to help achieve targeted weight loss and to prevent diseases. However, it is clearly stated that medications should be approved by the regulatory agencies, and clinicians should know what the benefits and health risks of the prescribed medication are. Medications work to reinforce lifestyle change and should be prescribed only as an adjunct to a good quality lifestyle intervention [1]. This issue should be mandatory, but it is not always taken into account by the companies developing antiobesity drugs when the clinical trials are designed to obtain drug approval. With few exceptions, indeed, the majority of the phase 2 and 3 trials and most of the non-sponsored studies include lifestyle intervention at low level of priority.

The regulatory point of view in this issue varies between US and European agencies. According to the American Food and Drug Administration (FDA) draft guidance, the efficacy of a 1-year treatment with an antiobesity drug should meet one of these two conditions: (I) the difference in weight change from the baseline between the treatment group and placebo is 5 %, and (II) the number of patients in the treatment group that obtains this weight gain is at least 35 % and approximately double the number of subjects in the placebo group. On the other hand, European Medicines Agency (EMA) require antiobesity drugs to satisfy the following two criteria: (I) a weight loss of at least 10 % of baseline weight and (II) a magnitude of weight loss significantly different from the placebo group treated with lifestyle intervention. However, after the position statement regarding the antidiabetic drugs issued by the Endocrinologic and Metabolic Drugs Advisory Committee in 2008, the FDA Advisory Committee established in March 2012 that the evaluation of antiobesity drugs should be made after their effectiveness in reducing cardiovascular risk had been assessed. Briefly, a two-step process is required to establish the cardiovascular safety of any antiobesity drug, consisting of a randomized cardiovascular event-driven trial before approval and a longer and larger trial after approval. Moreover, preliminary trials in the highest risk population are required to consolidate the findings.

23.3 Drugs Approved for Short-Term Use

Amphetamines and their analogues (phentermine, benzphetamine, phendimetrazine, and diethylpropion) were approved long time ago by the FDA.

In September 1999, the EMA recommended their withdrawal from the market because of their unfavorable risk to benefit ratio. However, the FDA still allows these drugs to be marketed in the USA, limiting their use to only the short term (<12 weeks) due to the risk of abuse in obese patients who do not respond to lifestyle modifications [2].

Among the analogues of amphetamine, phentermine represents the most prescribed antiobesity drug in the USA, and a meta-analysis of many randomized control trials (RCTs) showed that subjects treated with phentermine alone lost 3.6 kg compared to placebo [3]. Its use is now showing a novel rapid revival due to the new combo formulation with topiramate recently approved by the FDA (see below). Phentermine is commercially available in the USA in different formulations (hydrochloride salt, resin, or disintegrating tablets), and the recommended daily doses are up to 30 mg/day for the orally disintegrated tablets.

The major side effects of this class of drugs are insomnia, dry mouth, and anxiety. These effects are usually transient, and they do not differ between subjects receiving continuous versus intermittent therapy. More serious uncommon complications in prolonged use include primary pulmonary hypertension and cardiovascular or cerebrovascular events, hyperthyroidism, and glaucoma. Obviously, due to their mechanism of action, they are also contraindicated in individuals with psychiatric disorders, including anorexia, depression, or in patients at risk of drug dependency [2].

23.4 Drugs Approved for Long-Term Use

23.4.1 Orlistat

Orlistat is a gastrointestinal lipase inhibitor approved for use in adults and adolescents aged 12–16 years. It does not act directly on appetite, but decreases fat absorption to approximately 30 % of intake.

Orlistat's long-term efficacy (120 mg three times daily) was demonstrated in several RCTs of 2–4 years' therapy [4]. The results of these studies appear similar: orlistat reduces weight about 2.9 % more than placebo and increases the absolute percentage of participants achieving 5 % weight loss by about 21 %. Furthermore, the XENDOS study, a 4-year RCT of 3,305 nondiabetic obese patients, showed that orlistat reduced the risk of developing T2DM by 37.3 % compared to only lifestyle modification [5]. Orlistat has demonstrated its efficacy also in diabetic subjects: in a multicenter 57-week RCT, 120 mg orlistat or placebo was administered to 391 obese subjects with T2DM. The orlistat group lost about 2 kg more than the placebo group and twice as many patients receiving orlistat lost > or = 5 % of their initial body weight. Orlistat treatment was also associated with significant decreases in HbA1c, fasting plasma glucose, total cholesterol, LDL cholesterol, LDL/HDL cholesterol ratio, and triglycerides. The most commonly experienced side effects of orlistat are due to its mechanism of action and include diarrhea, fecal incontinence, flatulence, and abdominal pain [5]. Recently, FDA undertook a review of orlistat treatment safety, which identified a total of 13 cases of serious liver injury [2].

23.4.2 Lorcaserin

Lorcaserin is a selective serotonin (5HT) 2C receptor agonist, sharing characteristics similar to fenfluramine. The tolerability and efficacy of lorcaserin for the treatment of obesity were evaluated in three large RCTs, which provided the basis for FDA approval in June 2012.

In the BLOSSOM RCT, 4,008 obese or overweight patients with obesity-related comorbid conditions were randomized to receive either lorcaserin 10 mg/die (QD), lorcaserin 10 mg twice daily (BID), or placebo for 52 weeks. Weight loss was 4.7, 5.8, and 2.9 kg, respectively, similar among males and females, but higher in Caucasian patients than African-American or Hispanic patients. The percentages of subjects achieving 5 % or greater weight loss were 47.2, 40.2, and 25 % for lorcaserin BID, lorcaserin QD, and placebo, respectively [6].

The BLOOM RCT evaluated 3,182 patients for 2 years with similar results [7]. The BLOOM-DM RCT evaluated the safety and efficacy of lorcaserin in 604 patients with T2DM. Weight loss was approximately 5 kg for lorcaserin and 1.6 kg for placebo. The study found that 45 % of lorcaserin QD achieved at least a 5 % weight loss (16 % in the placebo group). Approximately half of the patients in the lorcaserin treatment arm obtained an HbA1c level <7 %, almost twice the rate in the placebo group [8]. Lorcaserin is generally well tolerated: the most frequent adverse reactions are headache, dizziness, and nausea. There was no increase in cardiac valvulopathy rate after a 2-year treatment with lorcaserin [6–8]. Considering its mechanism of action, extreme caution should be used when prescribing lorcaserin to patients taking a selective 5HT reuptake inhibitor or 5HT-NA reuptake inhibitor due to the potential for 5HT syndrome [6–8]. Lorcaserin was approved by the FDA as an antiobesity drug (Belviq®), whereas a few months later the marketing authorization application of lorcaserin in Europe was rejected by the EMA; the manufacturer of this drug then withdrew its application in Europe [9].

23.4.3 Topiramate and Phentermine Combo

Topiramate is an anticonvulsant drug approved for adjunctive treatment of partial onset and generalized tonic-clonic seizures. Its mechanism of action is not fully understood: it may include blockage of voltage-activated sodium channels, glutamate-receptor antagonism, inhibition of high-voltage-activated calcium channels, inhibition of carbonic anhydrase, and enhancing of gamma-aminobutyric acid-evoked currents [10]. For many years, topiramate alone has been demonstrated to be able to determine weight loss. A meta-analysis of 10 RCTs (3,320 individuals overall) showed that patients treated with topiramate lost an average of 5.34 kg more than with placebo [10]. Topiramate is quite well tolerated, especially at doses of 192 mg/die or less. Paresthesias are frequently experienced by patients. Other adverse effects are fatigue, depression, and difficulty with memory [10]. Finally, topiramate is contraindicated in pregnancy for its teratogenic effects [10].

The drug combination of phentermine and topiramate (Qsymia®) was approved by the FDA for the long-term treatment of obesity in 2012 [11]. However, this combo was not approved in Europe at two different marketing authorization applications due to the deficiency of long-term data on cardiovascular safety [11]. The manufacturer will probably resubmit the application when ad interim data from a cardiovascular outcome trial are available.

The tolerance and safety of this drug combination were evaluated in a series of phase III RCTs, respectively, named EQUATE, EQUIP, and CONQUER.

EQUATE was a 28-week study that included 756 patients treated with two doses of phentermine (7.5 or 15 mg), or two doses of topiramate (46 or 92 mg), or two doses of the combination phentermine/topiramate (PHEN/TPM) (7.5/46 or 15/92 mg) or placebo. The weight loss was 9.2 % for PHEN/TPM 15/92 mg, 8.5 % for PHEN/TPM 7.5/46 mg, 6.4 % for TPM 92 mg, 5.1 % for TPM 46 %, 6.1 % PHEN 15 mg, 5.5 % PHEN 7.5 mg, and 1.7 % placebo. In the combination therapy arm, the percentage of patients achieving a 10 % or greater weight loss was nearly sixfold that observed with placebo [12].

The EQUIP RCT included 1,267 patients with BMI ≥35 kg/m^2 and without T2DM. They were randomized to PHEN/TPM 15 mg/92 mg, PHEN/TPM 3.75 mg/23 mg, or placebo, for 52 weeks. The percentage of weight loss with high-dose PHEN/TPM was 10.9 % (−12.6 kg), compared with 5.1 % (−6 kg) in the low dose and 1.6 % (−1.8 kg) for placebo. The 66.7 % of 15/92 patients lost at least 5 % of baseline body weight vs 17.3 % in the placebo group [13].

The CONQUER RCT compared full-dose and mid-dose PHEN/TPM with placebo for 52 weeks. This study includes 2,487 obese or overweight adults with two or more related comorbidities (hypertension, T2DM, dyslipidemia). At the end of the study, weight loss was 9.8 % (−10.2 kg) for high-dose, 7.8 % (−8.1 kg) with mid-dose, and 1.2 % (−1.8 kg) for placebo. At least 5 % weight loss was achieved by 70, 62, and 21 % of the subjects, respectively [14]. This trial was followed by the SEQUEL study, an extension for one additional year: weight loss was maintained during the second year of treatment resulting in 10.5 % in PHEN/TPM 15/92 mg, 9.3 % in PHEN/TPM 7.5/46 mg, and 1.8 % in the placebo group [15]. In all studies, the 15/92 group had significantly greater changes relative to placebo for waist circumference, systolic and diastolic blood pressure, fasting glucose, HbA1c, triglycerides, and total LDL and HDL cholesterol. An RCT was recently performed to evaluate the effect of PHEN/TPM treatment on progression to T2DM and/or cardiometabolic disease in subjects with prediabetes and/or metabolic syndrome. Subjects were randomized to placebo, PHEN/TPM 7.5/46 mg, or PHEN/TPM 15/92 mg for 108 weeks. After this time, the annualized incidence rates of T2DM for those receiving 7.5/46 mg and 15/92 mg were reduced by 70.5 and 78.7 %, respectively, *vs* placebo [16]. The most common adverse reactions of PHEN/TPM therapy included paresthesias, dizziness, dysgeusia, insomnia, constipation, and mouth dryness. These side effects occurred in patients who received full and middle doses, but not in the low-dose group. Patients with previous history of major depression or suicidal ideation cannot use PHEN/TPM. However, the occurrence of depression-related adverse events in these trials was comparable in the 15/92 and the placebo groups [12–16]. A small increase in resting heart rate was observed in higher-dose PHEN/TPM treatment (56.1 %) than with placebo (42.1 %). This alteration led to some concerns regarding its potential long-term effect on cardiovascular events. For this reason, PHEN/TPM was approved with a requirement for a post-marketing trial to assess long-term cardiovascular safety [17]. The drug labeling recommends against prescription in patients with recent or unstable cardiac or cerebrovascular disease and suggests regular monitoring of resting heart rate [17].

In conclusion, three antiobesity drugs are currently approved for long-term obesity treatment: orlistat, Belviq, and Qsymia by the FDA, while only orlistat can be prescribed in Europe.

23.5 Drugs for Off-Label Use

23.5.1 Fluoxetine

Fluoxetine is a selective 5HT reuptake inhibitor which has been prescribed off-label for weight loss. In six double-blind, placebo-controlled studies, it was showed that maximum mean weight loss was around 5 kg and occurred at week 12–20 of therapy. Many studies also showed improvements in indices of glycemic control in obese diabetic patients treated with fluoxetine. Nevertheless, most RCTs did not show a significant difference when fluoxetine was compared to placebo at 52 weeks. Fluoxetine has a good safety profile: reported adverse events are mild and transient and are mainly headache, asthenia, nausea, diarrhea, and somnolence [18].

23.5.2 Metformin

Metformin, an antidiabetic drug used off-label in prediabetes and other insulin-resistant states, produces a weight loss of about 2 % in comparison with placebo. Metformin is rarely used as a monotherapy for obesity because it causes only a small weight loss, but its excellent safety profile makes it a good choice when other drugs are contraindicated. Metformin is also used to prevent or thwart weight gain due to atypical antipsychotic agents and mood stabilizers. A meta-analysis, examining antipsychotic weight gain, found an additional weight loss of approximately 3 kg with metformin compared to placebo [19].

23.5.3 Glucagon-Like Peptide-1 Analogues: Liraglutide and Exenatide

Liraglutide and exenatide are glucagon-like peptide-1 (GLP1) analogues developed and approved for the treatment of T2DM.

A meta-analysis of 21 studies including 6,411 patients demonstrated that GLP-1 agonists achieved a greater weight loss than control groups in all examined trials (weighted mean difference was −2.9 kg). Patients treated with liraglutide also showed a significant reduction in systolic and diastolic blood pressure, plasma cholesterol concentration, glycemic control, and prevalence of prediabetes (from 84 to 96 % in the different studies) [20]. Liraglutide was tested in two specific phase III trials in obese nondiabetic patients, and the results seem to be very promising [21, 22]. The most common adverse events with liraglutide are nausea and diarrhea, mainly mild and transient [23].

23.5.4 Bupropion

Bupropion is approved for the treatment of depression and smoking cessation. It inhibits reuptake of dopamine and noradrenaline resulting in a reduction of appetite and modest weight loss. A meta-analysis, including five studies, reported a mean weight loss of 2.8 kg [2]. The main adverse effects reported during the use of bupropion are mouth dryness, insomnia, anxiety, and palpitations. They are generally mild and transient [2].

23.5.5 Naltrexone

Naltrexone is a high affinity and long-acting opioid receptor antagonist which was originally produced for the treatment of opioid and alcohol dependence. In former narcotic addicts treated with naltrexone, many subjects experience a notable slimming effect, but RCTs have not demonstrated a statistically significant weight loss [2].

23.5.6 Zonisamide

Zonisamide is an antiepileptic medication, which also induces weight loss. A 12-month RCT found that a 400 mg dose led to significantly greater weight loss than placebo (6.8 % vs 3.7 %), and 54.7 % assigned to zonisamide 400 mg achieved 5 % or greater weight loss [24]. The most frequent side effects of zonisamide are gastrointestinal troubles, headache, dizziness, somnolence, and fatigue.

23.6 Drugs Awaiting FDA Reevaluation

23.6.1 Bupropion Plus Naltrexone (Contrave)

In an RCT named COR-I, 1,742 nondiabetic subjects were enrolled for 56 weeks to assess the efficacy of naltrexone plus bupropion. Participants were randomly assigned to receive: (1) sustained-release (SR) naltrexone 32 mg plus SR bupropion 360 mg (SR32) and (2) SR naltrexone 16 mg plus SR bupropion 360 mg (SR16) or (3) placebo. Mean change in body weight was −1.3 % in the placebo, −6.1 % in the

SR32 group, and –5.0 % in the SR16 group [25]. The improvement in cardiometabolic risk factors related to obesity was confirmed in the randomized, parallel-arm, placebo-controlled COR-II trial [26]. COR-Diabetes was a 56-week RCT of 505 overweight/obese with T2DM randomized to SR32 or placebo. A ≥5 % loss of body weight was achieved in 44.5 % of patients vs 18.9 % on placebo. A greater improvement in glycemic control was achieved in the treatment group with average baseline HbA1C reduced by 0.6 % compared to 0.1 % for placebo [27]. The most frequent adverse events detected in this combination therapy are nausea, constipation, vomiting, dizziness, headache, and dry mouth [27, 28].

The combination of naltrexone and bupropion is awaiting FDA approval. In December 2010, the FDA advisory panel voted in favor of approval of this combination, but the same agency declined to approve the drug in early 2011, necessitating additional studies on cardiovascular safety [17]. A phase 3 RCT (the Light Study) was therefore started in July 2012 and is still ongoing. This study is designed to assess the cardiovascular health outcomes of naltrexone/bupropion in overweight or obese patients with cardiovascular risk factors and is estimated to finish in 2017 [17].

Conclusion

Due to its unsuccessful history, research into new antiobesity drugs has recently clearly slowed down. The discrepancies in marketing authorization from the various agencies have not helped to promote efforts by pharmaceutical companies. Furthermore, a number of methodological problems in formulating clinical trials in obese patients limited the generalization of the results obtained in trials when extended to real life, increasing the vulnerability of this topic in the public opinion. Monotherapies too often offer moderate if not small weight loss benefits, while polytherapies, which seem to show more promising results in the management of obesity and related comorbidities, increase the hazard and the risk of severe side effects [28]. In conclusion, a prudent if not a pessimistic view about the future seems to surround the concept of tackling obesity by using pharmacological therapy; however, a constant and progressive understanding of the central and peripheral mechanisms that control energy homeostasis and cerebral hedonic pathways will probably pave the way for future drugs inducing more sustained benefits and less dangerous side effects.

References

1. Jensen MD, Ryan DH, Apovian CM et al (2013) AHA/ACC/TOS guideline for the management of overweight and obesity in adults. JACC. doi:10.1016/j.jacc.2013.11.004
2. Ioannides-Demos LL, Piccenna L, McNeill JJ et al (2011) Pharmacotherapies for obesity: past, current, and future therapies. J Obes 2011:179674. doi:10.1155/2011/179674, Epub 2010 Dec 12
3. Haddock CK, Poston WS, Dill PL et al (2002) Pharmacotherapy for obesity: a quantitative analysis of four decades of published randomized clinical trials. Int J Obes Relat Metab Disord 26:262–267

4. Hutton B, Fergusson D (2004) Changes in body weight and serum lipid profile in obese patients treated with orlistat in addition to a hypocaloric diet: a systematic review of randomized clinical trials. Am J Clin Nutr 80:1461–1468
5. Torgerson JSJ, Hauptman J, Boldrin MN et al (2004) XENical in the prevention of diabetes in obese subjects (XENDOS) study: a randomized study of orlistat as an adjunct to lifestyle changes for the prevention of type 2 diabetes in obese patients. Diabetes Care 27: 155–161
6. Fidler MC, Sánchez M, Raether B et al (2011) A one-year randomized trial of lorcaserin for weight loss in obese and overweight adults: the BLOSSOM trial. J Clin Endocrinol Metab 96:3067–3077
7. Smith SR, Weissman NJ, Anderson CM et al (2010) Behavioral Modification and Lorcaserin for Overweight and Obesity Management (BLOOM) Study Group, Multicenter, placebo-controlled trial of lorcaserin for weight management. N Engl J Med 363:245–256
8. O'Neil PM, Smith SR, Weissman NJ et al (2012) Randomized placebo controlled clinical trial of lorcaserin for weight loss in type 2 diabetes mellitus: the BLOOM-DM study. Obesity 20:1426–1436
9. Withdrawal of the marketing authorisation application for Belviq (lorcaserin). 2013. http://www.ema.europa.eu/docs/en_GB/document_library/Medicine_QA/2013/05/WC500143811.pdf
10. Kramer CK, Leitão CB, Pinto LC et al (2011) Efficacy and safety of topiramate on weight loss: a meta-analysis of randomized controlled trials. Obes Rev 12:338–347
11. European Medicine Agency (EMA), Questions and answers on the refusal of the marketing authorisation for Qsiva (phentermine/topiramate). 2012. EMA website, http://www.ema.europa.eu/docs/en_GB/document_library/Summary_of_opinion_Initial_authorisation/human/002350/WC500134085.pdf
12. Aronne LJ, Wadden TA, Peterson C et al (2013) Evaluation of phentermine and topiramate versus phentermine/topiramate extended-release in obese adults. Obesity 21:2163–2171
13. Allison DB, Gadde KM et al (2012) Controlled-release phentermine/topiramate in severely obese adults: a randomized controlled trial (EQUIP). Obesity 20:330–342
14. Gadde KM, Allison DB et al (2011) Effects of low-dose, controlled-release, phentermine plus topiramate combination on weight and associated comorbidities in overweight and obese adults (CONQUER): a randomised, placebo-controlled, phase 3 trial. Lancet 377:1341–1352
15. Garvey WT, Ryan DH, Look M et al (2012) Two-year sustained weight loss and metabolic benefits with controlled-release phentermine/topiramate in obese and overweight adults (SEQUEL): a randomized, placebo-controlled, phase 3 extension study. Am J Clin Nutr 95:297–308
16. Garvey WT, Ryan DH et al (2014) Prevention of type 2 diabetes in subjects with prediabetes and metabolic syndrome treated with phentermine and topiramate extended release. Diabetes Care 37:912–921
17. Di Dalmazi G, Vicennati V, Pasquali R et al (2013) The unrelenting fall of the pharmacological treatment of obesity. Endocrine 44:598–609
18. Li Z, Maglione M, Tu W et al (2005) Meta-analysis: pharmacologic treatment of obesity. Ann Intern Med 142:532–546
19. Mizuno Y, Suzuki T, Nakagawa A et al (2014) Pharmacological Strategies to Counteract Antipsychotic-Induced Weight Gain and Metabolic Adverse Effects in Schizophrenia: A Systematic Review and Meta-analysis. Schizophr Bull. Mar 17. [Epub ahead of print]
20. Visboll T, Christensen M et al (2012) Effects of glucagon-like peptide-1 receptor agonists on weight loss: systematic review and meta-analyses of randomised controlled trials. BJM 344:d7771. doi:10.1136/bmj.d7771
21. Astrup A, Rossner S, Van Gaal L et al (2009) NN8022-1807 Study Group, Effects of liraglutide in the treatment of obesity: a randomised, double-blind, placebo-controlled study. Lancet 374:1606–1616
22. Astrup A, Carraro R, Finer N et al (2012) Safety, tolerability and sustained weight loss over 2 years with the once-daily human GLP-1 analog, liraglutide. Int J Obes (Lond) 36:843–854

23. Lean ME, Carraro R, Finer N et al (2014) Tolerability of nausea and vomiting and associations with weight loss in a randomized trial of liraglutide in obese, non-diabetic adults. Int J Obes (Lond) 38:689–697
24. Gadde KM, Franciscy DM, Wagner HR et al (2003) Zonisamide for weight loss in obese adults: a randomized controlled trial. JAMA 289:1820–1825
25. Greenway FL, Fujioka K, Plodkowski RA et al (2010) Effect of naltrexone plus bupropion on weight loss in overweight and obese adults (COR-I): a multicentre, randomised, double-blind, placebo-controlled, phase 3 trial. Lancet 376:595–605
26. Apovian CM, Aronne L, Rubino D et al (2013) A randomized, phase 3 trial of naltrexone SR/bupropion SR on weight and obesity-related risk factors (COR-II). Obesity 21:935–943
27. Hollander P, Gupta AK, Plodkowski R et al (2013) Effects of naltrexone sustained-release/bupropion sustained-release combination therapy on body weight and glycemic parameters in overweight and obese patients with type 2 diabetes. Diabetes Care 36:4022–4029
28. Yanovski SZ, Yanovski JA (2014) Long-term drug treatment for obesity: a systematic and clinical review. JAMA 311:74–86

Bariatric Surgery

24

Nicola Basso, Emanuele Soricelli, Giovanni Casella, Alfredo Genco, and Adriano Redler

24.1 Introduction

Since several decades obesity is a "hot topic" making the front pages on worldwide media. Because of a variety of different reasons, both developed and developing countries confront obesity problems. While the opulent USA stand in pole position in China because of the rapid transition to a westernized way of life (less bicycles, more automobiles), the incidence of obesity in the general population is rapidly growing [1].

Obesity determines a significant reduction of life expectancy, with an inversely proportional relationship body weight/life span and is directly responsible for a mortality three times the combined mortality for colon and breast cancers. Obesity itself is correlated to an augmented frequency of different malignancies; the risk of breast cancer in obese women and of prostate cancer in obese men is roughly doubled when confronted with that of lean individuals both in USA and Italy [2, 3].

Nonsurgical therapies for obesity, such as diet, psychotherapy, drugs, etc., have a long-term success rate of less than 5 % [4] and, in most cases, it results in the so-called yo-yo syndrome. At present weight loss surgery appears the most effective tool to achieve a durable excess weight loss (EWL): mean 61.2 % with a significant effect on comorbidities and longer life [5, 6].

24.2 Laparoscopy and Bariatric Surgery

The late 80s of last century saw the birth of laparoscopic surgery. In 1991 the first bariatric procedure with this new technique was performed [7]. Since then laparoscopy enjoyed an unprecedented and enthusiastic continuous worldwide spreading

---

N. Basso, MD (✉) • E. Soricelli, MD • G. Casella, MD • A. Genco, MD • A. Redler, MD
Department of Surgical Sciences,
Policlinico "Umberto I", "Sapienza" – University of Rome, Rome, Italy
e-mail: nicola.basso@uniroma1.it

with ever increasing compliance not only by surgeons but, even more, by patients. At present it is the gold standard approach in bariatric surgery with more than 90 % of procedures performed with this technique.

Less pain, less hospital stay, less visible scars, and shorter convalescence have been greatly appreciated by the patients. On the other hand early mobilization, early intestinal functions, and less incisional hernias are of primary importance in augmented risk obese patients [8]. Laparoscopy played a major role in popularizing bariatric surgery: in the USA bariatric procedures, from around 10,000/year before laparoscopy, stepped up to more than 200,000/year in the last times.

24.3 Indications

Indications to bariatric surgery have been stated by national [9] and international societies [10–13] and have been accepted worldwide. Patients are considered morbidly obese and candidate to weight loss surgery when the BMI is >40 kg/m^2 or >35 kg/m^2 if comorbidities are present and when the age range is 18–55 years [14]. BMI score remains the major operative criterion although additional parameters have been suggested: waist circumference seems to have a significant relationship with mortality hazard ratio in obese patients [15].
Contraindications include:

1. <5 years of failed attempts at medical controlled management
2. Significant psychotic disorders: depression, eating disorders, etc.
3. Inability to participate in prolonged medical follow-up
4. Alcohol and/or drug dependencies
5. Major endocrinopathies
6. Unrealistic patients expectations
7. Patient's nonacceptance of surgery side effects
8. Malabsorption procedures in patients with liver cirrhosis

The indications based on the 35 kg/m^2 BMI and on the 18–55 age limits date back to 1991 and novel factors intervening in this long period of time suggest the need for revision.

24.3.1 Class I Obesity (BMI 30–34.9 kg/m^2)

There is increasing evidence that an augmented risk for developing weight-related diseases such as type 2 diabetes mellitus (T2DM), cardiovascular diseases, and cancers is present in Class I obesity patients [16]. In several randomized controlled trials (RCTs), nonsurgical management (diet programs, exercise, drug therapy, and behavioral therapy) of obese patients with BMI 30–35 kg/m^2 were not effective in achieving a substantial and durable weight loss [17]. On the contrary, a number of published RCTs and observational studies, support the hypothesis that in patients with BMI <35/kg/m^2, bariatric procedures provide an outcome in terms of weight loss, long-term quality of life, healthcare costs, and comorbidities' resolution comparable to that in morbidly obese patients [18]. In particular T2DM significantly improved after surgery, with significant reduction in cardiovascular medications when compared to the nonsurgical approach [19, 20].

24.3.2 Adolescent/Old Age

Age limits (18–55 years) conflict with the increasing rate of obesity in the adolescent age and with the percentage of people age 60 and over (10 % of the general population) who are obese (35 %).

The prevalence of obesity among children and adolescents is associated with an increased risk of cardiovascular and metabolic diseases and with cognitive deficits [21]. The most important concerns in the surgical management of obese children or adolescents are related to the psychological implications of complex surgical interventions in this age group and to the lack of knowledge about the long-term metabolic and growth consequences [22]. However, literature data favor weight loss procedures in carefully selected, extremely obese adolescents. The improvement in obesity-related comorbidities after bariatric surgery supports the concept of "early" intervention in this group of patients [23].

In the elderly population the potential health benefits of bariatric surgery have been reconsidered. A significant body of literature shows that the surgical management of obesity is not only safe, with morbidity and mortality rates comparable to those in the younger obese counterpart, but it can also provide long-lasting effects in terms of associated diseases' resolution, quality of life improvement, and longevity [24].

Another argument in favor of new guidelines for bariatric surgery indications is the increasing evidence that bariatric procedures have metabolic effects not solely dependent on weight loss and food restriction.

"Metabolic surgery" seems to be a very effective treatment for diabetes, and, at present, arguments are debated to extend surgery to simple obese (BMI 30–35) or just overweight (BMI <30) DMT2 patients [25].

24.4 Preoperative Workup

Surgery has its own costs in terms of complications and deaths: obese patients have higher anesthesiological and surgical risks. Specialized structures for overweight patients and a dedicated team with specific training and experience, encompassing the surgeon and different specialists such as endocrinologist, endoscopist, pneumologist, nutritionist, psychologist, anesthesiologist etc., are of outmost importance in the pre-, intra-, and postoperative management of obese patients. The surgeon is the main link among members of the team and mainly responsible for the overall results [27, 28].

Preoperatively the obesity team has to determine patients' indications to surgery; evaluate and treat, when appropriate, comorbidities; and evaluate the nutritional and psychological status. Routine preoperative studies include blood tests, cardiovascular and respiratory evaluation, sleep study when indicated, upper gastrointestinal (GI) tract endoscopy, and biliary ultrasound examination. An integral part of the preoperative workup and of outmost importance is the informed consent: it must exhaustively clarify anesthesiological and surgical risks, short- and long-term side effects, and underline realistic expectations.

Postoperatively the nutritionist is mainly responsible for diet education of the patient while, in diabetic patients, the endocrinologist must adapt the medical needs of the patient to the new situation.

24.5 Surgical Therapy

Several consensus conferences have recommended four standard types of surgical procedures: Adjustable gastric banding (AGB), Roux-en-Y gastric bypass (RYGBP), Sleeve gastrectomy (SG) and Biliopancreatic diversion (BPD) [9, 10, 26]. Because of insufficient evidence-based data, at present it is not possible to indicate specific procedures for specific patients; however, factors that may influence the choice can be summarized to three main ones:

- BMI and degree of desired and/or advisable EWL: different procedures have different EWL power, lowest after AGB, and highest after BPD.
- Presence of comorbidities differently affected by different procedures.
- Psychological profile by a psychiatrist experienced in obesity to foresee patient's compliance to follow-up and post-op dietary regimen.

An additional no less important factor to be considered is the surgeon's experience.

24.5.1 Intragastric Balloon

Introduction
The use of an intragastric balloon (IB) has been advocated since 1921 with the observation that patients with bezoar complained of postprandial fullness. Only in 1987, because of technical perfecting of the devices, it reached a worldwide consensus for the treatment of selected overweight/obese patients [29]. IBs are implanted by endoscopy. At present different types of IB exist, water filled, air filled [30], or IB attached to the abdominal wall by a combined endoscopy-surgery procedure [31]. Recently a self-administered swallowable balloon, not requiring endoscopy, has been devised and is under investigation [32].

Indications
IB is indicated for temporary use, associated with a specific dietary program under direct medical control, in patients with BMI <35 kg/m^2 when there are concurrent obese-related comorbidities (e.g., cardiovascular, orthopedic, metabolic, etc.), in patients with BMI >35 kg/m^2 who refuse bariatric surgical procedures or in patients

with BMI >50 kg/m² as a presurgical weight loss device, and as possible predictive role when used before laparoscopic adjustable gastric banding [33]. History of gastric surgery of any kind and serious psychological problems are absolute contraindication.

Technique

The Bioenterics intragastric balloon (BIB) is made up of a soft, transparent, silicone balloon connected, by means of a valve (radiopaque), to a "placement" catheter. Before BIB placement, a esophagogastroduodenoscopy is performed to rule out the presence of voluminous hiatal hernias (HHs) (>5 cm), severe esophagitis, and/or other diseases of the esophagus, stomach, and duodenum. Under conscious or unconscious sedation, the balloon is positioned with the valve under the cardia and is filled with 500–700 ml of physiological solution and 10 ml vital staining solution (methylene blue) to early identify balloon rupture or valve leaks (sudden appearance of blue-colored urine). BIB is deflated and removed no later than 180 days after its placement by endoscopy.

Mechanism of Action

BIB plays its weight loss action through different mechanisms:

- Elicitation of the satiety brain-gut axis through stimulation of the gastric wall baroceptors. This effect is particularly active in the first 2–3 months.
- Delayed gastric emptying owing to a reduced electric gastric activity and to mechanical sub-stenosis of the antral outlet.
- Reduction of gastric capacity of about 750 cm³.
- Sense of discomfort (nausea, vomiting, epigastric pain) when the patient fails to adhere to the prescribed dietary regimen.

Complications

- Mortality: 0.1 %

Major Complications

- *Impact of the balloon* in the antrum causing a gastric obstruction (0.5 %). The management can be conservative (insertion of a nasogastric tube) or may require removal of the device.
- *Intestinal obstruction (0.1%)*: due to passage of a deflated balloon from the stomach into the small bowel. This condition may require the surgical removal of the device.
- *Gastric ulceration*: removal of BIB is advisable.
- *Gastric perforation (0.15%)*: it is the most feared and life-threatening complication. It can occur early after BIB placement or few months later, presenting with a sudden acute abdominal pain. A marked dilation of the stomach, undetected gastric ulcers, or prior gastric surgeries are predisposing causes. Surgical treatment is mandatory.

Minor Complications

- *Intolerance (0.4 %)* to the sensation of discomfort determined by the device
- *Esophagitis (1.2 %)* mostly due to the discontinued use of proton pump inhibitors

Outcome

Weight Loss and Comorbidities
Data from the Italian Collaborative Study Group for Lap-Band and BIB (GILB), accounting 2,515 patients with a mean BMI of 44.4 kg/m^2, show an EWL of 33 ± 18.7 % and a BMI loss of 4.9 ± 12.7 kg/m^2 6 months after BIB placement. Comorbidities resolution and improvement occurred in 44.3 % and 44.8 % of patients, respectively [34]. Concerning the overweight population (BMI 25–30 kg/m^2), a recent European multicentre experience in 261 patients showed a mean %EWL of 55.6 and 29.1 at 6 months and 3 years of follow-up, respectively. The rate of patients with hypertension decreased from 29 % at baseline to 16 % at 3 years. Diabetes decreased from 15 to 10 %, dyslipidemia decreased from 20 to 18 %, and hypercholesterolemia decreased from 32 to 21 % [35].

Failure Rate
Fifty percent of BIB patients will not lose weight or will experience weight regain (WR). A careful selection, avoiding binge eaters, sweet eaters, and patients with important psychological problems will decrease the failure rate.

Advantages

- *Safe and not invasive*: endoscopic placement takes about 12 min and it can be performed in outpatients or day hospital.
- *Multiple indications*: intragastric balloon can be used either as a primary weight loss procedure or as a bridge to surgical interventions in patients with severe obesity (sequential treatment). It may, indicatively, test the compliance of patients eligible to dietary programs (BIB test). [33]. Placement of a second BIB, 30 days after the removal of the first one (multiple treatment) has been proposed in patients with weight loss of at least 15 % of the initial weight at first treatment, refusal of surgery, and failure to alter eating behavior (e.g., sweet eating).

24.5.2 Adjustable Gastric Banding

Introduction
The introduction of AGB by Kuzmack in 1986 promoted the worldwide diffusion of bariatric surgery [36]. Until 2008 laparoscopic AGB (LAGB) was the second most performed bariatric procedure after RYGBP, with a large prevalence in Europe and Asia, accounting about 150,000 interventions per year. More recently

Fig. 24.1 The procedure involves the placement of a silicone-made ring around the upper portion of the stomach in order to isolate a small (20–30 ml) proximal gastric pouch which communicates with the distal stomach through a narrow stoma. The inner volume of the ring can be augmented or reduced by injecting or aspirating saline solution from the subcutaneous port which is connected to the band through an intra-abdominal catheter

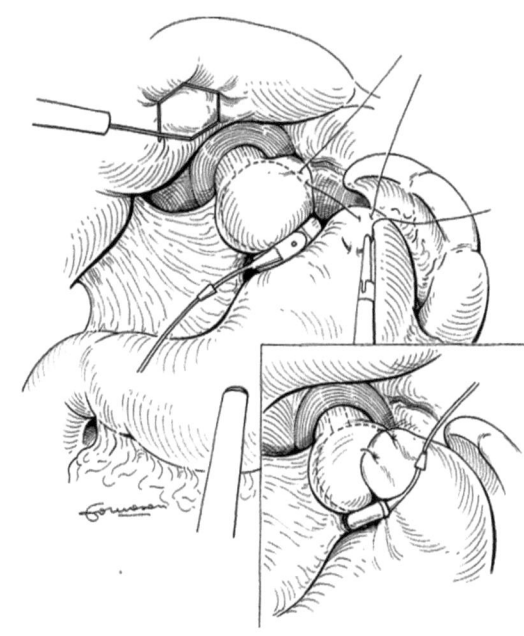

the prevalence of LAGB is decreasing, most of all because of the growing diffusion of laparoscopic SG (LSG) [37] (Fig. 24.1).

Mechanism of Action

LAGB is a pure restrictive procedure: the passage of food from the proximal small gastric pouch to the distal stomach is made difficult, with a consequent increase of the intraluminal pouch pressure. This mechanism promotes an early and prolonged sensation of satiety by stimulating of the gastric wall baroreceptors [38]. Thanks to the presence of the subcutaneous port, the surgeon is able to adjust the inner volume of the ring and then the degree of restriction, depending on both the clinical outcome and the comfort of the patient. This implies a close compliance to the follow-up program and the strict observation of dietary recommendations, which are mandatory for a successful LAGB. Solid foods should be preferred to semisolid or liquid ones, because the latter are often hyper caloric and get more easily through the band, without augmenting the pressure in the pouch.

Complications

- *Mortality*: 0.1–0.2 %

Major Complications

- *Slippage (0.2–12.5%)*: it is the prolapse of the gastric wall proximally through the band. Slippage-related symptoms are dysphagia, vomiting, and gastroesoph-

ageal reflux disease (GERD). It can be diagnosed by upper gastrointestinal contrast studies showing the improper placement of the band and the dilation of the gastric pouch. The management can be conservative (band deflation, fasting or liquid diet, stomach decompression by nasogastric tube). When the conservative management is not successful, the band must be removed.
- *Erosion (0–3.7 %)*: it is a process of chronic erosion of the band through the layers of the gastric wall until it penetrates into the gastric lumen. Clinical presentation may be at variance, epigastric pain, dysphagia, weight regain, and infection of the subcutaneous port. Removal of the band either laparoscopically or with a combined laparoscopic and endoscopic approach is indicated.
- *Band complications (up to 11 %)*: the most common ones are the infection of the subcutaneous port and the rupture or disconnection of the catheter. The former can be treated conservatively or through the substitution of the port; the latter is diagnosed by an abdominal x-ray and its management can require surgery.

Outcome

Weight Loss
It has been shown that LAGB can determine an EWL of 40–50 % with an average BMI loss of ten points. However, long-term outcomes are impaired by significant incidence of failures, because of insufficient weight loss (IWL) or WR or psychological intolerance to a "foreign body." These conditions may lead to revision operations. The best results occur in young women <45 years, BMI <45, no binge eating disorders or sweet eating, and good compliance to follow-up [39].

Comorbidities
After LAGB, arterial hypertension, obstructive sleep apnea syndrome (OSAS), and hyperlipidemia are resolved in 38.4, 94.6, and 71.1 % of patients, respectively. T2DM resolved in <50 % of cases [40].

Advantages

- *Safe and feasible*: LAGB is a simple procedure, with short operative time (about 30 min in high-volume centers) and hospital stay (1 or 2 days). Mortality and postoperative complication rates are very low.
- *Reversible*: the procedure does not involve any resection or anastomosis, thus restoring the original anatomy of the stomach is technically simple.

Disadvantages

- *Failure rates*: the incidence of IWL or WR after LAGB is up to 30 % in some series. When failure occurs, a revision procedure (band removal and conversion

to a RYGBP or SG) could be indicated to achieve a satisfying outcome. Revision procedures have higher rates of postoperative complications when compared with primary surgery.
- *Patients' compliance*: adherence to the follow-up program and observation of a hypocaloric diet play a crucial role to a successful LAGB. An accurate selection and education of the patients undergoing this procedure is mandatory.

24.5.3 Laparoscopic Roux-en-Y Gastric Bypass

Introduction
Gastric bypass (GB) as a bariatric intervention was first proposed by Mason in the 1960s, on the observation that in patients undergoing Billroth II procedures (partial gastrectomy with gastrojejunal anastomosis) a significant and durable weight loss was obtained [41]. Since then, several aspects of the surgical technique have been modified, entailing capacity of the small gastric pouch, Roux-en-Y reconstruction, and variations in the length of the alimentary limb. In 1994, Wittgrove first showed its feasibility with a laparoscopic approach [42] and nowadays laparoscopic RYGBP (LRYGB) represents the most performed bariatric procedure worldwide, accounting for about 50 % of all bariatric interventions [37] (Fig. 24.2).

Mechanisms of Action
RYGBP exerts its weight loss action through the reduction of caloric intake, achieved by means of concurrent mechanisms: the restrictive effect of the small gastric pouch (25–30 ml), the reduced sense of hunger, and the early feeling of satiety induced by significant changes in the secretion of neuro hormones. In particular it has been shown that RYGBP entails the decrease of ghrelin and the rise of peptide-YY (PYY) and of glucagon-like peptide-1 (GLP-1) serum levels [43]. Ghrelin is an orexigenic hormone which plays a role in both mealtime hunger and long-term regulation of body weight. Bypass surgery promotes the reduction of ghrelin secretion through the process of "override inhibition." It means that the exclusion of the greater part of the stomach from food passage elicits a persistent signaling that initially super stimulates, then exhausts the secretion of ghrelin. Release of GLP-1 and PYY from L cells of the small bowel is stimulated by the rapid transit of partially digested food in the ileum, eliciting an early sensation of satiety [44].

The abovementioned neurohormonal changes are very similar to those reported after LSG and are involved in the effects of LRYGB on diabetic patients. In fact, while ghrelin impairs both insulin secretion and sensitivity, GLP-1 improves insulin activity, promotes the growth of pancreatic beta-cells, and reduces hepatic glucose production through the inhibition of glucagon secretion [45].

Complications

- *Mortality*: 0.2–0.4 %

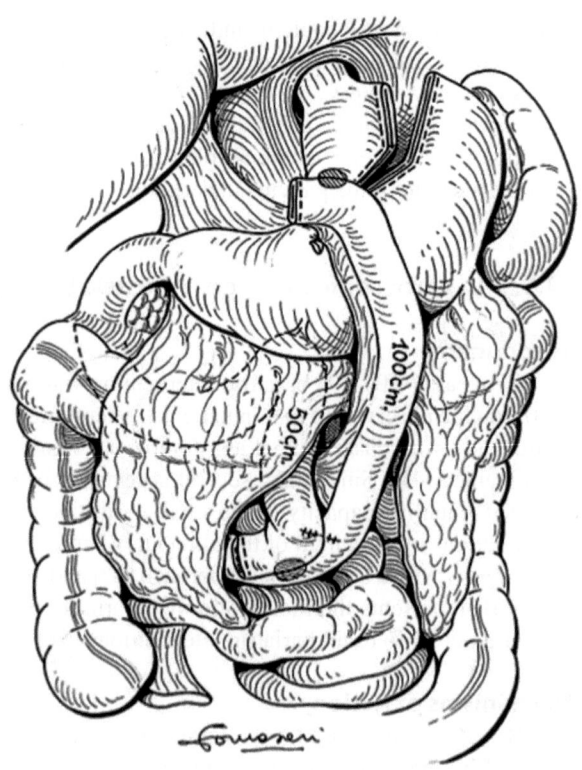

Fig. 24.2 The stomach is divided to form a small proximal gastric pouch of about 25–30 ml of volume. The transection begins about 6–8 cm below the esophageal gastric junction on the lesser curvature and proceeds first horizontally toward the great curvature, then vertically toward the angle of His. The jejunum is then divided below the ligament of Treitz and the proximal bowel segment (biliopancreatic limb) is connected to the alimentary limb 75–150 cm distal to the gastrojejunostomy. In patients with a BMI >50 kg/m^2, a 300 cm-long alimentary limb has been devised to improve the weight loss, by inducing a certain degree of malabsorption. The gastrojejunal anastomosis can be performed either by means of laparoscopic stapler (linear or circular) or by manual suture

Acute Complications (<30days)

- *Anastomotic leak (2%)*: in most cases occurs at the gastrojejunal anastomosis or at the gastric staple line of the pouch. The pathogenesis can be related to the presence of abdominal collections, to a deficient vascularization, or to abnormal tension on the anastomosis. The management can be conservative (percutaneous drainage, enteral/intravenous nutrition, broad-spectrum antibiotics). Uncontained leaks with systemic sepsis and cardiovascular instability require surgery.
- *Hemorrhage (1.9%)*: almost always from the gastrojejunal anastomosis and can occur either outside or inside the gastrointestinal lumen. It can be managed by interventional radiology (embolization) or by endoscopy. When these maneuvers fail, the surgical approach is recommended.

Late Complications (<30days)

- *Stenosis of the gastrojejunal anastomosis (5%)*: it can be successfully managed by means of one or more sessions of endoscopic dilation. The surgical intervention, entailing the revision of the anastomosis, should be considered only in selected cases when endoscopic approach has failed.

- *Internal hernia (3.7%)*: represents the most common cause of bowel obstruction after RYGBP. It is caused by lack or improper closure of the mesenteric defects during primary bypass surgery, in particular when the alimentary limb is transposed upward through the transverse mesocolon (transmesocolic reconstruction). The laparoscopic reduction of the hernia represents the approach of choice; however, the presence of adhesions and of inflated bowel loops may require conversion to open surgery.

Outcome

Weight Loss
Published data report a 60–70 % EWL at a 15-year follow-up [40]. However, up to 20 % of RYGBP patients may present with long-term weight loss failure or regain (%EWL <50).

Comorbidities
More than 75 % of patients undergoing LRYGB achieve the control of their obesity-related comorbidities. T2DM, hypertension, hyperlipidemia, and OSAS resolved in 83, 75, 93, and 86 % of cases, respectively [40].

Advantages

- *Effectiveness and safety*: due to its excellent clinical outcome and its low mortality and morbidity rates, the American Society for Metabolic and Bariatric Surgery (ASMBS) considers LRYGB the bariatric procedure of choice.
- *GERD improvement*: RYGBP improves esophageal reflux by reduced acid secretion from the small gastric pouch and by the diversion of the biliary esophageal reflux. Therefore, most authors perform LRYGB, rather than LAGB or LSG, when GERD and/or HH are present. Moreover LRYGB is considered the revision procedure of choice in patients developing a symptomatic reflux not controlled with medical therapy after LAGB or LSG.

Disadvantages

- *Complexity*: LRYGB is a technically demanding procedure; the available literature suggests an experience of 50–150 cases as a safe and proficient learning curve.
- *No standard approach in case of failure*: unlike patients with failed LSG, who may undergo the second stage of BPD with duodenal switch (BPD-DS) or bypass surgery, there is still no consensus about the surgical strategy to manage WR or IWL after LRYGB. Different revision procedures have been proposed (e.g., resizing or banding the pouch, modifying the length of the alimentary limb), but none of them is consistently supported by published data.

- *Presence of a "blind" gastric portion*: patients undergoing bypass surgery should be carefully informed that a major portion of their stomach, as well as the biliary tract, will be difficult to explore by endoscopy because of the anatomical changes consequent to the procedure.

24.5.4 Laparoscopic Biliopancreatic Diversion

Introduction

In the early 1970s the pioneer works by Scopinaro represented the most systematic scientific approach to the problem of malabsorption as therapy for obesity and were the physiopathological basis for a novel malabsorption procedure [46]. In 1976 Scopinaro performed the first BPD in a patient with morbid obesity. Today BPD is still the most effective bariatric procedure in terms of weight loss and resolution of obesity-related diseases [40]. In order to reduce the high rate of postoperative complications affecting Scopinaro's BPD, such as peptic ulceration at the anastomosis and malabsorption-related side effects, in 1988 Hess et al. proposed a modification of the original BPD, the BPD-DS (see surgical technique) [47]. According to the Survey of the International Federation for the Surgery of Obesity and Metabolic Disorders (IFSO), in 2011 BPD-DS has accounted for the 2.2 % of the overall bariatric procedures performed worldwide, with a prevalence of BPD-DS on BPD (5,271 vs. 2,324) [37] (Fig. 24.3).

Mechanism of Action

Scopinaro's BPD and BPD-DS exert their weight loss and metabolic actions by reducing dramatically the calories intake of the small bowel from the ingested nutrients. In fact, since bile salts and food blend only in the 50 cm of the common limb, the absorption of fats occurs in this short bowel segment. To the contrary the absorption of protein and starch, which is mediated by the enzymatic activity of the intestinal brush border, takes place in the entire intestinal segment comprised between the gastroenterostomy and the ileocecal valve. These changes in the pattern of nutrients absorption entails that, after biliopancreatic diversion, patients absorb an established amount of calories (about 1,700 Kcal in the man and 1,400 Kcal in the woman), irrespective of size and quality of their meals. The only limitation concerns the ingestion of monosaccharides and disaccharides, contained in fruits, candies, milk, sweet drinks, and alcohol, whose absorption is not impaired by BPD [48]. Despite a lower malabsorption effect, BPD-DS when compared to Scopinaro BPD, presents with similar weight loss and comorbidities resolution rates. The incidence of malabsorption-related side effects is lower.

BPD exerts a strong antidiabetic action, owing not only to the large weight loss and to the reduced nutrients absorption but also to the early and durable postoperative changes in the secretion of intestinal hormones. In fact after BPD a significant increase in the serum concentrations of PYY and GLP-1 has been demonstrated, entailing the improvement of both insulin sensitivity and secretion. These modifications are related either to the exclusion of the foregut (duodenum and jejunum) from the passage of food or to the rapid delivery of partially digested nutrients in the

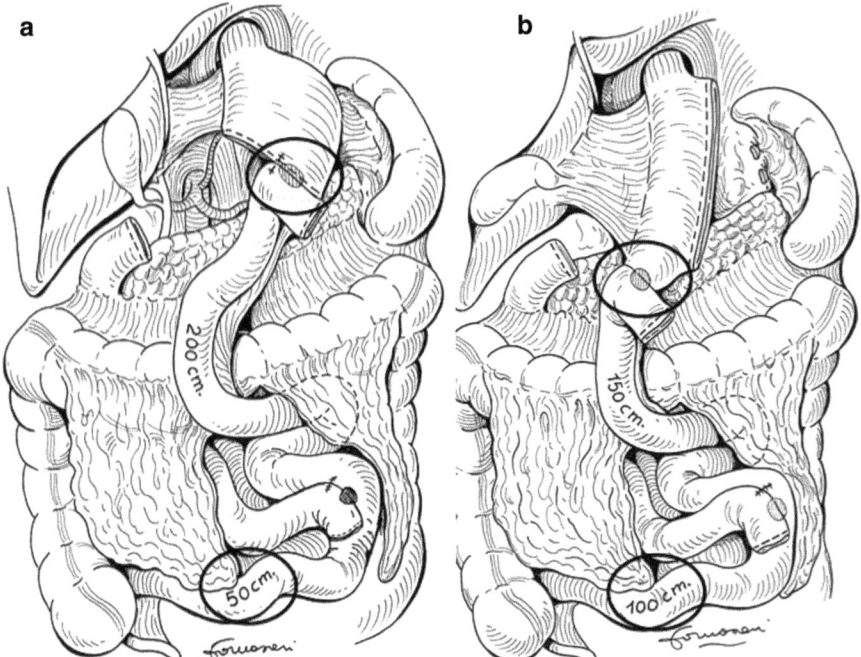

Fig. 24.3 (a) The Scopinaro's BPD entails a horizontal gastrectomy, performed by means of a linear stapler, leaving a 300–400 ml residual capacity of the stomach. Then the small bowel is measured from the ileocecal valve toward the ligament of Treitz and sectioned at 250–300 cm. The proximal stump (biliopancreatic limb) is anastomosed to the ileum at a distance of 50 cm from the ileocecal valve (common limb), while the distal stump (alimentary limb) is anastomosed to the gastric remnant. Cholecystectomy may be added. (b) In the BPD-DS, gastrectomy is performed in a vertical manner (sleeve gastrectomy) rather than horizontal, and the duodenum is divided 2–3 cm distal to the pylorus, and a duodenal-jejunal anastomosis is performed leaving in place the pylorus sphincter. The length of the common limb is 100 cm, twice as in the original Scopinaro procedure

distal ileum, stimulating the secreting activity of L cells. Concerning the plasma levels of ghrelin, they are unchanged or increased after Scopinaro's BPD, while they are significantly reduced after BPD-DS, due to resection of the gastric fundus (sleeve gastrectomy) [49].

Complications

- *Mortality*: 0–2.7 %

Early Complications (<30days)

- *Hemorrhage and leaks* (2–4 %): they can affect either the staple line of the gastric remnant and of the duodenal stumps or the anastomotic sites (gastroileal or duodenum-ileal). Bleeding can occur inside or outside the gastrointestinal lumen and is usually self-limited. Leaks can be managed conservatively by percutaneous drainage. Surgery is indicated in case of high-flow bleeding not responsive to embolization and in uncontained leaks in hemodynamically unstable patients.

Late Complications (<30days)

- *Peptic ulcer (3 %)*: affects the gastro-ileal anastomosis in the Scopinaro's BPD. The healing process can entail development of a fibrotic stenosis of the anastomosis which can be successfully treated by endoscopic dilation.
- *Nutritional deficiencies (4–6 %)*: they are related to the malabsorption effect of the procedure. Preventive lifelong oral integration of iron, calcium, and vitamins is the treatment of choice. These complications are less pronounced in BPD-DS patients.
- *Protein malnutrition (1 %)*: it is the most feared late complication of BPD. Poor compliance to postoperative follow-up, low proteins diet, or excessive malabsorption are the most frequent causes. Protein malnutrition can be managed by parenteral nutrition and dietary interventions. In severe cases surgical revision by means of common limb elongation or even suppression of the malabsorption effect is indicated.

Outcome

Weight Loss
It has been shown that BPD (both Scopinaro's procedure and BPD-DS) is the most effective procedure in terms of weight loss, with an EWL greater than 70 % at a very long follow-up (up to 15 years) [40].

Comorbidities
After BPD, hypertension, OSAS, and hyperlipidemia resolved in 83.4, 91.9, and 99 %, respectively [40].

T2DM
Almost all (97 %) diabetic patients definitively stop glucose-lowering drugs early soon after the procedure. The rate of resolution is lower in patients with a longer disease duration, because of a definitive impairment of pancreatic beta-cells function.

Advantages

- *Modulation of the malabsorptive effect*: since the BPD malabsorption depends on the length of the alimentary and common limbs, the degree of this effect can be tailored by modifying the length of the common limb or of the alimentary limb or both.
- *Long-term results*: clinical outcome from BPD series with a follow-up >15 years strongly supports its long-lasting effects in terms of weight loss and comorbidities' resolution.

- *Two-step surgery*: in high-risk super-obese patients, BPD-DS is usually performed in two subsequent surgical steps: SG first, then BPD-DS after 6–12 months, with a reduction in mortality and morbidity compared to single step BPD-DS.

Disadvantages

- *Complexity and safety*: laparoscopic BPD is a technically demanding procedure involving a partial gastrectomy (horizontal or vertical) and two anastomosis: gastroileal (or duodenojejunal) and jejunoileal. In addition the BPD-DS entails section of the duodenum 2–3 cm from the pylorus. Even if acceptable, the morbidity and mortality rates are higher when compared to other bariatric procedures.
- *Side-effects*: after BPD, patients could experience the development of malabsorption-related side effects, such as diarrhea with a daily number of evacuation up to ten and foul smelling stools, nutritional deficiencies, and flatulence. When these side effects are severe, they can impair the quality of life of the patient, even requiring a surgical correction.

24.5.5 Sleeve Gastrectomy

Introduction

LSG was initially performed as part of a hybrid malabsorptive procedure, the BPD-DS [47]. In early 2000s Micheal Gagner proposed a two-stage model of intervention, LSG first and then BPD-DS after an average 12 months interval, in order to reduce the high rate of complications and mortality registered after single-stage BPD-DS [50]. The good outcome of the first-stage LSG in terms of weight loss and comorbidities resolution encouraged a growing number of surgeons to perform LSG as a sole bariatric operation, and, in 2009, the ASMBS issued a position statement recommending LSG as an approved bariatric procedure [51]. Nowadays the LSG has the fastest growing rate and is the second most performed bariatric procedure worldwide after RYGBP [37] (Fig. 24.4).

Mechanisms of Action

Weight loss induced by LSG was initially ascribed solely to a restrictive action. However, it has been demonstrated that both the resection of the gastric fundus and the rapid emptying of the stomach promote significant neuro hormonal changes: in particular the former causes a significant decrease in the circulating levels of ghrelin, the hormone of appetite, while the latter entails an increased satiety through a food-mediated release of GLP-1 and PYY from the L cells of the small intestine. These changes persist 1 year after surgery, showing that LSG can be considered a "food-limiting" operation rather than a restrictive procedure [52]. These neuro hormones, also called incretins, are involved in the antidiabetic effect of LSG. In fact, while ghrelin acts by suppressing the insulin-sensitizing hormone adiponectin, blocking hepatic insulin signaling, and inhibiting insulin secretion, GLP-1 and

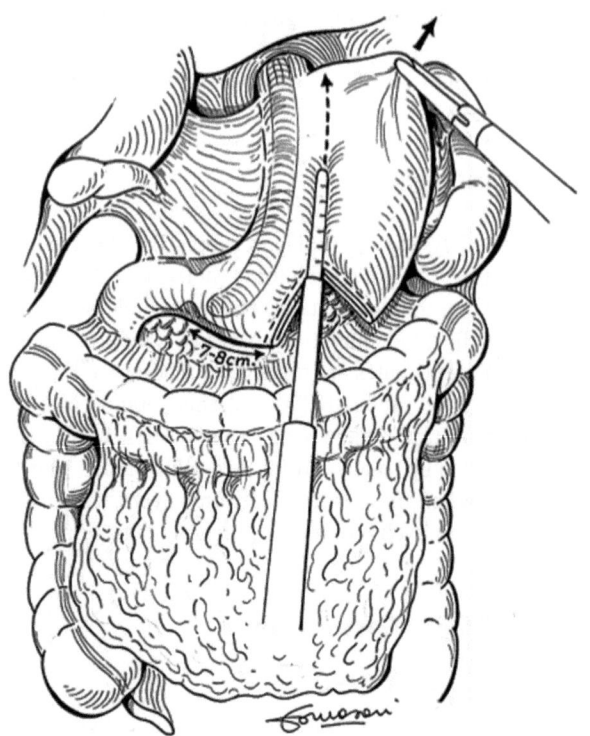

Fig. 24.4 The procedure entails the resection of the body and the fundus of the stomach by means of laparoscopic linear stapler. The capacity of the gastric remnant (60–100 ml) is tailored by the placement of a bougie alongside the lesser curvature of the stomach. The staple line could be reinforced by means of buttressing materials or by overlocking with absorbable suture in order to reduce the incidence of postoperative complications such as bleeding or leakage

PYY either improve insulin secretion and sensitivity or reduce hepatic glucose production through the inhibition of glucagon secretion. Serum levels of PYY and GLP-1 significantly augment just 72 h after LSG, before any weight loss or food passage through the alimentary tract has occurred. These early changes, which are associated with an immediate improvement of glucose homeostasis, suggest that there is an intrinsic neuro hormonal effect of the procedure and lead to the formulation of a "gastric hypothesis": the diminished hydrochloric acid production induced by the significant reduction of oxyntic cell mass stimulates the vagally innervated antral mucosa, left intact by SG, to secret gastrin-releasing peptide which induces the first early phase of GLP-1 secretion [53].

Complications

- *Mortality*: 0.1–0.5 %

Major Postoperative Complications

- *Hemorrhage (1–2 %)*: usually occurs within the first 24–48 h. The treatment is interventional radiology or, in fewer instances, open or laparoscopic surgical exploration.

- *Gastric leak (0–7 %)*: it is the most feared complication. It can occur within 7 days postoperatively (acute leaks) or within 1–6 weeks (early leaks); later leaks occur less frequently. In 90 % of cases, leaks occur at the upper portion of the gastric suture line suggesting an ischemic pathogenesis. The treatment is usually nonoperative (percutaneous drainage of the abdominal collection, endoscopic stents, and parenteral nutrition). Surgery is indicated in uncontained, symptomatic leaks with signs of general infection and hemodynamic instability.
- *Stenosis (0.6 %)*: usually occurs at the corpus-antrum transition zone (incisura angularis) of the gastric tubule. RYGBP reconstruction after failed conservative stricture treatment is a valid therapy.
- *GERD (6.5 %)*: published data are not so consistent to determine whether the preoperative diagnosis of GERD and/or HH should be considered a contraindication to LSG. However, it has been shown that the repair of an HH during LSG plays a beneficial role on GERD outcome: the hiatal area inspection should be performed always during LSG [54].

Outcome

Weight Loss
Data from a recent Consensus Summit accounting for more than 46,000 LSGs reported a mean EWL of 50 % at 6 years of follow-up. Long-term WR remains a controversial and largely insufficiently documented issue [55].

Comorbidities
The remission rate of arterial hypertension, OSAS, and hyperlipidemia after LSG ranges from 15 to 93 %, 39 to 100 %, and 5 to 75 %, respectively [55].

T2DM
In several studies [56–58] it has been shown that the remission of T2DM occurs in 60–80 % of patients undergoing LSG. The duration of the disease (>10 years) has been demonstrated to be an important prognostic factor for T2DM remission [59].

Advantages

- *Feasibility*: LSG is quite simple and does not involve anastomosis, entailing shorter learning curve (50 procedures) and operative time (about 60 min) when compared with LRYGBP and BPD. However, there are some technical aspects, such as the complete fundectomy and the accurate exploration of the hiatal area, whose proper execution is of paramount importance for a successful LSG.
- *Effectiveness and safety*: the clinical outcome of LSG in terms of weight loss and comorbidities resolution is comparable with those of RYGBP, while the incidence of major postoperative complication is lower, although not significantly, than in RYGBP and in BPD.

- *Lack of prosthesis and of "blind" gastric section*: LSG does not involve the placement of prosthesis and, unlike RYGBP, the whole gastric remnant is accessible by endoscopy.
- *Standardization in case of failure*: unlike after failed RYGBP, the management of WR or IWL after LSG is standardized, consisting in the second-stage BPD-DS or in the conversion to RYGBP.

Disadvantages

- *Staple-line leak*: its management could be very complex and long lasting, requiring a close cooperation with several different professional figures such as interventional radiologist, endoscopist, nutritionist, and infectious disease specialist. The timing of the treatment is a crucial prognostic factor; in fact, the earlier the diagnosis, the more conservative and successful is the management, avoiding difficult and often unsuccessful surgical reinterventions.
- *Long-term results*: most clinical results of LSG have a follow-up of 5–6 years. Few series with a longer follow-up (up to 8–9 years), although with small numbers, seem to confirm the good trend concerning EWL and comorbidities resolution [55, 56].

24.6 Outcome

In the Swedish Obesity Study (SOS) long term, prospective and controlled data from over 2,000 bariatric surgery patients and from over 2,000 matched control obese subjects were confronted. Primary end point was mortality rate in the two study groups, and secondary end points were incidence of cardiovascular diseases, diabetes, health-related quality of life, and biliary diseases [60].

At 10- and at 20-year follow-up, weight changes were −25 % in the operated patients and 0 % in the control group. At 16 years follow-up, the SOS study documented a significant reduction in the cumulative mortality of the operated patients (8 %) when compared to the control subjects (12.5 %). At the same time bariatric surgery induced dramatic positive effects on diabetes, cardiovascular diseases, cancer, and quality of life. In another clinical study on a very large sample (7,925 patients/group), the mortality in operated (RYGBP) patients was 40 % lower in confront to that of matched morbidly obese control subjects at a mean follow-up of 7.1 years [61]. The reduction was particularly pronounced for deaths from diabetes (−92 %) and cancer (60 %).

24.6.1 Patients' Satisfaction

Patients' satisfaction is of outmost importance in the correct evaluation of bariatric surgery results. Improved quality of life (QoL) and enhanced psychosocial functioning are important goals for bariatric surgery and should be actively pursued and evaluated. A crucial requirement to achieve patient's satisfaction is a comprehensive and exhaustive informed consent. The patient must be fully aware of the effects and possible side effects of the procedure and, most important, the postoperative expectations must be realistic in order to avoid disappointment and depression.

Although lifestyle intervention programs improve health-related quality of life (HRQoL) in morbidly obese subjects, bariatric surgery has a greater impact on the well-being of these patients.

Surgery outcomes were significantly better in terms of both weight reduction and psychological adjustment compared to highly motivated participants in a weight loss program which included vigorous physical exercises, behavior modification, and nutritional advice [62].

Several papers analyzed the topic of QoL after AGB, LSG, and RYGBP, using Medical Outcomes Survey Short Form 36 (SF-36) and Bariatric Analysis and Reporting Outcome System (BAROS) [63]. HRQoL changes after bariatric surgery compare very favorably with those in obese control groups, irrespective for the specific type of surgery and in all the five dimensions of HRQoL (physical, mental, emotional, obesity symptoms, and symptoms distress).

In a study on 83 LSG patients, BAROS score was "good" to "excellent" in 90 % of patients. In SF-36, "physical functioning" and "general health perception" only had scores significantly better in patients with an EWL >50 % than in patients with EWL <50, suggesting that weight loss is not the only factor influencing the results [64].

Sexual health is a relevant component of patients' satisfaction but it is infrequently well explored. In a recent prospective cohort study, 2 years following surgery (85 RYGBP and 21 AGB), women reported significant improvements in overall sexual functioning and specific domains of sexual functioning in addition to significant improvements in most domains of quality of life, as well as body image and depressive symptoms [65].

24.6.2 The Diabetes and the "Metabolic Surgery" Debate

The definition of "metabolic surgery" as "a set of gastrointestinal operations used with the intent to treat diabetes (diabetes surgery) and metabolic dysfunctions (which include obesity)" has been put forward by Rubino [66]. The term metabolic surgery describes surgical procedures that treat metabolic diseases, especially T2DM, with mechanisms that are, at least partly, independent by weight loss and it is comprehensive of conventional (AGB, RYGBP, SG, BPD) and of new procedures specifically aimed to determine metabolic effects: duodenojejunal bypass (DJB), mini-gastric bypass (MiniGBP), ileal interposition + SG etc.

The first Diabetes Surgery Summit was held in Rome in 2007 [67]. In 2008 surgical therapy for diabetes was mentioned by the American Diabetes Association (ADA) statement [68]. In 2011 a statement by the International Diabetes Federation (IDF) considered surgery as a reasonable therapeutic alternative for DMT2 patients with a 30–35 kg/m² BMI [69]. Although the official position of several important international societies testifies their attention to the potentialities of surgery in the therapy of the metabolic syndrome in general and of T2DM in particular, discussion on the appropriateness of considering surgery as "specific diabetes therapy" and on the "beyond weight loss" mechanisms of the metabolic effects of bariatric surgery is still going on [70].

Controlled trials confronted the effect of four standard bariatric procedures (AGB, RYGBP, SG, BPD) and of conventional or intensive medical therapy in obese diabetic patients [71–75]. Weight loss and glycemic control were significantly better in the surgical groups than in the control medical groups. In long-term non-controlled studies, T2DM remission occurred in 36.5 % at 5 years after AGB [76], in 97 % at 10 years after BPD [77], in 65 % at 6 years after RYGBP [78], and in 75 % at 5 years after SG [79].

In Table 24.1 the effect of surgery on the metabolic syndrome in RCTs has been summarized.

Accordingly, the conclusions of the 2011 IDF statement can be confidently accepted: "Bariatric surgery is an effective and cost-effective therapy for Type 2 diabetes and obesity with an acceptable safety profile. Bariatric surgery should be incorporated into Type 2 diabetes treatment algorithms" [69].

24.6.3 The Ultimate "Battle"

Obesity, commonly associated with hypertension, diabetes, dyslipidemia, sleep disorders, and low-grade inflammation, is considered a significant Cardiovascular (CV) risk factor predisposing to adverse cardiac events and premature death [80–82].

CV diseases, together with cancer [83], are the major causes of death in morbidly obese patients.

Obesity determines cardiac structure and function changes, especially increased left ventricular wall (LVW) thickness, mass, and diameters: the "obesity cardiomyopathy" [84–87].

Several Authors reported that bariatric surgery, irrespective of the type of procedure, has a remarkable positive influence on CV risk factors at a 2–10 years follow-up [88, 89].

Torquati observed a reduction of the 10-year Framingham coronary heart disease event risk score from 5.4 % in the control group to 2.7 % in the surgery group [90]. Heneghan, in a review of 52 studies involving 16,867 patients, found a 40 % reduction of the Framingham risk score [91].

The diminished CV risk score has been related to the positive effects of bariatric surgery on comorbidities such as hypertension, diabetes, etc.; however, an independent factor has been postulated by some investigators [92].

Heart structures, especially LV geometry, are influenced by bariatric surgery determining cardiac remodeling and improved cardiac function. Echocardiographic measures are a noninvasive, reproducible, and reliable index to monitor cardiac and

Table 24.1 Randomized controlled trials comparing the effect of surgery or medical treatment on T2DM and cardiovascular risk factors

Author	Year	Procedure	N Pts (surg vs. med treat)	Mean BMI	Study duration (years)	T2DM remission (%) at the end of FU — Surgery	T2DM remission (%) at the end of FU — Medical treatment	Mean glycemia (mg/dL) at the end of FU — Surgery	Mean glycemia (mg/dL) at the end of FU — Medical treatment	Mean HbA1c (%) at the end of FU — Surgery	Mean HbA1c (%) at the end of FU — Medical treatment	Mean HDL (mg/dL) at the end of FU — Surgery	Mean HDL (mg/dL) at the end of FU — Medical treatment	Mean triglycerides (mg/dL) at the end of FU — Surgery	Mean triglycerides (mg/dL) at the end of FU — Medical treatment	Stop antihypertensive medications in surgical group
Dixon [71]	2008	AGB	30 vs. 30	37	2	73	13	105	139	6.0	7.2	59	50	118	186	70 %
Mingrone [72]	2012	GBP + BPD	40 vs. 20	45	2	75 (GBP) 95 (BPD)	0	86	141	5.6	7.7	42 (GBP) 57 (BPD)	41	102 (GBP) 85 (BPD)	169	80 % (GBP) 85 % (BPD)
Ikramuddin [73]	2013	GBP	60 vs. 60	34.5	1	44[a]	9[a]	111	153	6.3	7.8	50	42	104	182	–
Liang [74]	2013	GBP	31 vs. 36	30.5	1	90	0	–	–	6.0	8.1	47	32	142	310	N. of medications −2.8 day/pt
Schauer [75]	2014	GBP + SG	100 vs. 50	36	3	38 (GBP) 24 (SG)[b]	5[b]	103	132	6.8	8.4	60	49	103	121	42 %

AGB adjustable gastric banding, *SG* sleeve gastrectomy, *GBP* gastric bypass, *BPD* biliopancreatic diversion, *FU* follow-up
[a]HbA1c <6.0 %
[b]Glycemic control (glycated hemoglobin level of 6.0 % with or without medications)

particularly LV shape changes and to follow cardiac remodeling after bariatric surgery. Decrease of LV mass and Dilation and its linear relationship to weight loss has been clearly documented [93–96].

Diminished CV risk factors and cardiac remodeling determine a significant reduction in cardiovascular diseases mortality. In a large cohort clinical study comparing 7,925 RYGBP patients to matched control subjects, Adams evidenced a 56 % decrease of CV mortality over a 10-year follow-up [61].

Christou matched 1,035 surgical patients to 5,746 obese controls. Mortality in the surgical cohort was 0.68 % at 5 years, as compared to 6.17 % for controls [97].

In the SOS, at a mean 10.9 years follow-up, the hazard ratio for mortality in the surgery group was 0.71 when compared with the no-surgery control group. CV deaths were also reduced, with 1.4 % CV mortality in surgery subjects versus 2.4 % in controls [98].

In conclusion, in obese patients bariatric surgery ameliorates CV risk factors and heart geometry, resulting in reduced mortality rate over 10 years [99].

Although at present there is a lack of RCT with mortality end point, it is reasonable to agree with the authors of the largest systematic review on this subject claiming "a marked beneficial effect of bariatric surgery on future CV risk" [100].

It would seem that bariatric surgery is favorably fighting the "ultimate battle" when confronting the obesity epidemic.

A very large number of data in extensive studies have demonstrated the beneficial and significant effects of bariatric surgery on most of the satellite comorbidities of obesity, suggesting that reduction of mortality rate and amelioration of quality of life and of comorbidities are the main target, consequently EWL achievement may be considered even as a "fringe benefit."

24.7 Microbiota

The participation of the gut microbiota in the genesis of obesity and obesity-related comorbidities has been extensively studied.

The gastrointestinal tract is known to be a complex and finely balanced ecosystem that hosts 10^{14} bacterial cells (gut microbiota) weighting 1–1.5 kg, with over three million genes (microbiome), 100 times the human genome: the microbiota organ [101]. Under normal conditions the gut microbiota and the human host enjoy a symbiotic relationship. When an imbalance occurs (dysbiosis), adverse effects may follow [102].

Recent studies have highlighted a role for gut microbiota in the genesis of obesity and of the metabolic syndrome. There are a number of linking arguments: dysbiosis occurs in diabetic and obese versus lean individuals; some components of the gut microbiota (e.g., lipopolysaccharides, LPS) play a harmful role in obesity and diabetes; the diet takes part in the modulation of the gut microbiome and microbiota composition/function in obesity and metabolic syndrome [103–108]. Experimental and clinical studies have shown that in obese individuals the gut microbiota has a higher proportion of the phylum Firmicutes and a lower proportion of the phylum Bacteroidetes than in lean subjects [105, 107]. In obese individuals the microbiota is capable of extracting extra energy from the food by fermenting, otherwise indigestible, carbohydrates to monosaccharides and to short-chain fatty acids (SCFAs) thus increasing fat storage [109]. Furthermore, microbiota may be responsible for increased gut permeability to LPS, thus inducing low-grade inflammation (metabolic endotoxemia), diminished insulin sensitivity, and, finally, metabolic syndrome. The two driving factors of the metabolic syndrome, energy harvest, and gut permeability are dependent on gut microbiota dysbiosis [110].

The development of obesity and dysglycemia can be influenced by antibiotics or prebiotics which determine changes in the intestinal flora with increased representation of the Bifidobacterium species, reduced intestinal permeability, and decreased endotoxemia [111]. Probiotics reduce body weight and adipose tissue in mice and slow down diabetes progression in rats [112].

In the last few years, it has become increasingly evident that microbiota changes induced by bariatric surgery may play an important role in the occurrence of the effects of surgery.

Bariatric surgery results in rapid weight loss, reduced adiposity, and improved glucose metabolism. These effects are not solely attributable to decreased caloric intake or absorption, but the mechanisms linking rearrangement of the gastrointestinal tract to these metabolic outcomes are largely unknown.

Preliminary data seem to suggest that bariatric surgery (RYGBP) affects the composition of the gut microbiota. These changes could be a consequence of anatomical rearrangement or environmental and systemic factors (use of antibiotics, changes in food, increase in mastication time, transit time, acid production and intestinal pH, enterohepatic cycle) [113, 114].

The important question is to establish whether these microbial changes play a fundamental role in the dramatic improvement of the metabolism after bariatric surgery or represent mere epiphenomena.

In a recent paper Liou et al. demonstrated that in mice the surgery-altered (RYGBP) microbiota, when transferred in an intact animal by gastric gavage or by intestinal infusion, induces in the host phenotypic and metabolic changes mimicking the effects of surgery in the operated subject, loss of weight and improvement of the metabolic syndrome parameters, thus confirming the direct involvement of the gut microbiota in the pathogenesis of bariatric surgery effects [115].

In man Vrieze et al. reported that transfer of gut microbiota from healthy lean subjects into nonmorbidly obese patients with metabolic syndrome resulted in improved hepatic and peripheral insulin resistance as well as reduced fasting lipid levels [116].

These findings suggest a potential role for the gut microbiota in glucose and lipid metabolism changes induced by bariatric surgery and, shedding new light on the genesis of obesity and related comorbidities, offer a new promising rationale for the therapy of the diabesity epidemic.

As a closing remark it needs to be said that, while gut microbiota functions have been extensively studied and clarified in the lab in mice and rats, at present their role in the clinical setup has been scarcely investigated and needs to be confirmed: additional studies are strongly needed.

Conclusions

The present generation is confronted by a new epidemic: globesity and consequently diabesity. Today surgery seems to be the most effective therapeutic tool in terms of % of success and of duration of the benefits. In all RCTs, with a 1–5 years follow-up, bariatric surgery patients have been found superior to medical no-surgery controls in terms of EWL. These results have been confirmed in nonrandomized trials with a longer, 15–20 years, follow-up. The same can be said when considering the effects of bariatric surgery on obesity comorbidities in general and on T2DM in particular. The improvement of the glycemic control, immediately after some bariatric procedures, has drawn the attention of surgeons and diabetologists worldwide, stimulating a new field of research and therapy: the metabolic surgery.

More widespread experiences with bigger numbers and longer follow-up are needed; however, at present, bariatric surgery is more than a promising tool.

The twenty-first century generation, for the first time in history, is confronted by an unprecedented threat, a life expectancy shorter than in the preceding generation. The cornerstone SOS study, demonstrating the significant mortality reduction in bariatric surgery patients when confronted to no-surgery controls, may suggest one possible mean to avoid this novel menace and/or open the search for new therapeutic means.

References

1. Stevens GA, Singh GM, Lu Y et al (2012) National, regional, and global trends in adult overweight and obesity prevalences. Popul Health Metr 10(1):22
2. Calle EE, Rodriguez C, Walker-Thurmond K, Thun MJ (2003) Overweight, obesity, and mortality from cancer in a prospectively studied cohort of U.S. adults. N Engl J Med 348(17): 1625–1638
3. Boru C, Silecchia G, Pecchia A et al (2005) Prevalence of cancer in Italian obese patients referred for bariatric surgery. Obes Surg 15(8):1171–1176
4. Stamler R, Stamler J, Grimm R et al (1987) Nutritional therapy for high blood pressure. Final report of a 4-year randomized controlled trial-the hypertension control program. JAMA 257:1484–1491
5. Sjostrom L, Lendroos A, Peltonen M et al (2004) Lifestyle, diabetes, and cardiovascular risk factors 10 years after bariatric surgery. N Engl J Med 351(26):2683–2693
6. Maggard MA, Shugarman LR, Suttorp M et al (2005) Meta-analysis: surgical treatment of obesity. Ann Intern Med 142(7):547–559
7. Broadbent R, Tracey M, Harrington P (1993) Laparoscopic gastric banding: a preliminary report. Obes Surg 3(1):63–67
8. Reoch J, Mottillo S, Shimony A et al (2011) Safety of laparoscopic vs open bariatric surgery: a systematic review and meta-analysis. Arch Surg 146(11):1314–1322
9. Società Italiana di Chirurgia dell'Obesità e delle malattie metaboliche (2008) Linee guida e stato dell'arte in Chirurgia bariatrica e metabolica in Italia. www.sicob.org/00_materiali/attivita_linee_guida.pdf

10. Sauerland S, Angrisani L, Belachew M et al (2005) Obesity surgery: evidence-based guidelines of the European Association for Endoscopic Surgery (EAES). Surg Endosc 19(2):200–221
11. SAGES Guidelines Committee (2009) SAGES guideline for clinical application of laparoscopic bariatric surgery. Surg Obes Relat Dis 5(3):387–405
12. International Federation for the Surgery of Obesity (1997) Statement on patient selection for bariatric surgery. Obes Surg 7(1):41
13. American Society for Bariatric Surgery. Society of American Gastrointestinal Endoscopic Surgeons (2000) Guidelines for laparoscopic and open surgical treatment of morbid obesity. Obes Surg 10(4):378–379
14. Hubbard VS, Hall WH (1991) Gastrointestinal surgery for severe obesity. Obes Surg 1(3):257–265
15. Cerhan JR, Moore SC, Jacobs EJ et al (2014) A pooled analysis of waist circumference and mortality in 650,000 adults. Mayo Clin Proc 89(3):335–345
16. Guh DP, Zhang W, Bansback N, Amarsi Z, Birmingham CL, Anis AH (2009) The incidence of co-morbidities related to obesity and over-weight: a systematic review and meta-analysis. BMC Public Health 9:88
17. Avenell A, Brown TJ, McGee MA et al (2004) What interventions should we add to weight reducing diets in adults with obesity? A systematic review of randomized controlled trials of adding drug therapy, exercise, behaviour therapy or combinations of these interventions. J Hum Nutr Diet 17:293–316
18. ASMBS Clinical Issues Committee (2013) Bariatric surgery in class I obesity (body mass index 30–35 kg/m^2. Surg Obes Relat Dis 9(1):e1–e10
19. Lee WJ, Chong K, Ser KH et al (2011) Gastric bypass vs sleeve gastrectomy for type 2 diabetes mellitus: a randomized controlled trial. Arch Surg 146:143–148
20. Abbatini F, Capoccia D, Casella G, Coccia F, Leonetti F, Basso N (2012) Type 2 diabetes in obese patients with body mass index of 30–35 kg/m^2: sleeve gastrectomy versus medical treatment. Surg Obes Relat Dis 8:20–24
21. Zhang Z, Kris-Etherton PM, Hartman TJ (2014) Birth weight and risk factors for cardiovascular disease and Type 2 diabetes in US children and adolescents: 10 year results from NHANES. Matern Child Health J 18:1423–32
22. Iqbal CW, Kumar S, Iqbal AD, Ishitani MB (2009) Perspectives on pediatric bariatric surgery: identifying barriers to referral. Surg Obes Relat Dis 5:88–93
23. Inge TH (2006) Bariatric surgery for morbidly obese adolescents: is there a rationale for early intervention? Growth Horm IGF Res 16(Suppl A):S15–S911
24. Dorman RB, Abraham AA, Al-Refaie WB, Parsons HM, Ikramuddin S, Habermann EB (2012) Bariatric surgery outcomes in the elderly: an ACS NSQIP study. J Gastrointest Surg 16(1):35–44
25. Cohen R, Pinheiro JC, Schiavon CA, Salles JE, Wajchenberg BL, Cummings DE (2012) Effects of gastric bypass surgery in patients with type 2 diabetes and only mild obesity. Diabetes Care 35:1420–1428
26. Buchwald H, Consensus Conference Panel (2005) Bariatric surgery for morbid obesity: health implications for patients, health professionals, and third-party payers. J Am Coll Surg 200(4):593–604
27. Statement by the American College of Surgeons (2000) Recommendations for facilities performing bariatric surgery. Bull Am Coll Surg 85(9):20–23
28. Collazo-Clavell ML, Clark MM, McAlpine DE et al (2006) Assessment and preparation of patients for bariatric surgery. Mayo Clin Proc 81(10 suppl):S11–S17
29. Yang Y, Kuwano H, Okudaira Y, Kholoussy AM, Matsumoto T (1987) Use of intragastric balloons for weight reduction. An experimental study. Am J Surg 153(3):265–269
30. Lecumberri E, Krekshi W, Matía P et al (2011) Effectiveness and safety of air-filled balloon Heliosphere BAG® in 82 consecutive obese patients. Obes Surg 21(10):1508–1512
31. Gaggiotti G, Tack J, Garrido AB Jr, Palau M, Cappelluti G, Di Matteo F (2007) Adjustable totally implantable intragastric prosthesis (ATIIP)-Endogast for treatment of morbid obesity: one-year follow-up of a multicenter prospective clinical survey. Obes Surg 17(7):949–956

32. Mion F, Ibrahim M, Marjoux S et al (2013) Swallowable Obalon® gastric balloons as an aid for weight loss: a pilot feasibility study. Obes Surg 23(5):730–733
33. Genco A, Lorenzo M, Baglio G et al (2014) Does the intragastric balloon have a predictive role in subsequent LAP-BAND® surgery? Italian multicenter study results at 5-year follow-up. Surg Obes Relat Dis 10:474–8
34. Genco A, Bruni T, Doldi SB et al (2005) BioEnterics Intragastric Balloon: the Italian experience with 2,515 patients. Obes Surg 15(8):1161–1164
35. Genco A, López-Nava G, Wahlen C et al (2013) Multi-centre European experience with intragastric balloon in overweight populations: 13 years of experience. Obes Surg 23(4):515–521
36. Kuzmak LI, Yap IS, McGuire L, Dixon JS, Young MP (1990) Surgery for morbid obesity. Using an inflatable gastric band. AORN J 51(5):1307–1324
37. Buchwald H, Oien DM (2013) Metabolic/bariatric surgery worldwide 2011. Obes Surg 23(4):427–436
38. O'Brien PE, Dixon JB (2003) Laparoscopic adjustable gastric banding in the treatment of morbid obesity. Arch Surg 138(4):376–382
39. Angrisani L, Di Lorenzo N, Favretti F et al (2004) The Italian group for LAP-BAND: predictive value of initial body mass index for weight loss after 5 years of follow-up. Surg Endosc 18(10):1524–1527
40. Buchwald H, Avidor Y, Braunwald E et al (2004) Bariatric surgery: a systematic review and meta-analysis. JAMA 292(14):1724–1737
41. Mason EE, Ito C (1969) Gastric bypass. Ann Surg 170(3):329–339
42. Wittgrove AC, Clark GW, Tremblay LJ (1994) Laparoscopic gastric bypass, Roux-en-Y: preliminary report of five cases. Obes Surg 4(4):353–357
43. Beckman LM, Beckman TR, Earthman CP (2010) Changes in gastrointestinal hormones and leptin after Roux-en-Y gastric bypass procedure: a review. J Am Diet Assoc 110(4):571–584
44. Cummings DE, Weigle DS, Frayo RS et al (2002) Plasma ghrelin levels after diet-induced weight loss or gastric bypass surgery. N Engl J Med 346(21):1623–1630
45. Romero F, Nicolau J, Flores L et al (2012) Comparable early changes in gastrointestinal hormones after sleeve gastrectomy and Roux-En-Y gastric bypass surgery for morbidly obese type 2 diabetic subjects. Surg Endosc 26(8):2231–2239
46. Scopinaro N, Adami GF, Marinari GM et al (1998) Biliopancreatic diversion. World J Surg 22(9):936–946
47. Hess DS, Hess DW (1998) Biliopancreatic diversion with a duodenal switch. Obes Surg 8(3):267–282
48. Scopinaro N (2006) Biliopancreatic diversion: mechanisms of action and long-term results. Obes Surg 16(6):683–689
49. Tsoli M, Chronaiou A, Kehagias I, Kalfarentzos F, Alexandrides TK (2013) Hormone changes and diabetes resolution after biliopancreatic diversion and laparoscopic sleeve gastrectomy: a comparative prospective study. Surg Obes Relat Dis 9(5):667–677
50. Regan JP, Inabnet WB, Gagner M, Pomp A (2003) Early experience with two-stage laparoscopic Roux-en-Y gastric bypass as an alternative in the super-super obese patient. Obes Surg 13(6):861–864
51. Clinical Issues Committee of the American Society for Metabolic and Bariatric Surgery (2010) Updated position statement on sleeve gastrectomy as a bariatric procedure. Surg Obes Relat Dis 6(1):1–5
52. Karamanakos SN, Vagenas K, Kalfarentzos F, Alexandrides TK (2008) Weight loss, appetite suppression, and changes in fasting and postprandial ghrelin and peptide-YY levels after Roux-en-Y gastric bypass and sleeve gastrectomy: a prospective, double blind study. Ann Surg 247(3):401–407
53. Basso N, Capoccia D, Rizzello M et al (2011) First-phase insulin secretion, insulin sensitivity, ghrelin, GLP-1, and PYY changes 72 h after sleeve gastrectomy in obese diabetic patients: the gastric hypothesis. Surg Endosc 25(11):3540–3550

54. Soricelli E, Iossa A, Casella G, Abbatini F, Calì B, Basso N (2013) Sleeve gastrectomy and crural repair in obese patients with gastroesophageal reflux disease and/or hiatal hernia. Surg Obes Relat Dis 9(3):356–361
55. Gagner M, Deitel M, Erickson AL, Crosby RD (2013) Survey on Laparoscopic Sleeve Gastrectomy (LSG) at the fourth international consensus summit on sleeve gastrectomy. Obes Surg 23(12):2013–2017
56. Abbatini F, Rizzello M, Casella G et al (2010) Long-term effects of laparoscopic sleeve gastrectomy, gastric bypass, and adjustable gastric banding on type 2 diabetes. Surg Endosc 24(5):1005–1010
57. Cottam D, Qureshi FG, Mattar SG et al (2006) Laparoscopic sleeve gastrectomy as an initial weight-loss procedure for high-risk patients with morbid obesity. Surg Endosc 20(6):859–863
58. Vidal J, Ibarzabal A, Romero F et al (2008) Type 2 diabetes mellitus and the metabolic syndrome following sleeve gastrectomy in severely obese subjects. Obes Surg 18(9):1077–1082
59. Casella G, Abbatini F, Calì B, Capoccia D, Leonetti F, Basso N (2011) Ten-year duration of type 2 diabetes as prognostic factor for remission after sleeve gastrectomy. Surg Obes Relat Dis 7(6):697–702
60. Sjöström L (2013) Review of the key results from the Swedish Obese Subjects (SOS) trial – a prospective controlled intervention study of bariatric surgery. J Intern Med 273(3):219–234
61. Adams TD, Gress RE, Smith SC et al (2007) Long-term mortality after gastric bypass surgery. N Engl J Med 357(8):753–761
62. Canetti L, Elizur Y, Karni Y, Berry E (2013) Health-related quality of life changes and weight reduction after bariatric surgery vs. a weight-loss program. Isr J Psychiatry Relat Sci 50(3): 194–200
63. Oria HE, Moorehead MK (1988) Bariatric Analysis and Reporting Outcome System (BAROS). Obes Surg 8:487–499
64. D'Hondt M, Vanneste S, Pottel H, Devriendt D, Van Rooy F, Vansteenkiste F (2011) Laparoscopic sleeve gastrectomy as a single-stage procedure for the treatment of morbid obesity and the resulting quality of life, resolution of comorbidities, food tolerance, and 6-year weight loss. Surg Endosc 25(8):2498–2504
65. Sarwer DB, Spitzer JC, Wadden TA et al (2014) Changes in sexual functioning and sex hormone levels in women following bariatric surgery. JAMA Surg 149(1):26–33
66. Rubino F, R'bibo SL, del Genio F, Mazumdar M, McGraw TE (2010) Metabolic surgery: the role of the gastrointestinal tract in diabetes mellitus. Nat Rev Endocrinol 6(2):102–109
67. Rubino F, Kaplan LM, Schauer PR, Cummings DE, Diabetes Surgery Summit Delegates (2010) The Diabetes Surgery Summit consensus conference: recommendations for the evaluation and use of gastrointestinal surgery to treat type 2 diabetes mellitus. Ann Surg 251(3): 399–405
68. American Diabetes Association, Bantle JP, Wylie-Rosett J et al (2009) Nutrition recommendations and interventions for diabetes: a position statement of the American Diabetes Association. Diabetes Care 31(Suppl 1):S61–S78
69. Dixon JB, Zimmet P, Alberti KG, Rubino F, International Diabetes Federation Taskforce on Epidemiology and Prevention (2011) Bariatric surgery: an IDF statement for obese Type 2 diabetes. Surg Obes Relat Dis 7(4):433–447
70. Arterburn DE, Bogart A, Sherwood NE et al (2013) A multisite study of long-term remission and relapse of type 2 diabetes mellitus following gastric bypass. Obes Surg 23(1):93–102
71. Dixon JB, O'Brien PE, Playfair J et al (2008) Adjustable gastric banding and conventional therapy for type 2 diabetes: a randomized controlled trial. JAMA 299:316–323
72. Mingrone G, Panunzi S, De Gaetano A et al (2012) Bariatric surgery versus conventional medical therapy for type 2 diabetes. N Engl J Med 366(17):1577–1585
73. Ikramuddin S, Korner J, Lee WJ et al (2013) Roux-en-Y gastric bypass vs intensive medical management for the control of type 2 diabetes, hypertension, and hyperlipidemia: the diabetes surgery study randomized clinical trial. JAMA 309(21):2240–2249

74. Liang Z, Wu Q, Chen B, Yu P, Zhao H, Ouyang X (2013) Effect of laparoscopic Roux-en-Y gastric bypass surgery on type 2 diabetes mellitus with hypertension: a randomized controlled trial. Diabetes Res Clin Pract. Epub ahead of print
75. Schauer PR, Kashyap SR, Wolski K et al (2012) Bariatric surgery versus intensive medical therapy in obese patients with diabetes. N Engl J Med 366(17):1567–1576
76. Segato G, Busetto L, De Luca M et al (2010) Weight loss and changes in use of antidiabetic medication in obese type 2 diabetics after laparoscopic gastric banding. Surg Obes Relat Dis 6(2):132–137
77. Scopinaro N, Papadia F, Camerini G, Marinari G, Civalleri D, Gian Franco A (2008) A comparison of a personal series of biliopancreatic diversion and literature data on gastric bypass help to explain the mechanisms of resolution of type 2 diabetes by the two operations. Obes Surg 18(8):1035–1038
78. Adams TD, Davidson LE, Litwin SE et al (2012) Health benefits of gastric bypass surgery after 6 years. JAMA 308(11):1122–1131
79. Abbatini F, Capoccia D, Casella G, Soricelli E, Leonetti F, Basso N (2013) Long-term remission of type 2 diabetes in morbidly obese patients after sleeve gastrectomy. Surg Obes Relat Dis 9(4):498–502
80. Madala MC, Franklin BA, Chen AY et al (2008) Obesity and age of first non-ST segment elevation myocardial infarction. J Am Coll Cardiol 52:979–985
81. Wolk R, Berger P, Lennon RJ et al (2003) Body mass index: a risk factor for unstable angina and myocardial infarction in patients with angiographically confirmed coronary artery disease. Circulation 108:2206–2211
82. Duflou J, Virmani R, Rabin I et al (1995) Sudden death as a result of heart disease in morbid obesity. Am Heart J 130:306–313
83. Poirier P, Giles TD, Bray GA et al (2006) Obesity and cardiovascular disease: pathophysiology, evaluation, and effect of weight loss: an update of the 1997 American Heart Association Scientific Statement on Obesity and Heart Disease from the Obesity Committee of the Council on Nutrition, Physical Activity, and Metabolism. Circulation 113:898–918
84. de las Fuentes L, Waggoner AD, Mohammed BS et al (2009) Effect of moderate diet-induced weight loss and weight regain on cardiovascular structure and function. J Am Coll Cardiol 54:2376–2381
85. Lakhani M, Fein S (2011) Effects of obesity and subsequent weight reduction on left ventricular function. Cardiol Rev 19:1–4
86. Wong CY, O'Moore-Sullivan T, Leano R et al (2004) Alterations of left ventricular myocardial characteristics associated with obesity. Circulation 110:3081–3087
87. Turkbey EB, McClelland RL, Kronmal RA et al (2010) The impact of obesity on the left ventricle: the Multi-Ethnic Study of Atherosclerosis (MESA). JACC Cardiovasc Imaging 3:266–274
88. Batsis JA, Sarr MG, Collazo-Clavell ML et al (2008) Cardiovascular risk after bariatric surgery for obesity. Am J Cardiol 102(7):930–937
89. Vogel JA, Franklin BA, Zalesin KC et al (2007) Reduction in predicted coronary heart disease risk after substantial weight reduction after bariatric surgery. Am J Cardiol 99(2):222–226
90. Torquati A, Wright K, Melvin W, Richards W (2007) Effect of gastric bypass operation on Framingham and actual risk of cardiovascular events in class II to III obesity. J Am Coll Surg 204(5):776–782
91. Heneghan HM, Meron-Eldar S, Brethauer SA, Schauer PR, Young JB (2011) Effect of bariatric surgery on cardiovascular risk profile. Am J Cardiol 108(10):1499–1507
92. See R, Abdullah SM, McGuire DK et al (2007) The association of differing measures of overweight and obesity with prevalent atherosclerosis: the Dallas heart study. J Am Coll Cardiol 50(8):752–759
93. Grapsa J, Tan TC, Paschou SA et al (2013) The effect of bariatric surgery on echocardiographic indices: a review of the literature. Eur J Clin Invest 43(11):1224–1230

94. Garza CA, Pellikka PA, Somers VK et al (2010) Structural and functional changes in left and right ventricles after major weight loss following bariatric surgery for morbid obesity. Am J Cardiol 105:550–556
95. Owan T, Avelar E, Morley K et al (2011) Favorable changes in cardiac geometry and function following gastric bypass surgery: 2-year follow-up in the Utah obesity study. J Am Coll Cardiol 57:732–739
96. Cavarretta E, Casella G, Calì B et al (2013) Cardiac remodeling in obese patients after laparoscopic sleeve gastrectomy. World J Surg 37(3):565–572
97. Christou NV, Sampalis JS, Liberman M et al (2004) Surgery decreases long-term mortality, morbidity, and health care use in morbidly obese patients. Ann Surg 240(3):416–423
98. Sjostrom L, Narbro K, Sjostrom CD et al (2007) Effects of bariatric surgery on mortality in Swedish obese subjects. N Engl J Med 357:741–752
99. Benraouane F, Litwin SE (2011) Reductions in cardiovascular risk after bariatric surgery. Curr Opin Cardiol 26(6):555–561
100. Vest AR, Heneghan HM, Agarwal S, Schauer PR, Young JB (2012) Bariatric surgery and cardiovascular outcomes: a systematic review. Heart 98(24):1763–1777
101. Ley RE (2010) Obesity and the human microbiome. Curr Opin Gastroenterol 26(1):5–11
102. Geurts L, Neyrinck AM, Delzenne NM, Knauf C, Cani PD (2014) Gut microbiota controls adipose tissue expansion, gut barrier and glucose metabolism: novel insights into molecular targets and interventions using prebiotics. Benef Microbes 5(1):3–17
103. Schwiertz A, Taras D, Schäfer K, Beijer S, Bos NA, Donus C, Hardt PD (2010) Microbiota and SCFA in lean and overweight healthy subjects. Obesity (Silver Spring) 18(1):190–195
104. Larsen N, Vogensen FK, van den Berg FW, Nielsen DS, Andreasen AS, Pedersen BK, Al-Soud WA, Sørensen SJ, Hansen LH, Jakobsen M (2010) Gut microbiota in human adults with type 2 diabetes differs from non-diabetic adults. PLoS One 5(2):e9085
105. Cox LM, Blaser MJ (2013) Pathways in microbe-induced obesity. Cell Metab 17(6):883–894
106. Tremaroli V, Bäckhed F (2012) Functional interactions between the gut microbiota and host metabolism. Nature 489(7415):242–249
107. Tilg H, Kaser A (2011) Gut microbiome, obesity, and metabolic dysfunction. J Clin Invest 121(6):2126–2132
108. Ley RE, Bäckhed F, Turnbaugh P, Lozupone CA, Knight RD, Gordon JI (2005) Obesity alters gut microbial ecology. Proc Natl Acad Sci U S A 102(31):11070–11075
109. Tremaroli V, Kovatcheva-Datchary P, Bäckhed F (2010) A role for the gut microbiota in energy harvesting? Gut 59(12):1589–1590
110. Turnbaugh PJ, Ley RE, Mahowald MA, Magrini V, Mardis ER, Gordon JI (2006) An obesity-associated gut microbiome with increased capacity for energy harvest. Nature 444(7122):1027–1031
111. Cani PD, Bibiloni R, Knauf C et al (2008) Changes in gut microbiota control metabolic endotoxemia-induced inflammation in high-fat diet-induced obesity and diabetes in mice. Diabetes 57:1470–1481
112. Lee HY, Park JH, Seok SH et al (2006) Human originated bacteria, Lactobacillus rhamnosus PL60, produce conjugated linoleic acid and show antiobesity effects in diet-induced obese mice. Biochim Biophys Acta 1761:736–744
113. Osto M, Abegg K, Bueter M, le Roux CW, Cani PD, Lutz TA (2013) Roux-en-Y gastric bypass surgery in rats alters gut microbiota profile along the intestine. Physiol Behav 119:92–96
114. Aron-Wisnewsky J, Doré J, Clement K (2012) The importance of the gut microbiota after bariatric surgery. Nat Rev Gastroenterol Hepatol 9(10):590–598
115. Liou AP, Paziuk M, Luevano JM Jr, Machineni S, Turnbaugh PJ, Kaplan LM (2013) Conserved shifts in the gut microbiota due to gastric bypass reduce host weight and adiposity. Sci Transl Med 5(178):178ra41
116. Vrieze A, Van Nood E, Holleman F et al (2012) Transfer of intestinal microbiota from lean donors increases insulin sensitivity in individuals with metabolic syndrome. Gastroenterology 143(4):913–916.e7

Reconstructive Plastic Surgery

25

Paolo Persichetti, Stefania Tenna, and Pierfranco Simone

25.1 Introduction

The advent of bariatric surgery had led to a new subspecialty in plastic surgery for contouring the skin and fat remaining after massive weight loss classified by Pittsburgh Weight Loss Deformity Scale [1, 2] (Table 25.1).

Patients in fact complain for a wide range of physical anomalies that do interfere with their quality of life often causing functional impairment.

According to Balagué et al., *body contouring* must be included in morbid obesity management as patients undergoing those procedures present better long-term weight control [3, 4].

As a general rule, contouring operations should be done after weight loss is complete, as wound complications tend to be higher when surgery is performed in patients who are still obese.

Given the opportunity to prioritize which parts of their bodies they would like to have addressed first by a plastic surgeon, the waist/abdomen is usually at the top of the list (46.2 %), followed by the upper arm (23.3 %), the chest/breast (12.3 %), and the rear/buttock (18.2 %) [5].

Performing multiple procedures in two or more stages should be considered if the patient has goals of reshaping different regions. The advantages of staging include less anesthetic time, reduced blood loss, less surgeon fatigue, avoidance of opposing vectors of pull on regions of the skin, and the chance to correct further irregularities [6–10].

The authors present a description of personal surgical approaches to the most requested interventions.

P. Persichetti, MD, PhD • S. Tenna, MD, PhD (✉) • P. Simone, MD
Plastic Surgery Unit, Campus Bio Medico University,
Via Alvaro del Portillo 200, 00128 Rome, Italy
e-mail: s.tenna@unicampus.it

© Springer International Publishing Switzerland 2015
A. Lenzi et al. (eds.), *Multidisciplinary Approach to Obesity:
From Assessment to Treatment*, DOI 10.1007/978-3-319-09045-0_25

Table 25.1 Pittsburgh Weight Loss Deformity Scale

Area	Scale	Preferred procedure
Arms	0 Normal	None
	1 Adiposity with good skin tone	ultrasound assisted lipoplasty (UAL) and/or standard assisted lipoplasty (SAL)
	2 Loose, hanging skin without severe adiposity	Brachioplasty
	3 Loose, hanging skin with severe adiposity	Brachioplasty ± UAL and/or SAL
Breasts	0 Normal	None
	1 Ptosis grade I/II or severe macromastia	Traditional mastopexy, reduction, or augmentation techniques
	2 Ptosis grade I/II or moderate volume loss or constricted breast	Traditional mastopexy ± augmentation
	3 Severe lateral roll and/or severe volume loss with loose skin	Parenchymal reshaping techniques with dermal suspension; consider autoaugmentation
Back	0 Normal	None
	1 Single fat roll or adiposity	UAL and/or SAL
	2 Multiple skin and fat rolls	Excisional lifting procedures
	3 Ptosis of rolls	Excisional lifting procedures
Abdomen	0 Normal	None
	1 Redundant skin with rhytids or moderate adiposity without overhang	Mini abdominoplasty, UAL and/or SAL
	2 Overhanging pannus	Full abdominoplasty
	3 Multiple rolls or epigastric fullness	Modified abdominoplasty techniques, including fleur-de-lis and/or upper body lift
Flank	0 Normal	None
	1 Adiposity	UAL and/or SAL
	2 Rolls	UAL and/or SAL
	3 Ptosis of rolls	Excisional lifting procedures
Buttocks	0 Normal	None
	1 Mild to moderate adiposity and/or mild to moderate cellulite	UAL and/or SAL
	2 Severe adiposity and/or severe cellulite	UAL and/or SAL ± excisional lifting procedure
	3 Skinfolds	Excisional lifting procedure
Mons	0 Normal	None
	1 Excessive adiposity	UAL and/or SAL
	2 Ptosis	Monsplasty
	3 Significant overhang below symphysis	Monsplasty

Table 25.1 (continued)

Area	Scale	Preferred procedure
Hips/lateral thighs	0 Normal	None
	1 Mild to moderate adiposity and/or mild to moderate cellulite	UAL and/or SAL
	2 Severe adiposity and/or severe cellulite	UAL and/or SAL ± excisional lifting procedure
	3 Skinfolds	Excisional lifting procedure
Medial thighs	0 Normal	None
	1 Excessive adiposity	UAL and/or SAL ± excisional lifting procedure
	2 Severe adiposity and/or severe cellulite	UAL and/or SAL ± excisional lifting procedure
	3 Skinfolds	Excisional lifting procedure
Lower thighs/ knees	0 Normal	None
	1 Adiposity	UAL and SAL ± excisional lifting procedure
	2 Severe adiposity	UAL and SAL ± excisional lifting procedure
	3 Skinfolds	Excisional lifting procedure

25.2 Abdominoplasty

Although *abdominoplasty* is a common procedure within plastic surgery, the management of the post massive weight loss of the abdomen is much more complicated [1, 2]. The aim is to reshape the abdominal wall by combining skin and subcutaneous tissue resection with musculoaponeurotic reinforcement. Conventional transverse resection is the first choice, but several and long scars may be necessary to give the patient the desired contour. The presence of a median or paramedian supraumbilical scar must be carefully considered especially after bariatric procedures. Vertical scars in the upper abdomen may impair vascularity or limit the advancement of the superior flap leading to unfavorable aesthetic results [11]. In those cases, transverse resection cannot guarantee adequate body contouring so the "*anchor-line*" abdominoplasty must be preferred [12].

25.2.1 Surgical Technique

Bowel preparation with enemas is carried out the day before surgery. Foley catheter is positioned preoperatively. Elastic stockings are applied to the legs to prevent venous stasis, and low-dose heparin is administered for deep venous thrombosis prophylaxis. Marking of the surgical incisions is made in the midline drawn from the xiphoid to the pubic symphysis with the patient in upright position. With the patient supine, a lower horizontal ellipsis plus an upper vertical medial triangle, which entails the supraumbilical scars, is marked. The upper components of the elliptical drawing run obliquely downward beneath the umbilicus, which is different from the conventional design. In this way, the final horizontal scars are placed as low as possible, in the natural suprapubic fold.

The width of the upper triangle is established by pinching, with the patient supine, so as to obtain the new abdominal silhouette. No excess tension must be exerted to avoid pubic hairline elevation.

Incisions are performed along the preoperative drawing, and an "en bloc" resection of skin and subcutaneous tissue is carried out. The umbilicus is resected in a triangular shape, with the base placed superiorly, isolating and preserving its stalk, which is left attached to the abdominal fascia.

The lateral flaps are elevated through sharp dissection in a prefascial plane in order to mobilize the flaps, sparing the lateral musculocutaneous perforators and being careful not to impair the vascular supply.

Plication of the rectus sheath is then performed; in most cases, it is vertical and sometimes vertical and horizontal depending on the myoaponeurotic laxity, and it is carried out with an inverted nonabsorbable suture such as Prolene 1-0.

In case of abdominal recurrent incisional or inguinal *hernias*, a Prolene mesh is placed in a preperitoneal position. The umbilicus, previously cut out in a triangular shape, with a superior base, is fixed to the aponeurosis and repositioned on the abdominal flap through a "Y"-shaped incision. Before advancing the abdominal flaps and starting the sutures, the operating table is flexed 30° to release tension on the sutures. Subcutaneous approximation is attained with absorbable polyglycolic acid sutures, followed by a running subcuticular nylon suture. Two suction drains are always placed, one in a supraumbilical position and the other in a lower position, beneath the umbilicus. The abdomen is padded with a cotton-wool bandage. An elastic pressure dressing is applied all over the area (Figs. 25.1 and 25.2).

25.2.2 Complications

For abdominal procedures, a multifactorial analysis of variance showed that the preoperative weight had a highly statistically significant effect on the incidence of complications, whereas previous bariatric surgery did not [13].

Patients with BMI over 35 have an increased risk to develop *seromas*, wound dehiscence, infection, and thrombosis [14].

Avoidance of pulmonary embolus is of utmost importance. Early mobilization and the use of low-molecular-weight heparin are commonly accepted even if with different schemes. The risk of seroma is high as well, and various techniques have been suggested to control its formation: mattress sutures, tissue sealants, and the use of doxycycline into the drains [15, 16].

Necrosis is less common and together with the recurrence of the upper abdominal excess or unsightly *scars* may depend on surgical planning and technique [17].

25 Reconstructive Plastic Surgery

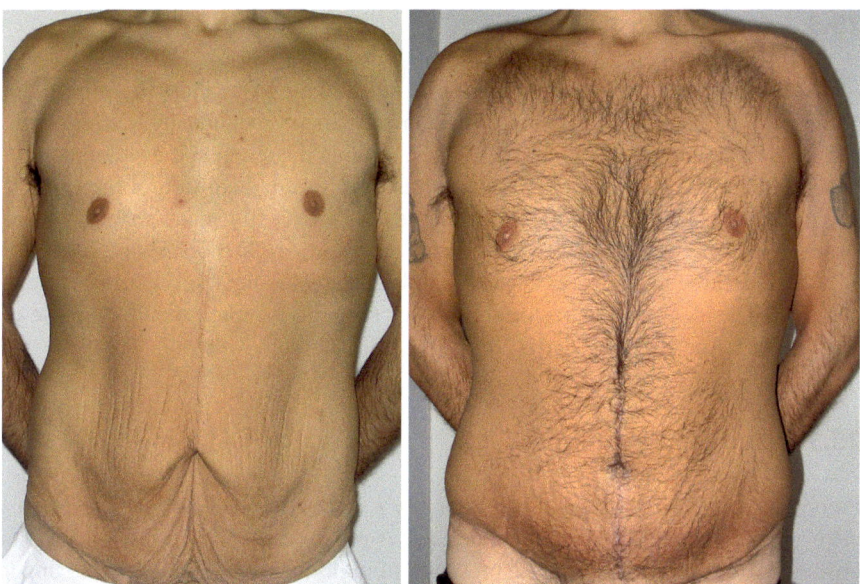

Fig. 25.1 Preoperative view of abdominal deformity after weight loss

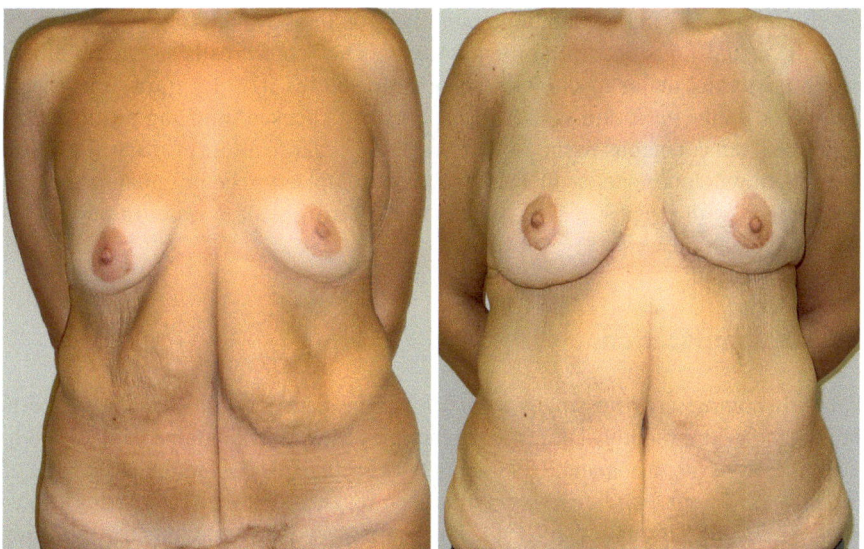

Fig. 25.2 Postoperative result after "anchor-line" abdominoplasty

25.3 Mastopexy

Breast reshaping after massive weight loss still remains a challenging procedure, because of the significant skin and subcutaneous tissues redundancy left following bariatric procedures [18, 19]. In such cases, volume depletion and development of skin/nipple-areola complex (NAC) ptosis result in severe distortion of breast morphology, and standard mastopexy techniques are frequently inadequate to reconstruct a pleasant breast. The use of implants to restore original breast volume is not advisable in these patients, because of skin laxity and the poor soft tissue coverage obtained. The ideal volume restoration in this scenario is represented by the use of autologous tissues (*AICAP flap*) [20].

25.3.1 Surgical Technique

Preoperative marking according to Pitanguy's inverted T superior pedicle *mastopexy* are obtained at the bed of the patient. A pinch test in the supine position is always performed to identify the presence of significant skin laxity in the upper abdominal wall. Under general anesthesia, disepithelization of the preoperative inverted-T pattern is performed. A flap is islanded on perforators from the anterior intercostal arteries and harvested to increase breast volume and correct abdominal skin laxity in a single step. The flap includes soft tissues above and below the inframammary fold, extending cranially 5–6 cm above the fold and inferiorly over the costal cage, according to skin laxity. The "auto-prosthesis" is stabilized to the pectoralis major fascia with absorbable sutures in order to prevent shearing forces on the perforators. Breast shape is then checked in sitting position, and abdominal subcutaneous tissue is undermined in order to allow primary closure of the abdominal donor site, as in a reverse abdominoplasty. The inframammary fold is redefined with nonabsorbable stitches to rib periosteum, in order to prevent its caudal dislocation.

25.3.2 Complications

A lightly compressive dressing is worn for 3–5 days and then patients wear a sports bra for the next 2 months. Drains are sometimes used and maintained at least 48 h. Complications are infrequent. Hematoma may occur especially in the lateral part of the breast. Minor *wound dehiscence* has been registered at the confluence of incisions along the inframammary fold. Dislocation of the inframammary fold may occur and need surgical revision [21, 22].

Mastopexy plus anterior intercostal artery perforator (AICAP) flap represents an evolution of conventional *mastopexy*; it is a versatile technique and proved to be a very good option to restore breast shape and projection in post-bariatric surgery patients.

The procedure can be easily standardized, and it is simple to perform, increases breast volume and projection, and corrects the upper abdominal skin laxity usually not responsive to classic *abdominoplasty* procedures (Figs. 25.3 and 25.4).

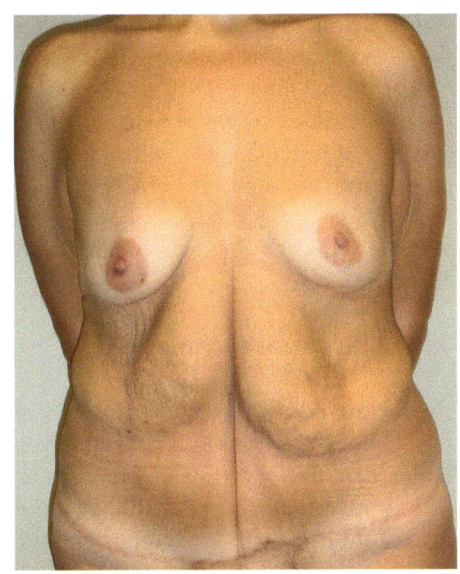

Fig. 25.3 Preoperative view of post-bariatric surgery breast ptosis and hypoplasia

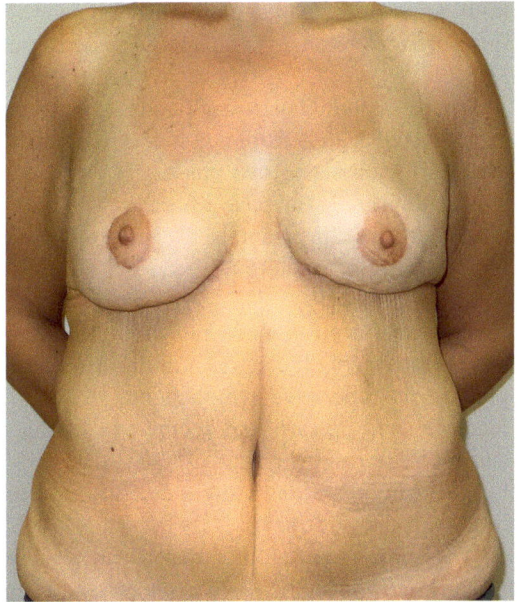

Fig. 25.4 Postoperative result after mastopexy plus AICAP flap

25.4 Inner-Thigh Lift

Post-bariatric skin redundancy and persisting fat deposits in the *inner-thigh* areas lead to severe friction between the inner surfaces of the thighs, with consequent functional impairment and reduced patient's mobility, intertriginous rashes, and chronic inflammation [23].

Correction of these deformities implies excision and redraping of excess medial thigh skin as well as persisting fat deposit removal.

The medial thigh lift was first described more than 50 years ago [24] but did not gain widespread acceptance due to frequent postoperative complications, such as caudal scar migration and widening, vulvar distortion, lymphatic impairment, and early recurrence of ptosis [25, 26].

In the authors' experience, best results and low complication rates are achieved with the surgical technique hereafter described.

25.4.1 Surgical Technique

Preoperative drawings are performed with the patient in standing position and legs abducted. The skin is pinched to assess cutaneous excess. A semicrescent component plus a vertical component are marked, entailing the redundant skin. The semicrescent is marked anteriorly as far as the medial one third of the groin fold and is prolonged posteriorly to include the medial one third of the subgluteal fold. The upper border of the semicrescent is 1 cm above the fold. The vertical triangular component is marked along the inner-thigh vertical midline, with the base lying on the inferior border of the semicrescent and the inferior apex along the inner-thigh vertical midline, below the distalmost skinfold.

The procedure is performed under general anesthesia. *Antibiotic prophylaxis* is administered with cefazolin at a dose of 2 g i.v. A urinary catheter is placed. The procedure consists of two phases. The first surgical phase is liposuction: in the medial thigh area, massive liposuction is performed on the subcutaneous tissue underlying the skin area to be excised. In the anterior thigh area and below the subgluteal fold, liposculpture is performed to remove fat deposits and improve contour.

The second phase is skin excision, including a thin layer of subcutaneous tissue, preserving the superficial fascia septa, in order to spare lymphatics and prevent postoperative lymphedema. After the excision, the flaps are moved medially and upward and secured to Colles' fascia with polydioxone (PDS) sutures. The resulting scar is a "T"-shaped scar, with a horizontal component lying in the groin and subgluteal fold and a vertical branch along the inner-thigh vertical midline.

Once final closure is completed and wounds are dressed, a semi-compressive bandage is applied. No drain is placed and resorbable sutures are used. The mean operation time is 3 h.

On the first postoperative day, the urinary catheter is removed, the surgical dressing is taken off, and wounds are checked and disinfected. A pressure garment is applied and the patient is mobilized.

Routinely, patients are discharged on the first postoperative day and are instructed to perform multiple daily wound irrigations with povidone-iodine.

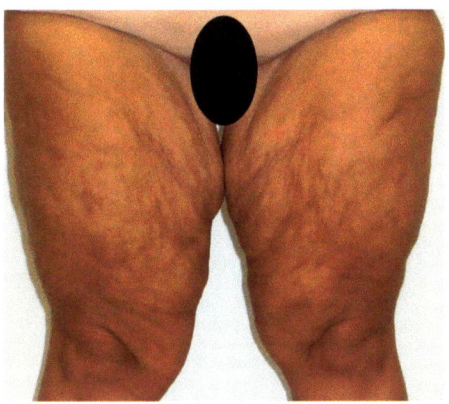

Fig. 25.5 Preoperative view of skin redundancy and persisting fat deposits in the inner thigh

Low-molecular-weight heparin is administered within 12 h after the surgery and for the following 5 days for thrombosis prophylaxis. Broad-spectrum antibiotics are administered for 7 days postoperatively. Panty hose is worn night and day for 2 months.

25.4.2 Complications

In our experience, postoperative complications are minimal: the superficial *dermolipectomy* allows to spare the lymphatic vessels, reducing the risk of postoperative lymphedema and *lymphocele* (30 % incidence reported in the medical literature); [26] the meticulous and multilayered closure with obliteration of dead spaces allows to avoid seroma (15 % incidence in some series) and hematoma and consequent delayed wound healing; postoperative management, in terms of early mobilization associated with LMWH administration and antibiotic therapy associated with multiple irrigations of wounds, drastically reduces, respectively, thromboembolic events and wound infections.

This thigh-lift technique, with a two-step approach (liposuction and dermolipectomy), allows to remove fat deposits and skin excess, reshaping circumferentially the thigh, which is narrowed and lifted. After surgery, patients obtain significant improvement of mobility and relief of symptoms due to severe chronic inflammation (Figs. 25.5 and 25.6).

25.5 Brachioplasty

The arm profile may be severely altered by massive weight loss, with skin redundancy resulting in a *"bat-wing"* deformity. As a consequence, post-bariatric surgery patients experience functional limitations and hampered movements. Moreover, the constant friction between the axillary and the arm tissues leads to chronic

Fig. 25.6 Postoperative result after inner-thigh lift

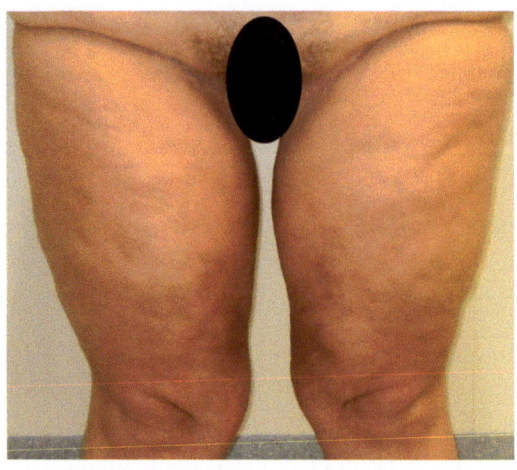

inflammation, often complicated by infection. Psychosocial issues are of paramount importance in such patients, too [27]. All these factors have made *brachioplasty* one of the most sought-after interventions in the post-bariatric surgery population: in 2012, 15,457 patients underwent upper arm lift in the USA alone, with a 4.4 % increase compared with 2000 [28]. The aim of the surgery is to solve functional and inflammatory issues as well as to restore a pleasant arm contour. Such goal is achieved by means of skin and subcutaneous tissue removal. Several techniques have been described, with ongoing debate regarding the placement of the scar, the area to be excised, the treatment of the axilla, and the concomitant use of liposuction [29, 30]. In the authors' experience, best results and low complication rates are achieved with the surgical technique hereafter described.

25.5.1 Surgical Technique

Preoperative drawings are performed with the patient in standing position and arms abducted. A line is drawn along the posteromedial arm surface, at the site of the future scar. The skin is pinched to assess the cutaneous excess. This maneuver allows to determine the upper and lower borders of the area to be excised. An ellipsis is then drawn, with the previously marked line as its major axis, along the posteromedial arm surface. A Z-plasty is planned in the axilla. The patient undergoes surgery under general anesthesia. Antibiotic prophylaxis is administered with cefazolin at a dose of 2 g i.v. The procedure consists of three phases. First, after infiltration with a solution of mepivacaine and epinephrine, liposuction of the subcutaneous tissue, underlying the marked area, and of persisting localized fat deposits is performed. Circumferential liposuction is sometimes indicated. This first phase allows fat debulking with preservation of vessels

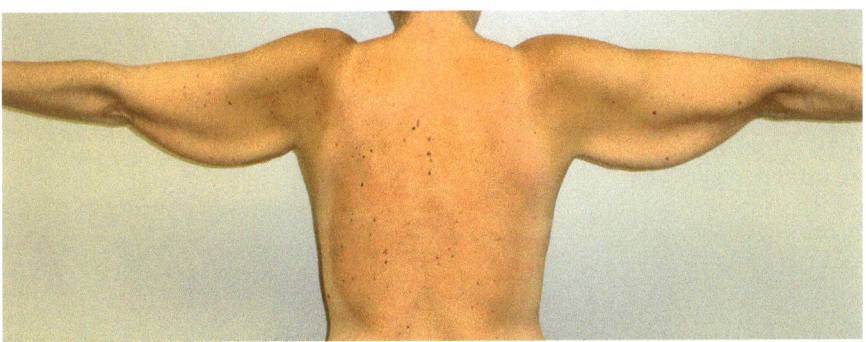

Fig. 25.7 Preoperative view of severe bat-wing deformity

and *lymphatics*. The second phase is surgical excision of the previously marked area. A progressive tailor-tucking technique is used to achieve proper skin resection. Subcutaneous septa, spared by liposuction, are visible during skin removal: these septa must not be excised with the cutaneous ellipsis, in order to spare lymphatics and prevent postoperative *lymphedema*. The third phase is the treatment of the axilla. A Z-plasty is performed to prevent retraction when the upper limb is lifted and to improve axillary contour by restoring medial convexity. No drain is placed, only resorbable sutures are used. The arm is then dressed with a compressive bandage. Mean operation time is 3 h. The patient is discharged on the first postoperative day and is instructed to limit arm movement and to disinfect the axillary wounds multiple times a day. Broad-spectrum antibiotics are administered for 7 days postoperatively. Patients wear a pressure garment for 2 months.

25.5.2 Complications

Several studies reported a high incidence of complications following *brachioplasty* (25–40 %), with 3–25 % of cases requiring a revisional procedure [31–33]. Possible complications are infection, hematoma, *seroma*, wound dehiscence, and hypertrophic scarring. Among these, wound dehiscence and hypertrophic scars are the most common, with a reported incidence of 7.3 and 24 %, respectively [33]. In our experience, these complications are dramatically reduced by debulking the arm with liposuction before surgical excision and by placing the scar on the posteromedial arm surface.

This brachioplasty technique, with a two-step approach (liposuction and dermolipectomy), allows to remove fat deposits and skin excess, reshaping the arm circumferentially. After surgery, patients obtain significant improvement in terms of mobility and preoperative symptoms (Figs. 25.7 and 25.8).

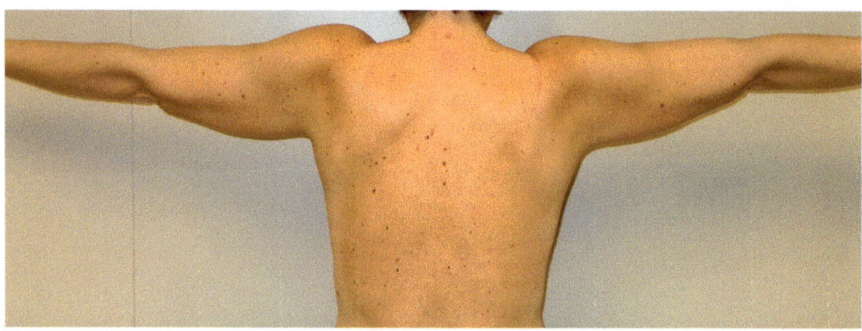

Fig. 25.8 Postoperative result after brachioplasty

References

1. Rubin JP, Matarasso A (2007) Aesthetic surgery after massive weight loss. Elsevier –Saunders. Philadelphia ISBN -13: 978-1-4160-2952-6
2. Ay S, Jean RD, Hurwitz DJ et al (2005) A classification of contour deformities after bariatric weight loss: the Pittsburgh rating scale. Plast Reconstr Surg 116:1535–1544
3. Jabir S (2013) Assessing improvement in quality of life and patient satisfaction following body contouring surgery in patients with massive weight loss: a critical review of outcome measures employed. Plast Surg Int 2013:515737
4. Balagué N, Combesure C, Huber O, Pittet-Cuénod B, Modarressi A (2013) A plastic surgery improves long-term weight control after bariatric surgery. Plast Reconstr Surg 132(4):826–833
5. Giordano S, Victorzon M, Stormi T, Suominen E (2014) Desire for body contouring surgery after bariatric surgery: do body mass index and weight loss matter? Aesthet Surg J 34(1):96–105
6. Aldaqal SM, Makhdoum AM, Turki AM, Awan BA, Samargandi OA, Jamjom H (2013) Post-bariatric surgery satisfaction and body-contouring consideration after massive weight loss. N Am J Med Sci 5(4):301–305
7. Singh D, Zahiri HR, Janes LE, Sabino J, Matthews JA, Bell RL, Thomson JG (2012) Mental and physical impact of body contouring procedures on post-bariatric surgery patients. Eplasty 12:e47, Epub 2012 Sep 12
8. Song AY, Rubin JP, Thomas V, Dudas JR, Marra KG, Fernstrom MH (2006) Body image and quality of life in post massive weight loss body contouring patients. Obesity (Silver Spring) 14(9):1626–1636
9. Torio-Padron N, Stark GB (2009) Body contouring after massive weight loss. Zentralbl Chir 134(1):57–65
10. Colwell AS (2010) Current concepts in post-bariatric body contouring. Obes Surg 20(8):1178–1182
11. Matarasso A, Swift RW, Rankin M (2006) Abdominoplasty and abdominal contour surgery: a national plastic surgery survey. Plast Reconstr Surg 117(6):1797–1808
12. Persichetti P, Simone P, Scuderi N (2005) Anchor-line abdominoplasty: a comprehensive approach to abdominal wall reconstruction and body contouring. Plast Reconstr Surg 116(1):289–294
13. Kim J, Stevenson TR (2006) Abdominoplasty, liposuction of the flanks, and obesity: analyzing risk factors for seroma formation. Plast Reconstr Surg 117(3):773–779; discussion 780–1
14. Le Lourne C, Pascal JF (2000) High superior tension abdominoplasty. Anesth Plast Surg 24:375–381

15. Vastine VI, Morgan RF, WilliAms GS et al (1999) Wound complications of abdominoplasty in obese patients. Ann Plast Surg 42(1):34–39
16. Pollock H, Pollock T (2000) Progressive tension sutures: a technique to reduce local complications in abdominoplasty. Plast Reconstr Surg 105(7):2583–2586
17. Matarasso A, Schneider LF, Barr J (2014) The incidence and management of secondary abdominoplasty and secondary abdominal contour surgery. Plast Reconstr Surg 133(1):40–50
18. Colwell AS, Driscoll D, Breuing KH (2009) Mastopexy techniques after massive weight loss: an algorithmic approach and review of the literature. Ann Plast Surg 63(1):28–33
19. Rubin JP (2006) Mastopexy after massive weight loss: dermal suspension and total parenchymal reshaping. Aesthet Surg J 26(2):214–222
20. Persichetti P, Tenna S, Brunetti B et al (2012) Anterior intercostal artery perforator flap autologous augmentation in bariatric mastopexy. Plast Reconstr Surg 130(4):917–925
21. Rubin JP, Khachi G (2008) Mastopexy after massive weight loss: dermal suspension and selective auto-augmentation. Clin Plast Surg 35(1):123–129
22. Losken A, Holtz DJ (2007) Versatility of the superomedial pedicle in managing the massive weight loss breast: the rotation-advancement technique. Plast Reconstr Surg 120(4):1060–1068
23. Bossert RP, Rubin JP (2012) Evaluation of the weight loss patient presenting for plastic surgery consultation. Plast Reconstr Surg 130:1361–1369
24. Lewis JR Jr (1957) The thigh lift. J Int Coll Surg 27:330–334
25. Lockwood TE (1988) Fascial anchoring technique in medial thigh lifts. Plast Reconstr Surg 82:299–304
26. Moreno CH, Neto HJ, Junior AH, Malheiros CA (2008) Thighplasty after bariatric surgery: evaluation of lymphatic drainage in lower extremities. Obes Surg 18:1160–1164
27. Sarwer DB, Fabricatore AN (2008) Psychiatric considerations of the massive weight loss patient. Clin Plast Surg 35(1):1–10
28. American Society of Plastic Surgeons (2012) Plastic surgery statistics report. http://www.plasticsurgery.org/Documents/news-resources/statistics/2012-Plastic-Surgery-Statistics/body-contouring-after-massive-weight-loss.pdf. Accessed 22 Feb 2014
29. Baroudi R (1975) Dermolipectomy of the upper arm. Clin Plast Surg 2:485–494
30. Symbas JD, Losken A (2010) An outcome analysis of brachioplasty techniques following massive weight loss. Ann Plast Surg 64:588–591
31. Gusenoff JA, Coon D, Rubin JP (2008) Brachioplasty and concomitant procedures after massive weight loss: a statistical analysis from a prospective registry. Plast Reconstr Surg 122(2): 595–603
32. Bossert RP, Dreifuss S, Coon D, Wollstein A, Clavijo-Alvarez J, Gusenoff JA, Rubin JP (2013) Liposuction of the arm concurrent with brachioplasty in the massive weight loss patient: is it safe? Plast Reconstr Surg 131(2):357–365
33. Zomerlei TA, Neaman KC, Armstrong SD, Aitken ME, Cullen WT, Ford RD, Renucci JD, VanderWoude DL (2013) Brachioplasty outcomes: a review of a multipractice cohort. Plast Reconstr Surg 131(4):883–889

26. Nutritional, Metabolic, and Psychological Rehabilitation

Paolo Capodaglio and Maria Letizia Petroni

Obesity is a long-term disease with high comorbidity with considerable impact on disability and quality of life. Rehabilitation of such patients requires a here-and-now multidimensional, comprehensive approach, where the intensity of rehabilitative treatments depends on the disability level and severity of comorbidities and consists of the simultaneous provision of physiotherapy, diet and nutritional support, psychological counseling, adapted physical activity, and specific nursing skills. A multidimensional approach able to provide frontline assessment and preventive strategies, risk stratification, and disease management is needed, and for that purpose, a team approach and the integration of several medical specialties, including clinical nutrition, endocrinology, psychiatry, and rehabilitation medicine encompassing different health professions, including dietitians, psychologists, physiotherapists, and nurses is required. This is in line with the indications of the Italian Society of Obesity [56], the 2010 consensus of the Italian Society of Obesity and the Italian Society of Eating Disorders [21], and the Italian Ministry of Health, who have recently acknowledged [34] the need for a rehabilitation pathway for severely obese patients with comorbidities. Those documents highlight the need for multiple rehabilitative settings according to the severity of disability, which calls for the need for multidimensional evaluation encompassing quality of life, disability, functioning, and participation. The Individual Rehabilitation Project should therefore encompass different interventions and short- and long-term goals:

P. Capodaglio (✉)
UO Riabilitazione e Laboratorio di Ricerca in Biomeccanica e Riabilitazione,
Ospedale S Giuseppe, Istituto Auxologico Italiano IRCCS, Piancavallo, Verbania, Italy

Rehabilitation, Istituto Auxologico Italiano, Via Cadorna 90, Oggebbio (VB), Italy
e-mail: p.capodaglio@auxologico.it

M.L. Petroni
Centro Obesità e Nutrizione Clinica, Ospedale Privato Accreditato Villa Igea,
Forlì 47122, Italy
e-mail: Marialetizia.petroni@gmail.com

© Springer International Publishing Switzerland 2015
A. Lenzi et al. (eds.), *Multidisciplinary Approach to Obesity:
From Assessment to Treatment*, DOI 10.1007/978-3-319-09045-0_26

(a) nutritional intervention, (b) motor/functional rehabilitation, (c) psychotherapeutic interventions, and (d) rehabilitative nursing. Intensive hospital-based rehabilitation for obese patients usually consists of a 4-week multidisciplinary program covering all those aspects. In a rehabilitation program for obese patients, weight loss is one of the main goal that has to be pursued through behavioral modification, diet, and exercise [2] even if the results of such interventions are often disappointing. In addition to optimize the compliance to pharmacologic treatment guidelines, the long timetable of rehabilitation programs allows us to choose drugs that have a favorable effect on weight [6]. Rehabilitation is a setting in which patient-centered care can be vigorously implemented, empowering patients who no longer delegate physicians, but become protagonist in their health management [3, 4]. Clinician–patient communication should be patient centered to include the patient perspective and the psychosocial context along with shared understanding and responsibility. Health literacy improvement is another goal of rehabilitation programs: low health literacy, quite habitual in the obese, can result in decreased adherence to medical recommendations, failure to engage in healthy behaviors, and inferior outcomes. Quality of life should be one of the standard outcome measures of rehabilitation and it should be measured by disease-specific, patient-reported measures [54].

26.1 Nutritional Intervention and Therapeutic Education

It is important that nutritional intervention may contribute to correct previous unhealthy eating habits on a permanent basis. For this purpose there is need of frequent professional contact with the patient aimed at assessing the level of understanding of the given dietary recommendations given, the eradication of bad eating behaviors related to so-called incorrect "dietary beliefs", and the verification of the satisfaction level of the dietary plan (meal organization to suit the patient's needs; as far as reasonably possible, respect of customary dietary habits and tastes while encouraging at the same time novel healthier choices) [7, 8].

As a matter of fact, the nutritional intervention should be included into a process of therapeutic education. This is an essential phase in the management of chronic patients: the aim is to implement the knowledge about the disease and its management and to change behaviors related to it for better management. In addition, therapeutic education allows to understand and to manage the psychological aspects related with the disease itself. Besides the role of providing the patient with information on practical aspects of disease management, therapeutic education also aims to help improve the patient's quality of life [56].

The nutritional intervention is therefore designed to:

- Inform about healthy nutrition and physical activity, with emphasis about regaining the physiological stimuli of hunger and satiety, recognizing the biological significance of food, and rediscovering a sense of comfort with physical activity.

- Train for managing and control nutrition and physical activity, even while under stress or in anxiety.
- Train in the management and control of simple clinical parameters (e.g., blood glucose, blood pressure).
- Increase the sense of responsibility in illness and care (illness behavior).
- Promote, strengthen, and maintain sufficient motivation to change.
- Contribute to the therapeutic compliance.

Therapeutic education for obesity must be guaranteed within the team by professionals (doctor, nurse, dietician, community health educator, psychiatrist, psychologist, exercise physiologists) specifically qualified and trained for educational activity [56].

Motivation is essential for obtaining adhesion to treatment and a stable weight loss. To this purpose, therapeutic education bases most of its intervention through techniques acting on conscious mental processes, some of which derived from cognitive–behavioral therapy, such as therapeutic alliance, problem solving, and empowerment [56].

Nutrition intervention will focus on:

(a) Achieving weight loss of at least 10 % from baseline body weight with a significant reduction in body fat and preservation of lean mass
(b) Reconstructing long-term healthy eating habits (quality, quantity, rate) based on the canons of the Mediterranean diet (www.piramidealimentare.it)
(c) Obtaining a patient's compliance adequate to achieve the established objectives

The procedures listed in Table 26.1 are suitable for most obese patients undergoing rehabilitation treatment. However, in elderly patients the mortality risks of muscle loss may outweigh the potential benefits of weight loss [31] (Miller 2008), and the risk to benefit ratio of treatment should be carefully evaluated. In these patients, whey protein and essential amino acids supplementation has been shown to limit lean tissue loss during hypocaloric diets and – in selected patients deemed adequate – it should be carried out, possibly coupled to strength training. Also, in these patients dynamometry should be routinely performed at the beginning and during weight-loss treatment as a proxy to evaluate changes in muscle mass.

Low-calorie diets (LCD), i.e., with energy content between 800 and 1,200 kcal/day (3,350–5,200 kJ/day) should be considered as first-line treatment subjects requiring fast and substantial weight loss for life-threatening conditions or to reduce anesthesiological and surgical risks. LCDs allow a more rapid loss of body fat with a favorable risk–benefit profile in absence of preexisting undernutrition. The LCD diet can be made of natural foods, meal replacements, and supplements. The LCD cycles usually last between 15 and 21 days alternating with same-duration cycles of standard moderately hypocaloric diets.

Also, there are patients with documented refractoriness to weight loss using conventional hypocaloric diets who represent a challenge for the nutrition rehabilitation

Table 26.1 Procedures for nutritional intervention

The following guidelines for hypocaloric diet composition have recently been published in the Italian standards for the treatment of obesity [56]
Hypocaloric diets should secure a caloric intake equal to ± 10 % of basal metabolism
Carbohydrates, mainly of complex type (fiber rich or containing slow absorption starch) should provide 65–70 % of nonprotein calorie intake ($\geq$150 g/day;, simple sugars should not exceed 10 % of total caloric intake (favoring the consumption of foods that contain natural sugars such as fruit and limiting the consumption of added sucrose)
Foods with low glycemic index are preferable, especially for weight maintenance after a hypocaloric diet
The remainder energy should be covered from fat, with an optimal 10 % monounsaturated, 10 % polyunsaturated, 10 % saturated fatty acids
The intake of polyunsaturated and in particular of n3 fatty acids (for a beneficial effect on the prevention of cardiovascular risk) is ensured through the introduction of at least 2 servings per week of fish
The daily intake of cholesterol should not exceed 300 mg/day in adults
The use of trans fatty acids must be drastically reduced ($\leq$2.5 g/day) because it is associated with increased body weight, waist circumference, and BMI in population-based studies
The recommended protein intake is 0.8–1 g/kg ideal body weight (which correspond to a BMI of 22.5 kg/m2)
Proteins must be of good biological value and must come equally from both animal and vegetable protein sources
Fiber intake is ideally around 30 g/day in order to obtain both functional-type effects (i.e., intestinal function) and metabolic-type effects (glucose and lipid metabolism)
Vitamin needs are generally covered by the consumption of fruits and vegetables generally prescribed in the diet (provided that calorie intake is at least 1,000–1,200 kcal/day)
Maximum sodium intake should approximately be 3 g/day (equivalent to 7.5 g of NaCl); this should further be reduced in patients with hypertension or a family history of hypertension
Calcium requirements are not generally covered by a low-calorie diet, unless two servings/day of dairy products plus if possible integration with calcium-rich waters is provided
Alcohol is not recommended during weight loss because it provides readily available energy (7 kcal/g), without satiating power nor significant advantages with regard to the provision of other nutrients

specialists and for whom no evidence-based treatment is available. In these refractory patients – once other known causes of low metabolic rate such as hypothyroidism, very low levels of 25-OH vitamin D, or significantly reduced fat-free metabolic active mass (sarcopenia) have been ruled out or corrected, a 15–21-day cycle of very-low-calorie diet (VLCD), i.e., energy content <800 kcal day (<3,350 kJ/day) can be attempted under close medical supervision, together with supplementation of vitamins, minerals plus ursodeoxycholic acid for gallstone prevention [23]. They can also be used as an alternative to LCDs or as an alternative to intragastric balloon positioning in patients with morbid obesity whose elective surgery had been postponed because of excessive weight. These diets have traditionally been linked to concern for renal and hepatic derangements, nevertheless a recent systematic review has been quite reassuring under this aspect [47].

Since very-low and low-calorie diets are associated with a greater risk of weight regain in the medium to long term as compared to standard diets, their coupling with an intensive cognitive–behavioral intervention [58] and the subsequent switch to a Mediterranean diet pattern are strongly recommended. Anti-obesity drugs, meal replacements, and high-protein diets may improve weight-loss maintenance after a VLCD/LCD period [28].

Multidisciplinary rehabilitation in *bariatric surgery* patients represents the newest frontier in obesity treatment. Specific protocols for this patient population have been described [22] and can be applied for:

- Assessment, eligibility, and planning
- Risk reduction and preparation to surgery
- Rehabilitation following surgery

26.2 Metabolic Rehabilitation: Adapted Physical Activity

A good activity program should entail both aerobic training, small bursts of anaerobic high-intensity activity and strength exercise. Aerobic activity consists of cycloergometer, recline ergometer, or arm ergometer (the choice depending on the presence of orthopedic problems). Based on the fact that a smaller muscle mass is used in cycling exercise to attain the same metabolic energy expenditure of walking [25] with a greater metabolic stress and energy requirement per unit of contracting muscle [38], it has been evidenced [26] that walking is a convenient mode of exercise, compared to cycling. Walking permits in fact to attain any given energy expenditure at a comparatively lower average heart rate (or in a shorter time), with lower lactic acid blood concentration and higher fat oxidation. In practice, by some reckoning from these data comparing the metabolic responses of the two modalities, to obtain the energy expenditure of 250 kcal with a bout of 25-min activity, cycling should be performed at an intensity requiring an average heart rate of about 160 b/min with 3 g of lipids oxidation, whereas it will be sufficient to walk at intensity requiring an average heart rate of about 130 b/min, with over 11 g of lipid oxidation. Under this perspective, for obese individuals, inherently limited in their work capacity, it is very attractive to devise forms of physical activity enabling the attainment of a considerable energy expenditure by preference promoting substantial fat oxidation with the lower subjective perception of effort and exercise intensity, which could ultimately allow a better tolerance and adherence to physical activity protocols.

The optimal duration of exercise is 30 min, or longer, to optimize fat oxidation [1].

The effects of regular aerobic and resistance training on cardiovascular risk and general well-being are clearly demonstrated [35–37, 39], and increasing both intensity and duration exerts a beneficial effect. Patients who are able to exercise to a level of 7.9 METs have lower rates of events. In our population, in a consecutive sample of 3,728 obese patients, 732 were not able to perform a treadmill exercise test; of the remaining 2,996 the vast majority reached a peak exercise level of less than 7.9 METs, and only 620 patients (21 %) exceeded that threshold. Exercise is safe and the risk of a cardiovascular event is very low in a cardiovascular rehabilitation setting [42–46]. Current guidelines recommend intensity range between 3 and 6 METs on most days of the week: this goal can be achieved by walking 30 min every day or walking 60 min every second day. Cycling also represents a good exercise mode for obese subjects: for those who complain of osteoarticular pain while standing or venous insufficiency, it may represent the first choice modality. Cycling in recline position is a safer mode of exercise, providing back support and relatively lower loading at knee level.

Target heart rate during exercise has to be based on resting heart rate and peak heart rate during a symptom-limited treadmill stress test. We use the formula Target HR = Resting HR + (Peak HR – Resting HR) × 0.7, i.e., resting heart rate + 70 % of the chronotropic reserve that level of effort is generally associated with a "comfortable fatigue" sensation.

Patients also undergo a strength exercise program that is individualized considering patient's characteristics. They work for 45–60 min on a daily basis at low intensity; the main purposes of this activity are to increase muscle strength, to balance muscle tone and mass, to reach a good equilibrium between flexor and extensor muscles, to improve joint stability and mobility, to improve motor coordination, to improve body and motor patterns, and to relax both physically and psychologically.

A significant improvement in quality of life, as well as in life expectancy, can be achieved independently of weight change only because of regular exercise [5]. Cardiac rehabilitation causes a significant improvement in the cardiovascular risk profile at all levels of BMI, independently of weight loss. The issue whether it is weight or fitness that makes the difference has been addressed by Lee and coworkers [27]: they studied over 14,000 men and found that, for each 1-MET improvement, a 19 % decrease in cardiovascular mortality was present, regardless of BMI or percent body fat change. Obese subjects who exercise regularly have a lower risk for metabolic abnormalities and their consequences than sedentary obese and represent the so-called fat-but-fit phenotype. Considering that obesity is a chronic disease and therefore a complete recovery is not foreseeable, we can try to adopt the same concepts that we use when we treat other chronic conditions such as hypertension or diabetes and set the "fat-but-fit" phenotype as a new target for obese subjects [55].

Moreover caution on promoting unconditional weight loss may be safe, since obesity has a complex relationship with all-cause mortality, and, in patients with congestive heart failure or coronary artery disease, the presence of obesity is associated with lower mortality when compared to normally weighting patients [24]. Therefore, our target, even if most of the features that characterize the obesity cardiomyopathy can be reversed by means of weight loss, should mainly focus on the adoption of an active lifestyle which has a great impact on the prognosis of obese patients. For a weight-loss intervention to be successful, a negative energy balance must be attained; in this view, energy expenditure in the form of physical activity is an important part in the management of obesity for losing weight and reducing associated risk factors for chronic disease. Many formulas are recommended, principally in the form of "moderate-intensity exercise" typically defined as 55–70 % of maximum heart rate, 30–60 min day, and 5–7 days a week [29, 30, 33]. Less is known about advisable heavier intensities of exercise. With regard to this last topic, it has been observed that bouts of exercise beyond anaerobic threshold added to a program of aerobic activity significantly increase the release of GH at a more extent than aerobic activity alone during physical exercise. This may be of some interest considering that GH is known as one of the most active substance able to ameliorate the ratio fat mass/fat-free mass [52].

Moreover, aerobic activity alone promotes a modest lowering of fat mass, a reduction in circulating nonesterified fatty acids, and an increase in circulating lactic acid, with a reduction in insulin resistance for glucose. Bouts of added anaerobic exercise to an aerobic program promote a significant more important lowering in fat mass, an increase in circulating nonesterified fatty acids, a decrease in circulating lactic acid, and no modification in insulin resistance for glucose.

The drop in circulating nonesterified fatty acids after aerobic training may be the result of an imbalance between a slow mobilization of fatty acids from adipose tissue and their rapidly increased extraction by skeletal muscle so demonstrating an increased oxidative capacity by the muscle. At the same time, the increase in lactic acid may be linked to the modified utilization of glucose due to the improvement in insulin sensitivity for it. The increase in circulating nonesterified fatty acids after aerobic plus anaerobic training may be due to an increased flow of substances with lipolytic activity after anaerobic stress (like GH, catecholamines, etc.) which causes an excessive mobilization of lipids that probably exceeds their dynamic utilization.

These observations may indicate the opportunity to initially prescribe aerobic with bouts of anaerobic training to decrease fat mass and subsequently aerobic training alone to maintain the weight loss and ameliorate the metabolic profile.

The exercise scheme "aerobic plus anaerobic" is probably inappropriate in obese patients with metabolic syndrome in view of the increase in serum nonesterified fatty acids and the lack of improvement in glucose metabolism [48–51, 53, 57, 59, 60].

Obese inpatients undergo daily functional rehabilitation exercises to optimize muscle strength and the lean to fat mass ratio, increase joint range of motion, and enhance cardiorespiratory conditioning. Since osteoarticular pain at spine, hip, and knee level is a major complaint and an obstacle to functional recovery in obese patients, physiotherapy focuses on joint unloading techniques, with the frequent use of taping and functional bandaging or sling therapy exercises [13–15, 17–20], passive and active lengthening and stretching of the muscular chains of the lower and upper limbs and the spine, strengthening and stabilizing of the lumbar trait, and active and passive mobilization of the dorsal spine [11, 12]. Manual lymphatic drainage and elastic compressive bandaging are also extensively used [13].

Resistance exercises aiming at muscle strengthening to reduce joint compression forces are performed 30–60 min daily. Their aim is also to improve balance by strengthening the heel stabilizer muscles [10]. Intensities of isotonic strengthening exercise are initially set at 40 % of the individual ten-repetition maximum during the first week, 50 % during the second week, and 60 % during the remaining rehabilitation period. The muscle groups to be trained are identified during the initial physiatrist evaluation. Strengthening-supervised exercises with arms and legs include dynamic standing and floor calisthenics using body weight as movement resistance. A major priority of exercise prescription is to focus on activities which contribute to muscular fitness and preserve muscle mass. This goal seems important also in view of the effects of caloric restriction, which result in reductions of both fat and fat-free mass. Water-based rehabilitation programs in a warm hydrotherapy pool are especially suitable for obese patients with osteoarthritis – since the buoyancy of water lightens body weight off the joints. This rehabilitation modality has been shown to be more effective than land-based programs in obese patients with chronic obstructive pulmonary disease [32].

Patients with severe motor limitations undergo physiotherapy and occupational therapy aimed at optimizing their capacities to cope with daily living activities through the use of walking aids, lifting, and transferring devices [9]. Respiratory rehabilitation is very often part of the rehabilitation program and includes adapting and training patients and caregivers to noninvasive ventilation [13]. Body awareness sessions which are carried out by trained therapists (using the Feldenkrais or the Courchinoux method), with a psychological supervision, typically represent an example of multidisciplinary treatment for obese patients with body scheme alteration and/or associated eating disorder.

26.3 Psychotherapeutic Intervention

As indicated in Cochrane systematic reviews, a psychological therapy, particularly cognitive–behavioral therapy (CBT) including psychoeducational approaches, could be functionally combined with a nutritional intervention and physical activity plan increasing weight loss, if compared with the only diet/exercise intervention.

The behavioral part of the therapy in obesity treatment is characterized by self-monitoring (e.g., using diaries), stimulus control (e.g., restricting quantities of food), and behavioral modification (e.g., chewing slowly, taking time to really taste and enjoy the food, maximizing the pleasure from it). According to other authors, components of behavioral therapy for obesity could be specifically self-monitoring, problem solving, contingency management, stimulus control, stress management, social support from family members and friends, and cognitive restructuring.

Moreover cognitive techniques could provide patients with useful strategies to accept realistic, but less-than-desired, weight losses. Relapse and weight regain could be generated by inappropriate feelings of failure after achieving modest but clinically important weight loss. It is focused on dysfunctional behaviors and cognitive processes, such as unrealistic weight goals and body image perceptions.

The mindfulness-based cognitive therapy (MBCT) represents the latter evolution of cognitive therapy for the psychological rehabilitation of obesity. This meditation-based approach was originally described by Kabat-Zinn for stress management and can be applied to weight management to control food cravings and to help patients to recognize internal cues in support of enhanced self-regulation [40].

The psychological intervention is a critical issue because the maintenance of weight loss after lifestyle modification, drug therapy, and weight-loss surgery is more likely to depend on behavior modification and enduring psychosocial support. Long-term behavioral therapy is more successful than short interventions.

Cognitive-behavioral approach represents the gold standard for the treatment of obesity, but other interventions are growing and are collecting new evidences. Hypnosis could supplementarily be used, with particular patients, enhancing them in correcting dysfunctional thoughts, attitudes, and beliefs.

Other promising psychotherapies used for the obesity treatment are the interpersonal approach, the systemic and strategic treatments, the psychodynamic approach, and the feminist-theories-based treatment. Especially for those patients in whom an emotive trauma triggered the onset of obesity, the EMDR (eye movement desensitization and reprocessing) approach could represent an interesting treatment.

Obese patients admitted to intensive rehabilitation programs are generally characterized by history of weight cycling and somatic comorbidities, which represent the main factors known to negatively influence psychological health [41]. Within a rehabilitation setting of a 4-week duration (which s generally considered too short to carry out proper "psychotherapy"), psychological interventions are generally represented by an initial psychodiagnostic assessment (plus a psychiatric evaluation if deemed necessary for drug prescription and/or monitoring) followed by both individual and group psychoeducational sessions. Group treatment helps patients benefit of peer support and problem solving and learn from others' success and difficulties [16]. Individual sessions with a therapist are often also essential – as well as offering an opportunity for experiencing empathic and nonjudgmental listening – to help the patient to focus on emotional vulnerability that may limit a proper adhesion to the strategies of weight control and nutrition and to select the tools best suited for support to long-term weight management. Obese patients with associated eating disorders or psychiatric conditions most likely will need to be referred to a psychotherapist or to mental care services following discharge at home.

References

1. Achten J, Jeukendrup AE (2004) Optimizing fat oxidation through exercise and diet. Nutrition 20:716–727
2. Ades PA, Savage PD, Harvey-Berino J (2010) The treatment of obesity in cardiac rehabilitation. J Cardiopulm Rehabil Prev 30:289–298
3. American College of Cardiology Foundation (2012) Health policy statement on patient-centered care in cardiovascular medicine: a report of the American College of Cardiology Foundation Clinical Quality Committee. J Am Coll Cardiol 59:2125–2143
4. Backholer K, Wong E, Freak-Poli R, Walls HL, Peeters A (2012) Increasing body weight and risk of limitations in activities of daily living: a systematic review and meta-analysis. Obes Rev 13:456–468
5. Byberg L, Mealhus H, Gedeborg R, Sundström J, Ahlbom A, Zethelius B, Berglund LG, Wolk A, Michaëlsson K (2009) Total mortality after changes in leisure time physical activity in 50 years old men: 35 year follow-up population based cohort. Br J Sports Med 43:482

6. Bray GA, Ryan DH (2012) Medical therapy for the patient with obesity. Circulation 125:1695–1703
7. Breland JY, Fox AM, Horowitz CR, Leventhal H (2012) Applying a common-sense approach to fighting obesity. J Obes 2012:710427
8. Brunani A, Liuzzi A, Sirtori A, Raggi A, Berselli ME, Villa V, Ceriani F, Tacchini E, Vicari V, Parisio C, Vismara L, Zanini A, Vinci C, Contini F, Braga E, Ricappi A, Camerlengo M, Ristea M, Leonardi M (2010) Mapping an obesity clinical evaluation protocol to the International Classification of Functioning, disability and health. Disabil Rehabil 32:417–423
9. Capodaglio P, Capodaglio EM (2008) La movimentazione del paziente obeso in ospedale. La Med Lav 99(6):466–477
10. Capodaglio P, Vismara L, Menegoni F, Baccalaro G, Galli M, Grugni G (2009) Strength characterization of knee flexor extensor muscles in Prader-Willi and obese patients. BMC Musculoskelet Disord 10(47):1–8
11. Capodaglio P, Castelnuovo G, Brunani A, Vismara L, Villa V, Capodaglio EM (2010) Functional limitations and occupational issues in obesity: a review. Int J Occup Saf Ergon 16(4):407–423
12. Vismara L, Menegoni F, Zaina F, Galli M, Negrini S, Capodaglio P (2010) Effect of obesity and low back pain on spinal mobility: a cross sectional study in women. J Neuroeng Rehabil 7(1):3
13. Capodaglio P, Vismara L, Tacchini E, Corsetti C, La fortuna C, Bozzoli E, Villa V, Parisio C, Mallone M, Baracchini M, Verzeni V, Precilios H, DeSouza S, Castelnuovo G (2011) Obesità e Riabilitazione. Il Fisioterapista 17(6):9–29
14. Capodaglio P, Liuzzi A, Faintuch J (eds) (2013) Disabling obesity: from determinants to health care models. Springer, Heidelberg
15. Capodaglio P, Cimolin V, Tacchini E, Precilios H, Brunani A (2013) Effectiveness of in-patient rehabilitation in obesity-related orthopedic conditions. J Endocrinol Invest 36(8):628–631. doi: 10.3275/8897
16. Cavill N, Hillsdon M, Anstiss T (2011) Brief interventions for weight management. National Obesity Observatory, Oxford
17. Cerretelli P, Di Prampero E (1987) Gas exchange in exercise. In: Farhi LE, Tenney SM (eds) Handbook of physiology, the respiratory system. Gas exchange. American Physiology Society, Bethesda, pp 307–309
18. Coker RH, Miller S, Schutzler S, Deutz N, Wolfe RR (2012) Whey protein and essential amino acids promote the reduction of adipose tissue and increased muscle protein synthesis during caloric restriction-induced weight loss in elderly, obese individuals. Nutr J 11:105
19. DeCaria JE, Sharp C, Petrella JP (2012) Scoping review report: obesity in older adults. Int J Obes 36:1141–1150
20. Donini LM, Brunani A, Sirtori A, Savina C, Tempera S, Cuzzolaro M, Spera G, Cimolin V, Precilios H, Raggi A, Capodaglio P, SIO-SISDCA Task Force (2011) Assessing disability in morbidly obese individuals: the Italian Society of Obesity test for obesity-related disabilities. Disabil Rehabil 33:2509–2518
21. Donini LM, Cuzzolaro M, Spera G, Badiali M, Basso N, Bollea MR (2010) Obesity and eating disorders. Indications for the different levels of care. An Italian expert consensus document. Eat Weight Disord 15(1–2 Suppl):1–31
22. Donini LM, Petroni ML (2013) Principles and protocols in nutritional rehabilitation. In: Capodaglio P, Liuzzi A, Faintuch J (eds) Disabling obesity: from determinants to health care models. Springer, Heidelberg
23. Festi D, Colecchia A, Larocca A, Villanova N, Mazzella G, Petroni ML, Romano F, Roda E (2000) Review: low caloric intake and gall-bladder motor function. Aliment Pharmacol Ther 14(Suppl 2):51–53
24. Fonarow GC, Srikanthan P, Costanzo MR, Cintron GB, Lopatin M, ADHERE Scientific Advisory Committee and Investigators (2007) An obesity paradox in acute heart failure: analysis of body mass index and inhospital mortality for 108,927 patients in the Acute Decompensated Heart Failure National Registry. Am Heart J 153:74–81

25. Hermansen L, Saltin B (1969) Oxygen uptake during maximal treadmill and bicycle exercise. J Appl Physiol 26:31–37
26. Lafortuna CL, Lazzer S, Agosti F, Busti C, Galli R, Mazzilli G, Sartorio A (2010) Metabolic responses to submaximal treadmill walking and cycle ergometer pedalling in obese adolescents. Scand J Med Sci Sports 20:630–637
27. Lee SL, Blair SN, Jackson AS (1999) Cardiorespiratory fitness, body composition, and cardiovascular disease mortality in men. Am J Clin Nutr 69:373–380
28. Johansson K, Neovius M, Hemmingsson E (2014) Effects of anti-obesity drugs, diet, and exercise on weight-loss maintenance after a very-low-calorie diet or low-calorie diet: a systematic review and meta-analysis of randomized controlled trials. Am J Clin Nutr 99(1):14–23
29. Matus CD, Klaege K (2007) Exercise and weight management. Prim Care Clin Off Pract 34:109–116
30. Malatesta D, Vismara L, Menegoni F, Galli M, Romei M, Capodaglio P (2009) Mechanical external work and recovery at preferred walking speed in obese subjects. Med Sci Sports Exerc 41(2):426–434
31. Miller SL, Wolfe RR (2008) The danger of weight loss in the elderly. J Nutr Health Aging 12(7):487–491
32. McNamara RJ, McKeough ZJ, McKenzie DK, Alison JA (2013) Obesity in COPD: the effect of water-based exercise. Eur Respir J 42:1737–1739
33. Menegoni F, Galli M, Tacchini E, Vismara L, Cavigioli M, Capodaglio P (2009) Gender-specific effect of obesity on balance. Obesity 17(10):1951–1956
34. Ministero della Salute (2011) Piano di Indirizzo per la Riabilitazione. Available at: http://www.salute.gov.it/imgs/C_17_pubblicazioni_1546_allegato.pdf
35. Mutlu GM, Rubinstein I (2005) The saga of obstructive sleep apnea syndrome and daytime hypercapnia: work in progress. Chest 127:698–699
36. Naimark A, Cherniack RM (1960) Compliance of the respiratory system and its components in health and obesity. J Appl Physiol 15:377–382
37. Kodama S, Saito K, Tanaka S, Maki M, Yachi Y, Asumi M, Sugawara A, Totsuka K, Shimano H, Ohashi Y, Yamada N, Sone H (2009) Cardiorespiratory fitness as a quantitative predictor of all-cause mortality and cardiovascular events in healthy men and women. J Am Med Assoc 301:2024–2035
38. Koyal SN, Whipp BJ, Huntsman D, Bray GA, Wasserman K (1976) Ventilatory responses to the metabolic acidosis of treadmill and cycle ergometry. J Appl Physiol 40:864–867
39. Kokkinos P, Myers J (2010) Exercise and physical activity. Clinical outcomes and applications. Circulation 122:1637–1648
40. O'Reilly GA, Cook L, Spruijt-Metz D, Black DS (2014) Mindfulness-based interventions for obesity-related eating behaviours: a literature review. Obes Rev 15:453–461
41. Petroni ML, Villanova N, Avagnina S, Fusco MA, Fatati G, Compare A, Marchesini G, QUOVADIS Study Group (2007) Psychological distress in morbid obesity in relation to weight history. Obes Surg 17:391–399
42. Pekkarinen T, Mustajoki P (1997) Use of very low-calorie diet in preoperative weight loss: efficacy and safety. Obes Res 5:595–602
43. Piper AJ, Wang D, Yee BJ, Barnes DJ, Grunstein RR (2008) Randomised trial of CPAP vs bilevel support in the treatment of obesity hypoventilation syndrome without severe nocturnal desaturation. Thorax 63:395–401
44. Precilios H, Brunani A, Cimolin V, Tacchini E, Donini LM, Fabris De Souza S, Capodaglio P, Precilios H (2012) Measuring changes after multidisciplinary rehabilitation of obese individuals. J Endocrinol Invest. doi: 10.3275/8240
45. Raggi A, Brunani A, Sirtori A, Liuzzi A, Berselli ME, Villa V, Ceriani F, ICF-Obesity Group, Leonardi M (2010) Obesity-related disability: key factors identified by the International Classification of Functioning, disability and health (ICF). Disabil Rehabil 32:2028–2034
46. Rognmo O, Moholdt T, Bakken H, Hole T, Mølstad P, Myhr NE, Grimsmo J, Wisløff U (2012) Cardiovascular risk of high- versus moderate-intensity aerobic exercise in coronary heart disease patients. Circulation 126:1436–1440

47. Rolland C, Mavroeidi A, Johnston KL, Broom J (2013) The effect of very low-calorie diets on renal and hepatic outcomes: a systematic review. Diabetes Metab Syndr Obes Targets Ther 6:393–401
48. Rosen CJ, Bouxsein ML (2006) Mechanism of disease: is osteoporosis the obesity of bone? Nat Clin Pract Rheumatol 2:35–43
49. Salvadori A, Fanari P, Mazza P, Agosti R, Longhini E (1992) Work capacity and cardiopulmonary adaptation of the obese subject during exercise testing. Chest 01:674–679
50. Salvadori A, Fanari P, Tovaglieri I, Giacomotti E, Nibbio F, Belardi F, Longhini E (2008) Ventilation and its control during incremental exercise in obesità. Respiration 75:26–33
51. Salvadori A, Fanari P, Palmulli P, Giacomotti E, Arreghini M, Bolla G, Miserocchi G, Longhini E (1999) Cardiovascular and adrenergic response to exercise in obese subjects. J Clin Basic Cardiol 2:229–236
52. Salvadori A, Fanari P, Marzullo P, Codecasa F, Tovaglieri I, Cornacchia M, Walker G, Brunani A, Longhini E (2010) Dynamics of GH secretion during incremental exercise in obesity, before and after a short period of training at different work-loads. Clin Endocrinol 73:491–496
53. Salvadori A, Fanari P, Marzullo P, Codecasa F, Tovaglieri I, Cornacchia M, Brunani A, Luzi L, Longhini E (2014) Short bouts of anaerobic exercise increase non-esterified fatty acids release in obesity. Eur J Nutr 53(1):243–249
54. Spertus JA (2008) Evolving applications for patient-centered health status measures. Circulation 118:2103–2110
55. Sui X, LaMonte MJ, Laditka JN, Hardin JW, Chase N, Hooker SP, Blair SN (2007) Cardiorespiratory fitness and adiposity as mortality predictors in older adults. J Am Med Assoc 298:2507–2516
56. Standard Italiani per la Cura dell'Obesità S.I.O./A.D.I. 2012/2013
57. Stucki A, Daansen P, Fuessl M, Cieza A, Huber E, Atkinson R, Kostanjsek N, Stucki G, Ruof J (2004) ICF core sets for obesity. J Rehabil Med 44(Suppl):107–113
58. Wadden TA, Sternberg JA, Letizia KA, Stunkard AJ, Foster GD (1989) Treatment of obesity by very low calorie diet, behavior therapy, and their combination: a five-year perspective. Int J Obes 13(Suppl 2):39–46
59. WHO (2008) The global burden of disease: 2004 update. WHO, Geneva
60. Zarich SW, Kowalchuk EA, Nesto RW (1991) Left ventricular filling abnormalities in asymptomatic morbid obesity. Am J Cardiol 68:377–381

Increasing Adherence to Diet and Exercise Through Cognitive Behavioural Strategies

27

Riccardo Dalle Grave, Simona Calugi, and Marwan El Ghoch

27.1 Introduction

Specifically designed cognitive behavioural principles are adopted in the management of obesity with a view to improving patients' long-term adherence to the changes in their eating and exercising habits. Originally, the treatment was based on learning theory (i.e. behaviourism), which postulates that the behaviours directly leading to obesity (overeating and under-exercising) are predominantly learned and can therefore be modified or relearned by associating re-education strategies with procedures designed to modify environmental cues (antecedents) and reinforce 'good' behaviour (consequences) [1]. However, since our understanding of the root causes of obesity has progressed, this approach to treatment has seen the integration of procedures derived from social cognitive theory [2] and cognitive therapy [3], as well as specific recommendations on diet and exercise. This complex combination is now known as 'weight loss lifestyle modification' [4], and here we describe the principal components, the short- and long-term outcomes, and recent developments in such treatment programmes.

27.2 Delivery of Weight Loss Lifestyle Modification Programmes

Losing weight is only half the story, and so weight loss lifestyle modification programmes are designed to feature both a weight loss phase, consisting of 16–24 weekly sessions over a 6-month period, and a phase targeted to weight maintenance.

R. Dalle Grave (✉) • S. Calugi • M. El Ghoch
Department of Eating and Weight Disorders, Villa Garda Hospital,
Via Montebaldo, 89, Garda (VR) 37016, Italy
e-mail: rdalleg@tin.it; si.calugi@gmail.com; marwan1979@hotmail.com

Fig. 27.1 The three components of weight loss lifestyle modification programmes

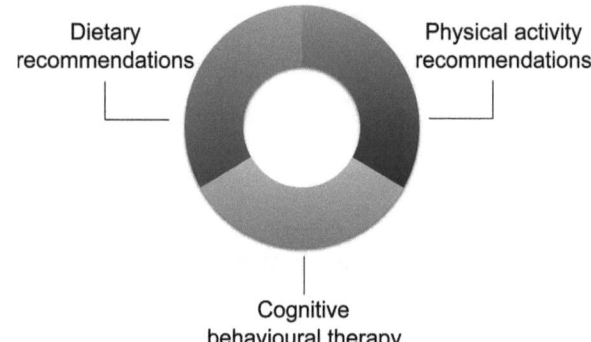

While there is general agreement about the length of the first phase – after 6 months weight loss tends to reach a plateau – no definitive data is yet available about the optimal duration and intensity of the weight maintenance phase [5].

The literature to date mainly derives from clinical research settings, in which the treatment has been tested in individual sessions, in group sessions comprising ~10–20 participants, and in various combinations of the two. In the real world, however, weight loss lifestyle modification programmes are delivered in various clinical environments, including primary care, private dietetics practices, inpatient rehabilitation units, and commercial clinics. Although the treatment can be delivered by a variety of professional figures, such as physicians, dieticians, physiotherapists, and psychologists trained in cognitive behavioural therapy for obesity, known as 'lifestyle modification counsellors', a multidisciplinary lifestyle modification team is best placed to manage the complex clinical problems often associated with obesity [5]. In these multidisciplinary teams, the physicians assess the patients, manage any medical complications, engage the patient in the treatment, and conduct periodic medical check-ups, and the other aspects of lifestyle modification are handled by the relevant experts in a fully orchestrated approach.

27.3 Lifestyle Modification Programme Components

Standard lifestyle modification programmes have three main components: (i) dietary recommendations, (ii) physical activity recommendations, and, last but by no means least, (iii) cognitive behavioural therapy to address weight loss and weight maintenance obstacles [4] (Fig. 27.1).

27.3.1 Dietary Recommendations

Weight loss lifestyle modification programmes recommend a low-fat, (relatively) high-carbohydrate, low-calorie diet aimed at inducing a calorie deficit of 500–1,000 kcal/day. This should produce a mean weight loss of 0.5–1.0 kg/week and eventually reduce cardiovascular risk markers [6]. Unfortunately, the main obstacle to reaching these goals is the patients themselves, and adherence is often an issue. However, empowering patients by training them to count their own calorie intake, with the aid of a purpose-designed booklet, can go some way to improving adherence, as can increasing dietary structuralization and limiting food choices. Providing comprehensive meal plans, including grocery lists, menus, and recipes, helps to add structure to the diet, and restricting the choice of food will reduce temptation and the opportunity to miscalculate energy intake [4]. The effectiveness of this strategy is supported by a study showing that the provision of both low-calorie food (free of charge or subsidized) and structured meal plans resulted in significantly greater weight loss than a diet with no additional structuralization [7]. Another useful strategy for increasing diet adherence is meal replacement, as confirmed by a meta-analysis of six RCTs, which showed that patients given liquid meal replacements lost 3 kg more on average than those on a conventional diet [8]. Finally, a similarly effective strategy for facilitating dietary adherence and weight loss is the use of portion-controlled servings of conventional foods [9].

27.3.2 Physical Activity Recommendations

The goal of lifestyle modification programmes is to help patients gradually achieve a level of physical activity sufficient to produce a calorie deficit of at least 400 kcal/day [10]. Patients are encouraged to check their baseline number of steps using a pedometer and then to add 500 steps at 3-day intervals up to a target value of 10,000–12,000 steps/day. Jogging (20–40 min/day), cycling, or swimming (45–60 min/day) may replace walking. Unlike diet adherence, exercise adherence tends to increase the less structure is imposed, presumably through a reduction in the barriers to exercising (e.g. lack of time or financial resources) [4]. This is supported by several studies, for example, one showing that patients tend to engage in more physical activity if instructed to do so on their own at home than if asked to attend on-site, supervised, group-based exercise sessions [11]. Interestingly, it has also been reported that increasing lifestyle activity (e.g. using stairs rather than elevators, walking rather than riding the bus or driving, and reducing the use of labour-saving devices) can produce comparable weight loss to structured exercise programmes, but greater weight maintenance over time [12]. It may also be helpful to suggest multiple short sessions of exercise (of 10 min each), as opposed to long workouts, an approach that seems to help patients accumulate more minutes of daily exercise [13].

27.3.3 Cognitive Behavioural Therapy

The cognitive behavioural therapy component of lifestyle modification programmes is based upon a set of procedures, which have been described in several recent reviews [4, 5, 14], aimed at addressing both weight loss and weight maintenance obstacles (see Table 27.1).

Table 27.1 Main cognitive behavioural procedures of weight lost lifestyle modification programmes

Procedures for addressing weight loss obstacles
Self-monitoring
Goal setting
Stimulus control
Practising alternative behaviours
Proactive problem solving
Cognitive restructuring
Involving significant others
Procedures for addressing weight maintenance obstacles
Providing continuous care
Encouraging patients to work on weight maintenance instead of weight loss
Establishing weight maintenance range and long-term self-monitoring
Building the long-term weight control mindset
Discontinuing self-monitoring
Devising a contingency plan
Building a weight maintenance plan

One of the main problems with traditional weight loss lifestyle modification programmes delivered in group sessions is that they are essentially a series of prepackaged lessons in which the clinicians teach all patients all the procedures involved in the programme. The lessons are delivered in the preplanned order, even if one or more patients have not yet had enough input to overcome their problems or have failed to understand entirely. These programmes therefore more resemble psycho-educational intervention than the cognitive behaviour therapy applied in the treatment of other psychological disorders, in which the approach is highly personalized and the procedures are introduced in such a way as to target the specific processes maintaining a patient's problems. The most recent developments in weight loss lifestyle modification programmes partly have made some steps to personalize delivery by introducing individual sessions with a case manager [15, 16], but the set lessons and uniformity of procedures still apply.

The Villa Garda lifestyle modification programme [5], on the other hand, has been designed to maximize the individualization of such treatment and is delivered in individual sessions that follow a structure similar to that of cognitive behavioural therapy for eating disorders (i.e. in-session weighing, reviewing self-monitoring, setting the agenda collaboratively, working through the agenda, setting homework, summarizing the session, and arranging the next appointment). The programme also benefits from the introduction of the personal 'cognitive behavioural formulation', a procedural tool specifically designed to further individualize the treatment. The formulation, widely used in other areas of cognitive behavioural therapy [17], but not in standard weight loss lifestyle modification programmes, is a visual representation (a diagram) of the main cognitive behavioural processes that are hindering adhesion to weight loss and lifestyle change in a particular patient. Led by the clinician, but with the active involvement of the patient, the formulation is constructed

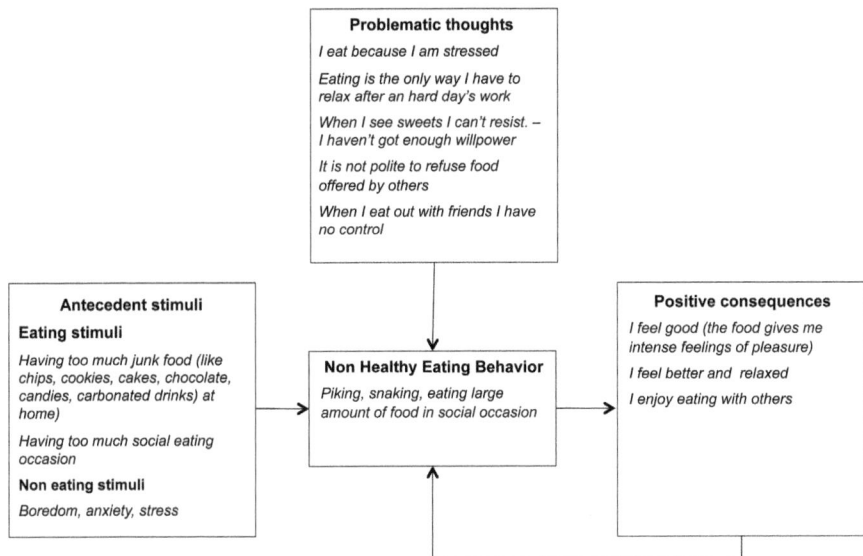

Fig. 27.2 An example of personal cognitive behavioural formulation, featuring a patient's main obstacles to weight loss (based on this formulation, the treatment was focused on reducing eating stimuli; addressing boredom, anxiety, and stress; challenging problematic thoughts; and finding alternatives to food as a reward) (From Dalle Grave et al. [5]:1–11. Copyright © 2013 Springer-Verlag GmbH)

step by step, without haste. A natural first step in this process is to elicit from the patient which, if any, stimuli are associated with eating (i.e. the sight of food, social eating situations) and/or do not (i.e. life events and changes of mood) influence their eating behaviour. The clinician can then assess whether overeating is maintained by any positive emotional and/or physical consequences of food intake and/or bring to light any problematic thoughts (see Fig. 27.2). In this way the formulation helps the clinician to select the specific procedures most likely to help the patient and to implement a targeted, fully individualized treatment. Once the formulation has been drawn up, the clinician can discuss its implications with the patient, emphasizing that control of eating is not wholly dependent on their willpower, but can be improved through specific strategies designed to counteract the processes hampering adhesion to the eating changes necessary to lose weight. The clinician should also stress that the formulation is provisional and will be custom modified as needed during the course of the treatment.

27.4 Outcomes of Weight Loss Lifestyle Modification Programmes

A recent systematic review on the outcome of weight loss lifestyle modification programmes found that at 1 year, about 30 % of participants had a weight loss of ≥10 %, 25 % of between 5 % and 9.9 %, and 40 % of ≤4.9 % [18]. As mentioned, weight loss reaches its peak after 6 months of treatment, and in the absence of a weight maintenance programme, the trend starts to reverse, with half of patients returning to their original weight after about 5 years [19]. However, trials of the latest incarnations of weight loss lifestyle modification programmes that include the most innovative and powerful procedures have shown better long-term results. The most striking example is the Look AHEAD (Action for Health in Diabetes) study, which assessed the effects of intentional weight loss on cardiovascular morbidity and mortality in 5,145 overweight/obese adults with type 2 diabetes, randomly assigned to intensive lifestyle intervention (ILI) or usual care (i.e. diabetes support and education – DSE). At year 8, 88 % of both groups completed an outcomes assessment, which revealed that ILI and DSE participants lost, on average, 4.7 % and 2.1 % of their initial weight, respectively ($P<0.001$). Among the ILI and DSE participants, 50.3 and 35.7 %, respectively, lost ≥ 5 % ($P<0.001$), and 26.9 and 17.2 %, respectively, lost ≥ 10 % ($P<0.001$) [20]. These impressive figures show that well-conducted lifestyle modification programmes can produce clinically meaningful weight loss long-term.

27.5 New Avenues

In recent years, major efforts have been devoted to improving weight loss lifestyle modification programme outcomes by integrating pharmacotherapy, residential treatment, and/or bariatric surgery.

27.5.1 Combining Weight Loss Lifestyle Modification with Pharmacotherapy

One of the main factors implicated in the long-term failure of weight maintenance is the biological pressure to regain weight. Pharmacological therapies may be able to alleviate this pressure, and it is therefore vital to consider their integration into weight loss lifestyle modification programmes. The most significant study on this issue to date is a randomized controlled trial that compared the effects of group-based weight loss lifestyle modification and sibutramine (15 mg/day), alone or in combination. This revealed that, after 1 year, participants treated with the combined approach lost nearly twice as much weight as those receiving either therapy alone [21]. Unfortunately, sibutramine has now been taken off the market due to an unfavourable safety record in individuals with pre-existing cardiovascular diseases or diabetes mellitus. Nonetheless, the availability of new weight loss drugs (i.e. lorcaserin hydrochloride or a combination of phentermine and extended-release topiramate), recently approved by the US Food and Drug Administration, may prove effective in combination with lifestyle modification in the management of obese patients.

27.5.2 Combining Lifestyle Modification with Inpatient Rehabilitation

Inpatient rehabilitation treatment has been developed in Italy to manage patients with morbid obesity and severe comorbidities and/or disability who do not respond to standard outpatient treatment. A recent randomized controlled trial assessed the effect on 88 morbidly obese patients of high-protein (HPD) and high-carbohydrate diets (HCD), of identical energy content and percentage fat and saturated fat, combined with individualized weight loss cognitive behavioural procedures based on the principles described in this chapter [22]. The treatment was divided into two stages: stage one (inpatient treatment, 3 weeks) comprising 15 group cognitive behavioural sessions (5 per week), regular scheduled aerobic exercise, and 6 physiotherapist-led callisthenics sessions and stage two (outpatient treatment, 40 weeks) comprising 12 individual sessions of 45 min each with a dietician trained in lifestyle modification, held over a period of 40 weeks. In completers ($N=69$), weight loss was 15.0 % for HPD and 13.3 % for HCD at 43 weeks, with no significant difference between the arms observed throughout the study period (Fig. 27.3). Both diets also produced a similar improvement in cardiovascular risk factors and psychological profiles. The percentage weight loss achieved by these treatments was much higher than the mean 8–10 % seen in conventional lifestyle modification programmes, and, furthermore, no tendency to regain weight was observed between months 6 and 12. These findings indicate that inpatient rehabilitation treatment followed by individual outpatient sessions can increase the positive effect of lifestyle modification on weight loss and maintenance.

27.5.3 Combining Lifestyle Modification with Bariatric Surgery

Bariatric surgery makes no claims to modify a patient's lifestyle, instead achieving weight loss through the biological alteration of gastrointestinal function; hence, long-term maintenance is by no means guaranteed. However, it is likely that combining bariatric surgery with a weight loss lifestyle modification programme may improve the patient outcomes. Confirmation of this hypothesis comes from a trial of 144 Hispanic Americans randomized, 6 months after gastric bypass surgery, to comprehensive nutrition and lifestyle educational intervention ($n=72$) or not ($n=72$) [23]. Twelve months after the surgery, both groups had lost significant weight, but those who also received weight loss lifestyle modification showed greater excess weight loss (80 % vs. 64 % of preoperative excess weight; $P<0.001$) and were significantly more involved in physical activity than comparison group participants. Another study randomized 60 consecutive morbidly obese patients who had undergone gastric bypass surgery into low-exercise or multiple-exercise groups, finding that the latter patients had a significantly more rapid reduction of body mass index, excess weight loss, and fat mass compared with the former [24].

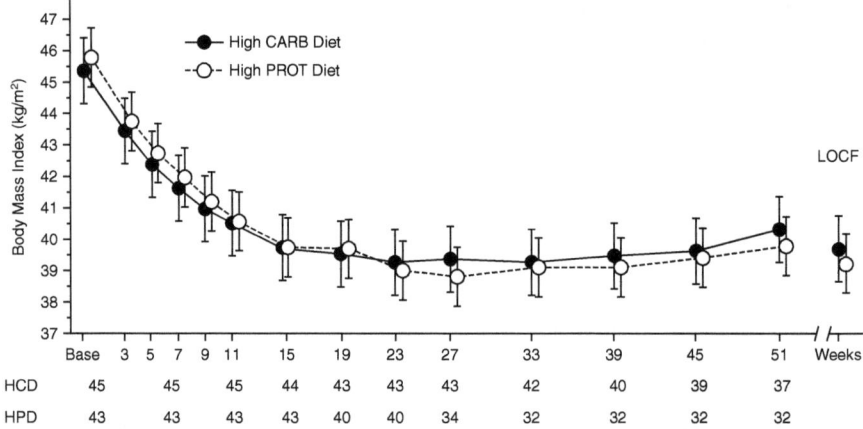

Fig. 27.3 Mean body weight of participants on the high-protein or high-carbohydrate diet combined with an intensive weight loss lifestyle modification programme. Error bars represent 95 % confidence intervals (From Dalle Grave et al. [22]. Copyright © 2013 The Obesity Society)

As a whole, these findings indicate that bariatric surgery may be more effective if integrated in a broader strategy of obesity management including education and lifestyle modifications.

Conclusions

Lifestyle modification is the cornerstone of obesity management. Programmes based on lifestyle modification have been dramatically improved over recent years, and we now have data proving their efficacy in producing long-term weight loss. Very promising results have been achieved by individualizing the treatment and integrating innovative cognitive behavioural procedures. Recent data also show that weight loss outcomes are improved when pharmacotherapy, inpatient treatment, and bariatric surgery are combined with lifestyle modification, indicating that such programmes should be at the forefront of an individualized multidisciplinary treatment for obesity.

References

1. Stuart RR (1967) Behavioral control of overeating. Behav Res Ther 5:357–365
2. Bandura A (1986) Social foundations of thought and action: a social cognitive theory. Prentice-Hall, Englewood Cliffs
3. Beck AT, Rush AJ, Shaw BF, Emery G (1979) Cognitive therapy of depression: a treatment manual. Guilford Press, New York
4. Fabricatore AN (2007) Behavior therapy and cognitive-behavioral therapy of obesity: is there a difference? J Am Diet Assoc 107:92–99
5. Dalle Grave R, Calugi S, El Ghoch M (2013) Lifestyle modification in the management of obesity: achievements and challenges. Eat Weight Disord 18:339–349

6. Clinical guidelines on the identification, evaluation, and treatment of overweight and obesity in adults-the evidence report. National Institutes of Health (1998). Obes Res 6(Suppl 2): 51S–209S
7. Wing RR, Jeffery RW, Burton LR, Thorson C, Sperber-Nissimoff K, Baxter JE (1996) Food provision vs. structured meal plans in the behavioral treatment of obesity. Int J Obes Relat Metab Disord 20:56–62
8. Heymsfield SB, van Mierlo CA, van der Knaap HC, Heo M, Frier HI (2003) Weight management using a meal replacement strategy: meta and pooling analysis from six studies. Int J Obes Relat Metab Disord 27:537–549
9. Metz JA, Stern JS, Kris-Etherton P, Reusser ME, Morris CD, Hatton DC, Oparil S, Haynes RB, Resnick LM, Pi-Sunyer FX, Clark S, Chester L, McMahon M, Snyder GW, McCarron DA (2000) A randomized trial of improved weight loss with a prepared meal plan in overweight and obese patients: impact on cardiovascular risk reduction. Arch Intern Med 160:2150–2158
10. Dalle Grave R, Centis E, Marzocchi R, El Ghoch M, Marchesini G (2013) Major factors for facilitating change in behavioural strategies to reduce obesity. Psychol Res Behav Manag 6:101–110
11. Perri MG, Martin AD, Leermakers EA, Sears SF, Notelovitz M (1997) Effects of group – versus home-based exercise in the treatment of obesity. J Consult Clin Psychol 65:278–285
12. Andersen RE, Wadden TA, Bartlett SJ, Zemel B, Verde TJ, Franckowiak SC (1999) Effects of lifestyle activity vs structured aerobic exercise in obese women: a randomized trial. JAMA 281:335–340
13. Jakicic JM, Wing RR, Butler BA, Robertson RJ (1995) Prescribing exercise in multiple short bouts versus one continuous bout: effects on adherence, cardiorespiratory fitness, and weight loss in overweight women. Int J Obes Relat Metab Disord 19:893–901
14. Wadden TA, Webb VL, Moran CH, Bailer BA (2012) Lifestyle modification for obesity: new developments in diet, physical activity, and behavior therapy. Circulation 125:1157–1170
15. The Diabetes Prevention Program (DPP): description of lifestyle intervention (2002). Diabetes Care 25:2165–2171
16. Ryan DH, Espeland MA, Foster GD, Haffner SM, Hubbard VS, Johnson KC, Kahn SE, Knowler WC, Yanovski SZ (2003) Look AHEAD (Action for Health in Diabetes): design and methods for a clinical trial of weight loss for the prevention of cardiovascular disease in type 2 diabetes. Control Clin Trials 24:610–628
17. Fairburn CG, Cooper Z, Shafran R, Bohn K, Hawker DM, Murphy R, Straebler S (2008) Enhanced cognitive behavior therapy for eating disorders: the core protocol. In: Fairburn CG (ed) Cognitive behavior therapy and eating disorders. Guilford Press, New York, pp 45–193
18. Christian JG, Tsai AG, Bessesen DH (2010) Interpreting weight losses from lifestyle modification trials: using categorical data. Int J Obes 34:207–209
19. Wing RR (2002) Behavioral weight control. In: Wadden TA, Stunkard AJ (eds) Handbook of obesity treatment. The Guildford Press, New York, pp 301–316
20. Eight-year weight losses with an intensive lifestyle intervention: the look AHEAD study (2014). Obesity 22:5–13
21. Wadden TA, Berkowitz RI, Womble LG, Sarwer DB, Phelan S, Cato RK, Hesson LA, Osei SY, Kaplan R, Stunkard AJ (2005) Randomized trial of lifestyle modification and pharmacotherapy for obesity. N Engl J Med 353:2111–2120
22. Dalle Grave R, Calugi S, Gavasso I, El Ghoch M, Marchesini G (2013) A randomized trial of energy-restricted high-protein versus high-carbohydrate, low-fat diet in morbid obesity. Obesity 21:1774–1781
23. Nijamkin MP, Campa A, Sosa J, Baum M, Himburg S, Johnson P (2012) Comprehensive nutrition and lifestyle education improves weight loss and physical activity in Hispanic Americans following gastric bypass surgery: a randomized controlled trial. J Acad Nutr Diet 112:382–390
24. Shang E, Hasenberg T (2010) Aerobic endurance training improves weight loss, body composition, and co-morbidities in patients after laparoscopic Roux-en-Y gastric bypass. Surg Obes Relat Dis 6:260–266

Interdisciplinary Approach to Obesity

28

Stefania Mariani, Mikiko Watanabe, Carla Lubrano,
Sabrina Basciani, Silvia Migliaccio, and Lucio Gnessi

28.1 Introduction

Obesity is a complex disease of multifactorial origin. Genes, socioeconomic status, dietary patterns, and psychological profile are only some of the factors that may lead to excess body weight and its deleterious outcomes.

The management and treatment of obesity have wider objectives than weight loss alone or fat mass reduction and include mortality risk decrease and health and quality of life improvement. Appropriate treatment of obesity comorbidities in addition to weight loss should include glyco-insulinemic and lipid profile control, blood pressure management, evaluation of respiratory disorders (such as sleep apnea syndrome), pain control and mobility needs in osteoarthritis, management of psychosocial disturbances, including affective disorders, eating disorders, and body image disturbance. The socioeconomic context of patients also needs to be taken into account in establishing the correct treatment strategy.

Appropriate goals of weight management should be a realistic weight loss in order to achieve a reduction in health risks and should include promotion and maintenance of weight loss. Patients should understand that, since obesity is a chronic disease, weight management will need to be lifelong [1].

S. Mariani • M. Watanabe • C. Lubrano • S. Basciani • L. Gnessi (✉)
Department of Experimental Medicine, Section of Medical Pathophysiology,
Food Science and Endocrinology, Sapienza University of Rome,
Viale del Policlinico, Rome 00161, Italy
e-mail: stefaniamariani@yahoo.com; mikiko.watanabe@gmail.com;
carla.lubrano@uniroma1.it; sabrinabascaini@yahoo.it; lucio.gnessi@uniroma1.it

S. Migliaccio
Department of Movement, Human and Health Sciences, Unit of Endocrinology,
University of Rome "Foro Italico", Largo Lauro De Bosis 15, Rome 00195, Italy
e-mail: silvia.migliaccio@uniroma4.it

28.2 Multidimensional Evaluation

Obese patients should be evaluated in a multidimensional manner covering six fields of interest [2–5]:

- Body composition: Not only weight or body mass index (BMI) but also fat mass and fat-free mass amount and distribution evaluated by anthropometry (weight, stature, waist circumference, skinfold thickness) and/or bioelectrical impedance analysis. DEXA is currently only recommended for research purposes [6].
- Biochemical parameters: Lipid profile (total cholesterol, low-density lipoprotein (LDL) cholesterol, high-density lipoprotein (HDL) cholesterol, and triglycerides), glucose metabolism (fasting glucose levels, oral glucose tolerance test), insulin resistance, serum proteins, and uric acid are the most important markers of obesity comorbidities.
- Energy balance: Evaluation of dietary intake via direct observation, dietary recall or food diaries; calculation of basal metabolic rate by indirect calorimetry and assessment of physical activity level in order to have total energy expenditure.
- Clinical condition and comorbidities assessment: Cardiovascular, respiratory, endocrinological, hepatic, musculoskeletal, and gastroenterologic pathologies should be looked for.
- Physical fitness and physical disability: Assessment of motor function via a 6-min walk test [7, 8] and Borg's Perceived Exertion Scale [9], muscular strength of the forearm flexor muscles via handgrip dynamometry [10], evaluation of articular mobility, osteoarticular diseases, and any other condition that could hinder physical activity.
- Psychological/psychiatric status: Assessment of psychiatric comorbidities (e.g., binge-eating disorder, bulimia nervosa, substance-related disorders, depressive and anxiety disorders), psychosocial factors influencing physical activity and food intake, body image disturbances, health-related quality of life, and motivational attitude toward treatment.

Given overweight's multifactorial origin, only an individually tailored, comprehensive management can be effective [11]. This must be accomplished by an appropriate obesity management team which is multidisciplinary and comprises different professionals able to tackle the different aspects of obesity and its related disorders, providing a wide spectrum of clinically proven treatment options and combinations of them, such as lifestyle change based on diet, physical activity and functional rehabilitation, educational therapy, cognitive behavior therapy, and bariatric surgery [12–14]. An obesity multidimensional *equipe* should thus include different medical specialists such as a clinical nutritionist, an endocrinologist, a psychiatrist, a bariatric surgeon, and a physiatrist together with other health professionals (i.e., dietitian, psychologist, physiotherapist, nurse). This team should be ideally led and coordinated by an endocrinologist, gastroenterologist, or clinical nutritionist that would take into consideration the whole team's evaluations in order to plan an optimal weight loss strategy for the single patient.

In overweight and obese individuals in whom weight loss is indicated and who wish to lose weight, comprehensive lifestyle interventions consisting of diet, physical activity, and behavior therapy (all three components) produce average weight losses of up to 8 kg in 6 months of frequent (i.e., initially weekly), on-site treatment provided by a trained team in group or individual sessions. Such losses (which can approximate reductions of 5–10 % of initial weight) are greater than those produced by usual care (i.e., characterized by the limited provision of advice or educational materials). Comparable 6-month weight losses have been observed in treatment comparison studies of comprehensive lifestyle interventions, which did not include a usual care group [6]. Moreover, comprehensive approach led to a lower rate of dropouts and longer treatment duration compared to diet-only approaches [15].

After initial weight loss, some weight regain can be expected, on average, with greater regain observed over longer periods of time. Continued provision of a comprehensive weight loss maintenance program (on-site or by telephone), for periods of up to 2.5 years following initial weight loss, reduces weight regain, as compared to the provision of minimal intervention (e.g., usual care). The optimal duration of weight loss maintenance programs has not been determined and is reasonably to be considered lifelong [6].

In addition to the three abovementioned main approaches, other interventions appear to be useful in selected cases, such as pharmacologic, pshychotherapeutic, and bariatric surgery approaches. These interventions are, however, always to be considered as a complementary add-on in a multidisciplinary context. For example, according to the latest guidelines, bariatric surgery is considered the right approach in morbidly obese subjects resistant to various treatment and rehabilitation attempts conducted following optimal standards. Such approach, however, cannot be considered a resolutive, self-standing treatment and is always to be associated with a psychiatric and nutritional support both before and after surgery [2].

A brief outline of the steps of the take on responsibility of the obese patient is depicted in Fig. 28.1.

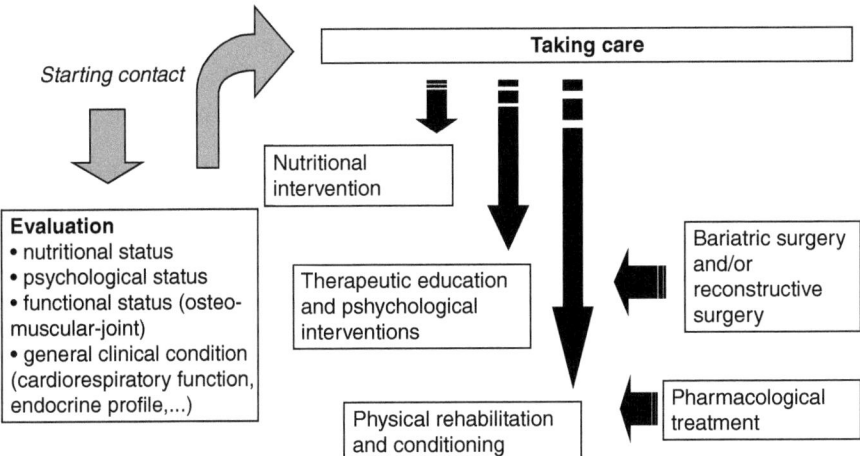

Fig. 28.1 Schematic presentation of the basic interventions in the take charge process of the obese patient

28.3 Levels of Care

The management of obese patients should be articulated in five levels of care [16]:

- Primary care (i.e., general practitioner)
- Outpatient clinics held by a multidisciplinary *equipe*
- Day hospital
- Residential rehabilitation treatment
- Hospitalization

Primary care, although not capable of treating obesity according to literature [6], is crucial in preventing the development of overweight and its comorbidities by educating patients to correct lifestyle and behavior and, where this is proven inefficacious, in directing the patient to the right level of care avoiding delays.

All the levels of care may prove beneficial at some point in the management of a single obese subject. Intensive care levels such as day hospital, day care, and residential approaches represent an essential step when obesity and its comorbidities have reached a high level, when the impact on quality of life is heavy, when many interventions are needed in order to treat the patient's condition, or when lower levels of care have proven ineffective. Taking advantage of these approaches will prevent acute events to be treated via hospitalization with evident advantages in terms of health, quality of life, and economic expenses.

28.4 Advantages and Disadvantages of a Multidisciplinary Approach to Obesity

The advantages of a multidisciplinary team approach have been outlined. Yet, there are some disadvantages to be considered. Compared to a single-clinician approach, a multidisciplinary one may bring to fragmentation, resulting in the patient receiving different and at times conflicting advice from the different components of the team. In addition, in the absence of excellent and constant communication among health professionals, there may be no clinician aware of the full clinical picture of the patient.

The major difficulties are thus substantially caused by education of the single health professionals, still not sufficiently teamwork-oriented in most countries [17, 18].

In order to prevent the abovementioned drawbacks, the whole team should be trained to apply a complex model of multidimensional treatment, to have a consistent approach to patients. The therapeutic roles and areas of intervention of each member should be well defined at the beginning and coordinated within the team. In addition, it is essential that clinicians, while maintaining their specific professional roles, share the same basic rationale and use a similar language with patients. It is crucial to have team meetings at regular times in order to evaluate and discuss treatment processes, strategies, and issues. Every health care professional should have a comprehensive view of the patient's clinical management and condition, identify his own role in the therapeutic plan, correctly establish the timing of his intervention, and coordinate it with those performed by others.

Moreover, team members should be helped to reflect on their attitudes toward obese patients and to counteract widespread weight biases that are relevant for an effective therapeutic relationship and management of obesity.

From a patient's perspective, multidisciplinary approach is not always seen as the best choice. The main reason why many patients still prefer traditional dietetic interventions is that the latter is much less time-consuming. Thus, only people with flexible schedules or a lot of spare time can reasonably take advantage of a multidisciplinary treatment. Moreover, obesity is still merely seen by many patients, health care professionals, and institutions as a benign condition caused by a lack in willpower, thus making a demanding treatment very difficult to be accepted [15].

References

1. Tsigos C, Hainer V, Basdevant A et al (2008) Management of obesity in adults: European clinical practice guidelines. Obes Facts 1:106–116
2. Donini LM, Dalle Grave R, Caretto A, Lucchin L (2013) From simplicity towards complexity: the Italian multidimensional approach to obesity. Eat Weight Disord. doi:10.1007/s40519-013-0097-9
3. Donini LM, Cuzzolaro M, Spera G et al (2010) Obesity and eating disorders. Indications for the different levels of care. An Italian expert consensus document. Eat Weight Disord 15(1–2 Suppl):1–31
4. Sbraccia P, Vettor R (2012) SIO, Societa' Italiana dell'Obesita' e ADI, Associazione Dietetica Italiana. Standard italiani per la cura dell'obesita' 2012–2013. SIO, Societa' Italiana dell'Obesita', Roma
5. Expert Panel on the Identification, Evaluation, and Treatment of Overweight in Adults (1998) Clinical guidelines on the identification, evaluation, and treatment of overweight and obesity in adults: executive summary. Am J Clin Nutr 68(4):899–917
6. Jensen MD, Ryan DH, Apovian CM, Ard JD et al (2013) AHA/ACC/TOS guideline for the management of overweight and obesity in adults: a report of the American College of Cardiology/American Heart Association Task Force on Practice Guidelines and The Obesity Society. Am Coll Cardiol 63(25 Pt B):2985–3023. doi:10.1016/j.jacc.2013.11.004
7. Enright PL, McBurnie MA, Bittner V, Tracy RP et al (2002) Cardiovascular health study: the 6-min walk test: a quick measure of functional status in elderly adults. Chest 122:387–398
8. ATS Committee on Proficiency Standards for Clinical Pulmonary Function (2002) ATS statement: guidelines for the six-minute walk test. Am J Respir Crit Care Med 166:111–117
9. Borg G (1990) Psychophysical scaling with applications in physical work and the perception of exertion. Scand J Work Environ Health 16(Suppl 1):55–58
10. Andrews AW, Thomas MW, Bohannon RW (1996) Normative values for isometric muscle force measurements obtained with hand-held dynamometers. Phys Ther 76:248–259
11. Donini LM (2013) Debate on obesity medicine. Endocr Pract 19(1):169
12. Dalle Grave R, Calugi S, El Ghoch M (2013) Lifestyle modification in the management of obesity: achievements and challenges. Eat Weight Disord 18(4):339–349
13. Wing RR, Bolin P, Look AHEAD Research Group et al (2013) Cardiovascular effects of intensive lifestyle intervention in type 2 diabetes. N Engl J Med 369(2):145–154

14. Sjostrom L, Lindroos AK, Peltonen M et al (2004) Lifestyle, diabetes, and cardiovascular risk factors 10 years after bariatric surgery. N Engl J Med 351(26):2683–2693
15. Donini LM, Savina L, Castellaneta E, Coletti C et al (2009) Multidisciplinary approach to obesity. Eating Weight Disord 14:23–32
16. Donini LM, Cuzzolaro M, Spera G, Badiali M (2010) Obesity and eating disorders. Indications for the different levels of care. An Italian expert consensus document. Eating Weight Disord 15(1–2 Suppl):1–31
17. Upshur R, Tracy S (2008) Chronicity and complexity. Is what's good for the diseases always good for the patients? Can Fam Phys 54:1655–1658
18. Stans S, Stevens J, Beurskens A (2013) Interprofessional practice in primary care: development of a tailored process model. J Multidiscip Healthc 6:139–147

Index

A
Acetazolamide, 138
Adiponectin, 8, 85, 101, 112
Adipose tissue
  adipokines, 8
  adipose cell differentiation, 6
  BAT, 3
  in bone marrow, 3–4
  cytokines, 8
  MAT, 4
  multi-depot adipose organ, 4–5
  transdifferentiation process, 6–8
  UCP1 immunoreactive brown
    adipocytes, 3
  WAT, 3
Adjustable gastric banding (LAGB).
    See Laparoscopic adjustable
    gastric banding (LAGB)
Adrenal hormones
  cortisol (see Glucocorticoid functions)
  mechanism of action, 64
Adrenal stimulation test, 69
Adverse metabolic effects, 34
Aerobic activity, 319, 321
Aerobic plus anaerobic exercise
    scheme, 321
Aerobic threshold (AerT), 208
Alanine transaminase (ALT), 164
Amphetamines, 262
Anorexia, 22
Anterior intercostal artery perforator
    (AICAP), 306, 307
Antibiotic prophylaxis, 308
Apnea-hypopnea index (AHI), 136
Atherogenic dyslipidemia (AD)
  lipoprotein metabolism,
    123–124
  metabolic abnormalities, 122
  VLDL, 122–123

B
BA. *See* Brown adipocytes (BA)
Bariatric surgery
  adjustable gastric banding (*see*
    Laparoscopic adjustable gastric
    banding (LAGB))
  adolescent/old age, 273
  class I obesity, 272–273
  diabetes, 289–290
  GH/IGF-1 axis, 59–60
  intragastric balloon
    advantages, 276
    complications, 275–276
    failure rate, 276
    indications, 274–275
    use of, 274
    weight loss and comorbidities, 276
  laparoscopic biliopancreatic diversion (*see*
    Biliopancreatic diversion with
    duodenal switch (BPD-DS))
  laparoscopy, 271–272
  lifestyle modification, 333–334
  LRYGB (*see* Laparoscopic Roux-en-Y
    Gastric Bypass (LRYGB))
  metabolic syndrome, 290, 291
  microbiota, 292–294
  patients' satisfaction, 288–289
  PCOS, 79–80
  preoperative management, 274
  sleeve gastrectomy
    advantages, 287–288
    comorbidities, 287
    complications, 286–287
    disadvantages, 287–288
    hybrid malabsorptive procedure, 285
    mechanisms of action, 285–286
    T2DM, 287
    weight loss, 287
  SOS, 288

Basal energy expenditure (BEE), 172
Basal metabolic rate (BMR), 172, 173
BAT. *See* Brown adipose tissue (BAT)
Behaviour therapy, 223–224, 228
Bi-level positive airway pressure (BPAP), 137
Biliopancreatic diversion with duodenal switch (BPD-DS)
    advantages, 284–285
    comorbidities, 284
    complications, 283–284
    disadvantages, 285
    mechanism of action, 282–283
    peptic ulceration, 282
    prevalence, 282
    T2DM, 284
    weight loss, 284
Binge eating disorder (BED), 194–195
    behaviour therapy, 223–224
    CBT, 226
    DBT, 228
    IPT, 227
Bioelectrical impedance analysis (BIA), 91, 158
Bioenterics intragastric balloon (BIB), 275
    advantages, 276
    complications, 275–276
    esophagogastroduodenoscopy, 275
    failure rate, 276
    mechanism of action, 275
    weight loss and comorbidities, 276
BMD. *See* Bone mineral density (BMD)
Body composition
    biological variables, 173
    fat-free mass (FFM)
        air-displacement plethysmography, 175
        anthropometry-based methods, 177
        BIA, 179
        bi-compartmental model, 174
        BMC, 175
        BMI, 177
        body weight, 177
        circumference measurement, 178
        CT and MRI, 180
        dilution methods, 177
        DXA, 179–180
        hip circumference, 179
        lean tissue mass (LTM), 175
        molecular model, 175
        MUAC, 179
        overweight, 177, 178
        skinfold equations, 175, 176
        skinfold thickness, 177
        underwater weighing, 175
        visceral organs, 174
        waist circumference (WC), 179
        waist-hip ratio, 179
    fat mass (FM)
        air-displacement plethysmography, 175
        anthropometry-based methods, 177
        bi-compartmental model, 174, 175
        BMI, 177
        BMR, 174
        body impedance assessment (BIA), 179
        body weight, 177
        circumference measurement, 178
        CT and MRI, 180
        dilution methods, 177
        DXA, 179–180
        hip circumference, 179
        molecular component, 175
        molecular model, 175
        MUAC, 179
        overweight, 177, 178
        skinfold equations, 175, 176
        skinfold thickness, 177
        underwater weighing, 175
        visceral organs, 174
        waist circumference (WC), 179
        waist–hip ratio, 179
Body impedance assessment (BIA), 179
Bombesin-like peptides, 19
Bone mineral content (BMC), 175
Bone mineral density (BMD), 84
Brain amino acid sensing, 25
Brain glucose sensing, 24
Brain lipid sensing, 24
Breast cancer, 80
Brown adipocytes (BA), 44
Brown adipose tissue (BAT), 3, 5, 7
Bupropion, 267

C

CARDIA study, 257
Cardiopulmonary exercise testing, 207–208
Cardiovascular disease (CVD), 102
Children obesity, 35, 36
Cholecystokinin (CCK), 20–21
Cholesteryl ester transfer protein (CETP), 123
Ciliary neurotrophic factor (CTNF), 23
Circadian clock, 14–15
Clinical evaluation
    arterial hypertension, 161
    BMI, 157–158
    cardiovascular risk factors, 163
    diabetes and prediabetes in adults, 161
    fat distribution
        fatty infiltrations, 160
        visceral fat accumulation, 159–160
    hepatic function, 164
    metabolic syndrome, 162–163
    respiratory function, 164–165

SCORE system, 163
staging, 166–167
Clinician–patient communication, 316
Cognitive–behavioural therapy (CBT), 225–227, 329–331
Continuous positive airway pressure (CPAP), 137
CTNF. *See* Ciliary neurotrophic factor (CTNF)
Cushing's syndrome, 22
CVD. *See* Cardiovascular disease (CVD)

D
Dialectical behaviour therapy (DBT), 228
Dietary data, 36
Dietary intervention
  balanced diet
    BMR, 240–241
    dietary plan, 240, 242
    DRVs, 244, 245
    macronutrients, 243
    physical activity level (PAL), 241, 242
    protein intake level, 242
  high-protein *vs.* standard-protein diets, 234–235
  low-fat diet/normal-fat diet
    ketogenic diet, 238–240
    VLED, 237–238
  low *vs.* standard carbohydrate diets, 235–236
Dietary reference values (DRVs), 244, 245
Disabilities, 31
Dopamine signalling, 24
Dual-energy x-ray absorptiometry (DEXA), 158
Dyslipidemia, 162
  AD (*see* Atherogenic dyslipidemia (AD))
  healthy diet, 126
  physical exercise, 125–126
  treatment targets, 124–125
  weight loss, 125
Dyspnea, 135

E
Edmonton obesity staging system (EOSS), 167
Empathy, 220
Endogenous cannabinoids, 19–20
Energy balance
  BMR predictive equations, 184, 185
  calorimetry techniques
    direct calorimetry, 188
    indirect calorimetry, 188–190
  definition, 180
  energy expenditure evaluation, 183

energy intake
  longitudinal methods, 182
  retrospective methods, 181
energy storage, 182–183
non-calorimetric approaches, 187
physical activity levels (PALs), 184, 186
TEE, 186
Energy intake regulation
  agouti-related protein (AgRP), 17
  arcuate nucleus (ARC), 15–16
  brain amino acid sensing, 25
  brain glucose sensing, 24
  brain lipid sensing, 24
  cannabinoid system, 19–20
  cocaine-and amphetamine-regulated transcript (CART), 17–18
  CTNF, 23
  dual-centre hypothesis, 13
  energy metabolism control, 14–15
  gastrointestinal tract signals, 20–21
  glucocorticoids, 22–23
  insulin receptors, 22
  lateral hypothalamus (LH), 13
  leptin, 22
  monoamine neurotransmitters, 23–24
  neuropeptide Y (NPY), 16
  neuropeptide YY (PYY), 16
  peptides mediating appetite stimulation, 17–18
  peptides mediating appetite suppression, 18
  pro-inflammatory cytokines, 23
  pro-opiomelanocortin (POMC), 17
  sex steroids, 23
  ventromedial hypothalamus (VMN), 13
Energy metabolism and fertility, 73, 75
Environmental factors, 36–37
Epidemiology
  adverse metabolic effects, 34
  mortality, 34, 35
  prevalence rates, 33, 34
  risks, 33–34
  weight category classification, 32–33
Epworth sleepiness scale (ESS), 137
Estrogen receptors (ERs), 74
European Food Safety Authority (EFSA), 234
Excessive daytime sleepiness (EDS), 137
Exenatide, 266–267
Expiratory reserve volume (ERV), 133

F
Fat-but-fit phenotype, 320
Fat mass and obesity-associated (FTO) gene, 110
Fatty acid-binding proteins (FABPs), 110

Fluoxetine, 266
Free fatty acids (FFA), 109
Functional evaluation
   cardiopulmonary exercise testing, 207–208
   disability evaluation, 208
   joint and muscle problems, 206–207
Functional residual capacity (FRC), 133

G
GABA, 19
Ghrelin, 21
GHRH+arginine test, 56, 57
Glucagon-like peptide-1 (GLP-1), 21, 266–267
Glucagon-like peptide-2 (GLP-2), 21
Glucocorticoid functions
   adrenal stimulation test, 69
   agouti-related peptide (AgRP), 68
   11-β-HSD activity, 68, 70
   11-β-HSD2 activity, 70
   fatty acid metabolism, 65
   ghrelin, 68
   HPA axis, 63, 69, 70
   in vitro studies, 66
   in vivo studies, 67
   leptin, 68
   lipid uptake, 65
   lipolysis, 65, 66
   metabolic effects, 64, 68
   neuropeptide Y (NPY), 68
   transcriptional regulation, 67
Glucose metabolism
   abdominal fat mass, 108
   diabetes, 108
   epidemiology, 107–108
   MAO, 108
   MNO, 108
   pathophysiology
      adiponectin, 112
      FABPs, 110
      FFA, 109
      FTO gene, 110
      GLUT4, 110–111
      IL6, 112
      MCP-1, 112
      oxidative stress, 111
      PPAR-γ, 110
      resistin, 112
      sex hormones, 112–113
   physical exercise, 108
   prevalence, 107
   RANKL system
      glucose homeostasis, 113
      osteocalcin, 113–114

GLUT4, 110–111
Growth hormone/insulin-like growth factor 1 (GH/IGF-1 axis)
   adipose tissue
      anabolic action, 54
      hormone-sensitive lipase activity, 54
      hypothetical maladaptive mechanisms, 55, 56
      NF-kB activity regulation, 54
      pathophysiological mechanism, 55
      proinflammatory mediators, 55
   bariatric surgery, 59–60
   low GH status diagnosis, 55–57
   metabolic consequences, 57–58
   treatment effectiveness, 58–59

H
Health-related quality of life (HRQL)
   chronic diseases treatment, 214
   generic instruments, 212–213
   HSP scale, 213
   IWQOL scale, 213
   Moorehead-Ardelt Quality of Life, 213
   ORWELL 97, 213
   QUOVADIS study, 214
   treatment interventions, 212
Health State Preference (HSP) scale, 213
High-protein diets (HPD), 234
HRQL. *See* Health-related quality of life (HRQL)
Hyperandrogenism, 77
Hyperinsulinaemia, 100
Hyperthyroidism, 47, 48
Hypocaloric diet, 44
Hypothalamic endocannabinoids, 20
Hypothalamic–pituitary–adrenal (HPA) axis, 63
Hypothyroidism, 47–48

I
Impact of Weight on Quality of Life (IWQOL) scale, 213
Incorrect "dietary beliefs," 316
Individual Rehabilitation Project, 315–316
Inpatient rehabilitation treatment, 333, 334
Insulin resistance (IR), 74
Insulin tolerance test (ITT), 56
Intensive hospital-based rehabilitation, 316
International Federation for the Surgery of Obesity and Metabolic Disorders (IFSO), 282
Interpersonal psychotherapy (IPT), 227

Intravaginal ejaculatory latency time (IELT), 151
IR. *See* Insulin resistance (IR)
Italian Ministry of Health, 315
Italian Society of Eating Disorders, 315
Italian Society of Obesity, 315
ITT. *See* Insulin tolerance test (ITT)
IWQOL scale. *See* Impact of Weight on Quality of Life (IWQOL) scale

K
Ketogenic diets (KD)
    macronutrient composition, 239
    pediatric epilepsy, 239
    pharmacological therapy, 238
    very low-calorie ketogenic diet, 239–240

L
Laparoscopic adjustable gastric banding (LAGB)
    advantages, 278
    comorbidities, 278
    complications, 277–278
    disadvantages, 278–279
    mechanism of action, 277
    prevalence, 276–277
    weight loss, 278
Laparoscopic Roux-en-Y Gastric Bypass (LRYGB)
    advantages, 281
    bariatric interventions, 279, 280
    Billroth II procedures, 279
    comorbidities, 281
    complications, 279–281
    disadvantages, 281–282
    mechanisms of action, 279
    weight loss, 281
LCD. *See* Low-calorie diets (LCD)
LCKD. *See* Low-calorie ketogenic diet (LCKD)
Learning theory, 327
LFDs. *See* Lower-fat diets (LFDs)
LGIDs. *See* Low glycemic index or load diets (LGIDs)
Light–dark cycle, 15
Liraglutide, 267
Lorcaserin, 264
Low-calorie diets (LCD), 236, 317, 319
Low-calorie ketogenic diet (LCKD), 239, 240
Low-carbohydrate diets (LChoDs), 235–236
Lower-fat diets (LFDs), 236–237

Low glycemic index or load diets (LGIDs), 236
LRYGB. *See* Laparoscopic Roux-en-Y Gastric Bypass (LRYGB)

M
Male obesity secondary hypogonadism (MOSH), 100–101
Malnutrition, 31
MAO. *See* Metabolically abnormal obese (MAO)
Marrow adipose tissue (MAT), 4
MCP-1, 112
Medications
    amphetamines, 262–263
    bupropion plus naltrexone, 267–268
    lifestyle intervention, 262
    long-term use
        lorcaserin, 264
        orlistat, 263
        phentermine, 263, 265
        topiramate, 264–265
    off-label use
        bupropion, 267
        exenatide, 266–267
        fluoxetine, 266
        liraglutide, 267
        metformin, 266
        naltrexone, 267
        zonisamide, 267
Mediterranean diet, 236, 237
Medroxyprogesterone, 138
Menarche, 75
Menopause, 78
Metabolically abnormal obese (MAO), 108
Metabolically normal obese (MNO), 108
Metabolic rehabilitation, 319–322
Metabolic syndrome (MetS), 102
Metformin, 266
Midlife overweight, 35
Mid-upper arm circumference (MUAC), 179
MNO. *See* Metabolically normal obese (MNO)
Monoamine neurotransmitters, 23–24
Monounsaturated fatty acids (MUFA), 125
Moorehead-Ardelt Quality of Life, 213
MOSH. *See* Male obesity secondary hypogonadism (MOSH)
Motivational interview, 224–225
MUAC. *See* Mid-upper arm circumference (MUAC)
Multidisciplinary rehabilitation, 319
Multinodular goiter, 47
Myosteatosis, 93

N

Naltrexone, 267
National Health and Nutrition Examination Survey, 33
Neurotensin, 19
Nonalcoholic fatty liver disease (NAFLD), 164
Nonalcoholic steatohepatitis (NASH), 164
Nonenzymatic antioxidant capacity (NEAC), 111
Non-exercise activity thermogenesis (NEAT), 173
Noninvasive positive pressure ventilation (NIPPV), 137
Non-resting energy expenditure, 172–173
Nutritional counseling, 244–247
Nutritional intervention
  goals, 317
  LCD, 317, 319
  mortality risks, 317
  procedures, 317, 318
  therapeutic education, 316–317
Nutritional status
  biochemical laboratory data, 173
  body composition (*see* Body composition)
  cardio-metabolic risk, 174
  energy balance, 173
    BMR predictive equations, 184, 185
    definition, 180
    energy expenditure evaluation, 183
    energy storage, 182–183
    longitudinal methods, 182
    non-calorimetric approaches, 187
    physical activity levels (PALs), 184, 186
    retrospective methods, 181
    TEE, 186
  energy expenditure, 172
  total energy expenditure (TEE), 172–173
  visceral adipose tissue, 173–174

O

Obesity hypoventilation syndrome (OHS), 137–138
Obesity paradox, 35
Obesity-Related Well-Being (ORWELL 97), 213
Obstructive sleep apnea (OSA), 135, 136
Orexigenic peptides, 22
Orexins A and B, 18
Orlistat, 263
Osteocalcin (OCN), 113–114

Osteoporosis
  adiponectin, 85
  BMD, 84
  causes, 83
  evidence-based observations, 84–85
  gene microarrays, 86
  leptin, 85
  resistin, 85
  visceral white adipose tissue (VAT), 85
  Wnt signaling pathway, 86
Oxidative stress, 111

P

PCOS. *See* Polycystic ovary syndrome (PCOS)
Peroxisome proliferator-activated receptor (PPAR-γ), 110
Pharmacotherapy, 332
Phentermine, 263, 265
Physical activity
  body weight control, 257
  duration, 255–256
  energy balance, 254–255
  health benefits, 257
  intensity, 256
  mode of exercise, 255–256
Physician communication style, 220
Pittsburgh Weight Loss Deformity Scale, 301–303
Polycystic ovary syndrome (PCOS)
  in adolescents, 77–78
  bariatric surgery, 79–80
  bisphenol A (BPA), 77
  cardiovascular risk, 76
  diagnosis, 76
  endocrine disturbances, 75
  hyperandrogenism, 77
  non-pharmacological treatment, 78–79
  pharmacological treatment, 79
  physical examination, 76
  2-h oral glucose tolerance test, 76
Polysomnography (PSG), 136, 165
Prader-Willi syndrome (PWS), 57
Psychiatric and psychological evaluation
  anxiety and depression, 196
  bariatric surgery candidates, 197–198
  BED, 194–195
  food addiction, 195–196
  food craving, 195
  lifestyle education, 193–194
  negative body image and social stigma, 196–197
  night eating disorder, 195

psychometric instruments, 199–200
serious mental illnesses, 199
Psychological factors, 221–223
Psychotherapeutic intervention, 322–323
Psychotherapeutic treatments, 228
Pulmonary complications
   airway resistance, 133
   anesthesia, 140
   asthma, 139
   COPD, 139–140
   dyspnea, 135
   fat distribution, 132
   lung volumes, 133
   OHS, 137–138
   pulmonary physiology, 134
   SDB, 135–137

Q
Quality of Life. *See* Health-related quality of life (HRQL)

R
Reconstructive plastic surgery
   abdominoplasty
      "anchor-line," 303
      complications, 304
      musculoaponeurotic reinforcement, 303
      surgical technique, 303–305
   brachioplasty
      "bat-wing" deformity, 309
      complications, 311, 312
      surgical technique, 310–311
   inner-thigh lift
      complications, 309, 310
      surgical technique, 308–309
   mastopexy
      auto-prosthesis, 306
      complications, 306, 307
   Pittsburgh Weight Loss Deformity Scale, 301–303
Resistance exercises, 321
Resistin, 112
Respiratory rehabilitation, 322
Resting energy expenditure, 172

S
Sarcopenic obesity
   clinical characteristics, 89
   cutoff points, 91
   definition, 90–91
   diagnostic criteria, 90
   dietary protein intake, 92–93
   disability, 93
   imaging systems, 91
   pathogenetic and functional role, 92
   physical performance evaluation test, 92
   pre-sarcopenia, 91
   relative sarcopenia, 93
   severe sarcopenia, 91
   significant findings, 89–90
   6MWT, 93
   treatment, 94–95
   TSD-OC test, 93
   weight cycling, 92
Secondary hypogonadism (SH), 99
Serotonin (5-HT), 24, 264
Sex hormones, 112–113
Sexual distress
   alimentation and sexuality, 145–146
   psychosocial factors, 150
   reproductive hormones, 150
   sexual dysfunction
      erectile dysfunction (ED), 147, 148
      IWQOL-Lite sexual life responses, 148, 149
      premature ejaculation, 147, 148
      sexual desire, 148
   treatment, 150–151
   weight-related comorbidities, 149–150
SH. *See* Secondary hypogonadism (SH)
Single-nucleotide polymorphisms (SNP), 37
6-minute walking test (6MWT), 93
Sleep-disordered breathing (SDB), 135–137
Sleeve gastrectomy
   advantages, 287–288
   comorbidities, 287
   complications, 286–287
   disadvantages, 287–288
   hybrid malabsorptive procedure, 285
   mechanisms of action, 285–286
   T2DM, 287
   weight loss, 287
SNP. *See* Single-nucleotide polymorphisms (SNP)
Standard-protein diets (SPD), 234
STOP-Bang questionnaire, 165
Strengthening-supervised exercises, 322
Strength exercise program, 320
Study 36-Item Short Form Health Survey (SF-36), 208, 212
Subfertility, 74
Swedish Obesity Study (SOS), 288
Systemic coronary risk estimation (SCORE) system, 163

T

T2DM. *See* Type 2 diabetes mellitus (T2DM)
Testosterone deficiency syndrome (TDS)
 CVD, 102
 endocrinometabolic disturbances, 100, 101
 hyperinsulinaemia, 100
 leptin, 100
 MetS, 102
 MOSH, 100–101
 secondary hypogonadism (SH), 99
 signs and symptoms, 99–100
 T2DM, 102
 TRT, 102–104
 visceral adiposity, 99
Testosterone replacement therapy (TRT), 102–104
Therapeutic patient education (TPE), 221
Thermic effect of food (TEF), 172
Thyroid cancer, 47
Thyroid function
 assessment, 46
 hyperthyroidism, 47, 48
 hypothyroidism, 47–48
 leptin regulation, 45
 nutritional status, 44–45
 pharmacological treatment, 48–49
 thyroid volume, 46–47
 thyroxine (T4), 43
 3,5,3'-triiodothyronine (T3), 43, 44
 ultrasound, 47
Thyrotropin releasing hormone (TRH), 18
Topiramate, 264–265
Total daily energy intake (TDEI), 233
Total energy expenditure (TEE), 172–173
TRH. *See* Thyrotropin releasing hormone (TRH)
TRT. *See* Testosterone replacement therapy (TRT)
Type 2 diabetes mellitus (T2DM), 99, 101, 102, 284, 287

U

Uncoupling protein (UCP1) immunoreactive brown adipocytes, 3
Upper airway resistance syndrome (UARS), 135
Urocortins, 18
Uvulopalatopharyngoplasty, 137

V

Very-low-calorie diet (VLCD), 237–238
Very-low-density lipoproteins (VLDL), 122–123
Vitamin D treatment, 86

W

WAT. *See* White adipose tissue (WAT)
Water-based rehabilitation programs, 322
Weight category classification, 32–33
Weight loss lifestyle modification programmes
 bariatric surgery, 333–334
 cognitive behavioural therapy, 329–331
 counsellors, 328
 dietary recommendations, 328–329
 duration, 327–328
 inpatient rehabilitation treatment, 333, 334
 pharmacotherapy, 332
 physical activity recommendations, 328, 329
 treatment outcomes, 331–332
Weight-lowering agent, 49
White adipose tissue (WAT), 3, 7

Y

Yale Food Addiction Scale (YFAS) scores, 169

Z

Zonisamide, 267

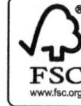

MIX
Papier aus verantwortungsvollen Quellen
Paper from responsible sources
FSC® C105338

If you have any concerns about our products,
you can contact us on
ProductSafety@springernature.com

In case Publisher is established outside the EU,
the EU authorized representative is:
**Springer Nature Customer Service Center GmbH
Europaplatz 3, 69115 Heidelberg, Germany**

Printed by Libri Plureos GmbH
in Hamburg, Germany